PSYCHOSOCIAL ASPECTS OF CANCER

Psychosocial Aspects of Cancer

Editors

Jerome Cohen, Ph.D.

Professor
School of Social Welfare
University of California, Los Angeles
Los Angeles, California

Joseph W. Cullen, Ph.D.

Deputy Director
Jonsson Comprehensive Cancer Center
University of California, Los Angeles
Los Angeles, California

L. Robert Martin, M.D.

Professor and Chairman
Department of Family and Community Medicine
School of Medicine
University of Nevada
Reno, Nevada

Raven Press ■ New York

Raven Press, 1140 Avenue of the Americas, New York, New York 10036

Made in the United States of America

International Standard Book Number 0–89004–494–5
Library of Congress Catalog Card Number 80–5057

Great care has been taken to maintain the accuracy of the information contained in the volume. However, Raven Press cannot be held responsible for errors or for any consequences arising from the use of the information contained therein.

Dedications

This book is dedicated to three individuals who initiated, enhanced, and enriched the contents:

Robert F. Murphy
(1919–1977)

Humanitarian, educator, and administrator, who, as the Executive Vice-President of the American Cancer Society, California Division, had the foresight and commitment to initiate and facilitate the development of this book.

Leo G. Reeder, Ph.D.
(1921–1978)

Sociologist who was dedicated to the behavioral concerns of people and who met an untimely death during the preparation of this book. His presence and his contributions are sorely missed.

Margaret M. Martin
(b. 1921)

Mother, wife, and individual whose battle with cancer epitomizes the needs and concerns expressed in this book. Her indominable will overcame and her courage placed in sharp focus the many psychosocial barriers confronting the cancer patient.

Preface

The National Cancer Act of 1971 sanctioned the efforts of a dedicated cadre of oncologists and allied health professionals who have long labored in the study and management of cancer patients by establishing guidelines for an all-out war on cancer and infusing into the effort a marked increase in federal dollars. Since that time, there have been dramatic gains made in the comprehensive care and treatment of cancer patients nationwide. When one considers, however, that cancer has attendant psychological, social, and economic sequellae that affect not only the patient but the patient's significant others, thereby having an impact on a considerable multiple of the nearly 800,000 people now afflicted with the disease each year, it stands out that cancer management implies more than medical intervention. In fact, the psychosocial dimensions of this disease may, for any given patient, family, or complex of individuals, be more relevant, require more attention, and cause more "pain" and morbidity than do the physical ravages of the disease.

In order to address the psychosocial dimensions of the complex of diseases subtended by the term "cancer," one must have an armamentarium of facts, intervention strategies, trained and concerned professional personnel, and other varied resources. Yet each of these important ingredients is in short supply. Indeed, the facts related to the definition of the psychosocial issues and variables of interest are disappointingly sparse; most experts agree that the intervention strategies related to these issues and variables are virtually unexplored. Furthermore, these strategies need to be considered in relationship to the patient, the patient's significant others, the health care provider, and the complex medical care system into which these elements converge. Whereas there is a literature base already available to draw on for some insight, that base is diffuse, difficult to identify, and almost consistently lacking in research data. Although studies have been carried out that have engendered data comparable in objectivity with some of the best basic biomedical research, they are the exception. Furthermore, due to the paucity of dollars previously spent in examining the psychosocial dimensions, much of the work already performed has been done by individuals whose primary function and intent is clinical (service) rather than research (scientific). This is not a criticism; these highly dedicated individuals had neither the resources nor the time for research.

With these facts in mind, this book explores research issues related to all interventions in the cancer management spectrum from prevention through detection, diagnosis, treatment, rehabilitation, and continuing care. This book also attempts to relate these issues to the patient and the complex of individuals surrounding him, the provider, and the medical care system. Consequently, this text should be of interest not only to social/behavioral scientists but also to other allied health professionals including social workers, nurses, health educators, and economists, as well as physicians, particularly oncologists and those who manage oncology patients. It will be only through an integration of all these disciplines that the important psychosocial dimensions in cancer ultimately will be understood for the benefit of those who are potentially at risk for the disease as well as those who are already attempting to cope with it.

Jerome Cohen
Joseph W. Cullen
L. Robert Martin

Foreword

To enlighten, to replace ignorance with knowledge—this is the primary challenge to all societies. Our society seeks to enlighten the public so that it may benefit from discovery. This is especially true in matters of public health. People are healthier, not simply because they know more, but because they choose to use their knowledge for the betterment of all society.

The American Cancer Society is the leader in informing and educating the public about the nature of cancer. This enlightenment has not uniformly led to increased early detection or prevention of cancer, and of itself, it has not materially changed our ability to cope with the emotional and social stresses of the diagnosis. Either through ignorance or in spite of enlightenment, the philosophy of "It won't happen to me" all too often prevails. Subsequently, when it *does* happen, a perplexed and thoroughly fearful and frustrated patient asks, "Why me?"

This book provides an intensive inquiry into the emotional and social behavior of the public confronting the threat of cancer and into the individual facing his diagnosis. Several chapters in this volume discuss behavioral research that is essential in the application of the knowledge that discontinuation of smoking *really* does aid in the prevention of lung cancer and that breast self-examination and the Pap smear *really* do detect early and curable cancer. Also included are studies on the emotional and social responses to surgical alteration, the depression often associated with the occasional, severe side effects of chemotherapy, and the almost overwhelming impact of the realization of economic hardship, permanent disability, or impending death. Some chapters in this volume tell us with rare clarity that even when we have the knowledge, we may fail to take the appropriate action. Why don't we prevent? Why don't we detect? Why don't we cope?

The answers to these questions are within reach of the behavioral, social, and psychosocial sciences. The work presented and discussed in these pages must be extended through the support of research scientists and increased psychosocial investigations. Deliverance from ignorance alone is not enough: Enlightenment and the utilization of knowledge will answer the "why's" and ultimately lead to real progress toward the prevention, early detection, and management of cancer.

Louis A. Leone

Acknowledgments

In 1976, Robert Murphy, then Executive Vice-President of the American Cancer Society, California Division, approached me with the request that I assume the responsibility of Chairman of the Ad Hoc Task Force Committee to study the psychosocial aspects of cancer with the objective of encouraging the American Cancer Society to identify and study the emotional and social needs of cancer patients and to subsidize the research that would validate them. This overture was made partially in response to a number of forceful presentations which were made by Dr. J. Cullen, one of the editors of this book, that recognized the growing concern about the psychosocial aspects of cancer and the need for support of quality research in this field.

The California Division, under the guidance and leadership of Robert Murphy, Helen Brown, and Alan Jonas, felt that the American Cancer Society, as the one voluntary organization dedicated to the interest and concerns of patients suffering from all types of cancer, should assume the leadership role in identifying the social problems confronting the cancer patients and searching for resolutions to these problems through valid research methodology. The Board of Directors of the California Division approved the formation of the Ad Hoc Committee and provided appropriate funding for its activity; this support has continued.

The responsibility of the Chairman was lightened considerably through the tireless efforts of Dr. Jerome Cohen and Dr. Joseph Cullen, both of whom contributed freely of their professional knowledge and expertise, of their time, and of themselves to the success of this effort. Mere words cannot reflect the magnitude of their support.

The papers that are contained within this monograph are edited versions of the presentations given at the first scientific session of the Ad Hoc Committee in San Diego, the purpose of which was to identify the psychosocial problems related to cancer and the research issues that these problems generated. The planning and implementation of this scientific session was supported and funded by the California Division of the American Cancer Society.

The editors of this monograph and the authors of the papers presented herein wish to express their sincere appreciation to the American Cancer Society, California Division, for their staff support and financial subsidy that has led to the publication of this volume.

L. Robert Martin

Contents

Introduction

Psychosocial/Behavioral Issues in Cancer Prevention

Cancer Control

Contributors

Joan R. Bloom, R.N., Ph.D.
Department of Social and Administrative
   Health Sciences
School of Public Health
University of California, Berkeley
Berkeley, California 94720

Jerome Cohen, Ph.D.
School of Social Welfare
University of California, Los Angeles
Los Angeles, California 90024

Marie M. Cohen, M.S.W.
Wright Institute
Los Angeles, California 90035

Catherine S. Cordoba, M.S.W.
Service and Rehabilitation
American Cancer Society, California
   Division
San Francisco, California 94102

Joseph W. Cullen, Ph.D.
Jonsson Comprehensive Cancer Center
University of California, Los Angeles
Los Angeles, California 90024

Carol N. D'Onofrio, Dr.P.H.
School of Public Health
University of California, Berkeley
Berkeley, California 94720

Frances Lomas Feldman, M.S.W.,
   A.C.S.W.
School of Social Work
University of Southern California
Los Angeles, California 90007

Jean S. Felton, M.D.
Department of Community Medicine
University of Southern California Medical
   School
Los Angeles, California 90033
and
University of California, Irvine
Irvine, California 92717

Patricia Fobair, M.S.W., M.P.H.
Lawrence Berkeley Laboratory
Berkeley, California 94720

Bernard H. Fox, Ph.D.
National Cancer Institute
National Institutes of Health
Bethesda, Maryland 20205

Ellen R. Gritz, Ph.D.
Veterans Administration Center,
   Brentwood
and
The Neuropsychiatric Institute
School of Medicine
University of California, Los Angeles
Los Angeles, California 90024

Jill Gregory Joseph, Ph.D.
Program in Epidemiology
School of Public Health
University of California, Berkeley
Berkeley, California 94720

David M. Kaplan, Ph.D.
Department of Family, Community, and
   Preventive Medicine
Stanford University
Stanford, California 94305

S. Stephen Kegeles, Ph.D.
Department of Behavioral Sciences and
   Community Health
University of Connecticut Health Center
Farmington, Connecticut 06032

Richard S. Lazarus, Ph.D.
Department of Psychology
University of California, Berkeley
Berkeley, California 94720

Louis A. Leone, M.D.
Division of Biology and Medicine
Brown University
Department of Medical Oncology
Rhode Island Hospital
Providence, Rhode Island 02902

Thomas A. MacCalla, Ed.D.
International Institute for Urban and
  Human Development
San Diego, California 92110

Joanne E. Mantell, M.S.S.W.,
M.S.P.H.
Division of Behavioral Sciences and Health
  Education
School of Public Health
University of California, Los Angeles
Los Angeles, California 90024

L. Robert Martin, M.D.
Department of Family and Community
  Medicine
University of Nevada
School of Medicine
Reno, Nevada 89507

Nelda McCall, M.A.
Stanford Research Institute
Menlo Park, California 94025

Daphne M. Panagis, Ph.D.
West Coast Cancer Foundation
San Francisco, California 94133

Robert D. Ross, Ph.D.
SRI International
Menlo Park, California 94025

Arthur H. Schmale, M.D.
Psychosocial Medicine Unit
University of Rochester Cancer Center
Rochester, New York 14627

Stuart O. Schweitzer, Ph.D.
Division of Health Services
School of Public Health
University of California, Los Angeles
Los Angeles, California 90024

John J. Spinetta, Ph.D.
Department of Psychology
San Diego State University
San Diego, California 92182

S. Leonard Syme, Ph.D.
Program in Epidemiology
School of Public Health
University of California, Berkeley
Berkeley, California 94720

Psychosocial Aspects of Cancer,
edited by Jerome Cohen et al.
Raven Press, New York © 1982.

Chapter 1

Overview of the Psychosocial Aspects of Cancer

L. Robert Martin

*Department of Family and Community Medicine, University of Nevada,
Reno, Nevada 89507*

The quest to identify the cause or causes of cancer has been a long and tedious one. Scientists have identified environmental, genetic, and acquired causal agents. This monumental work has been translated into therapeutic modalities consisting of surgery, radiation, and chemicals, all designed to remove, destroy, or inhibit the growth of the cancer cell. Great emphasis has been placed on increasing the velocity and productivity of this quest for new knowledge in the field of biocellular research.

Using the same data base, assessment and management (diagnostic, therapeutic, patient education, and future planning) of the psychosocial issues are at least equal to or more complex than the biomedical assessment and management. Despite this fact, projects related to psychosocial aspects of cancer are few in number and inadequately funded. The psychosocial arena is on the verge of losing whatever research expertise is presently available because of the general lack of interest of the established medical profession and the difficulty in obtaining grant subsidy funds.

This chapter is written not from the point of view of the professional social or behavioral scientist, but from the perspective of a family physician who has had a lifelong interest in the problems of early diagnosis, prevention, and treatment and psychosocial issues arising in the ambulatory office, the home, and the hospital. The ambulatory health care center is the most frequent point of patient entry into the health care system. It is the focal point of family-oriented health care and is the site of comprehensive care, patient education, preventative medicine, consultation and referral, and continuing care for all members of the family. It is from such family/individual/continuity oriented settings that patients are referred to the oncology specialist and it is to such a setting that many patients return for routine post-therapy health care and in cases of terminal illness and death. Frequently, it is the family physician who first confronts the patient with the diagnosis of cancer, makes arrangements for definitive care, consults with the family, becomes the interpreter of the

1

oncologist's therapy to the patient and to the family, and manages the patient's terminal illness and death.

In addition to these challenges with their multiple clinical expressions, which are usually found in a family physician's practice, this chapter has taken on a very personal note. During the preparation of this paper, the author's wife was found to have metastatic carcinoma and is presently undergoing chemotherapy. In addition, the prospect of possible cobalt therapy and a second-look abdominal procedure have challenged her with definition of wellness and the quality of life and, realistically, with the concern of death. This experience has provided another dimension of personal involvement. Self-observation of the psychosocial impact of medical decisions and the opportunity to observe intimately and to experience personally such emotional body blows have emerged. Most physicians have an awareness of such psychosocial issues, but this personal experience has enhanced the author's sensitivity to these issues.

This chapter will discuss a multiplicity of concerns regarding the psychosocial support system available to the cancer patient and his family, based on personal observation of the behavioral aspects associated with the diagnosis and treatment of cancer. Concern for the maintenance of a state of good health or "wellness" despite the presence of cancer and the right of the patient to consider rejection of the therapeutic protocol will also be considered. A theoretical framework, depicting the relationships among the family, the physician, and the patient in what the author terms as the "core health-concern unit" will be presented. The potential relationships that exist between this core unit and an impacting "peripheral health-concern unit" consisting of all of the identifiable forces which impact on the care of the patient will also be discussed.

INITIAL IMPACT OF CANCER

The diagnosis or suspicion of cancer results in a number of emotional responses such as fear of life and death, vulnerability, and an admixture of hopefulness and hopelessness. Because of these emotional responses, a flurry of biomedical questions spring from the patient and the nuclear family to the physician. Most of these questions are related to the stage of disease, potential length of life, available treatment, curability, type of therapy, complications, and on occasion, the economics of care. Few, if any, of the initial questions relate to the psychosocial issues of cancer, such as the quality of life while undergoing therapy, the potential problems of coping, the availability of community resources, the need for communication with spouse and family, and among other issues, the right to make the decision to live with therapy or die without it.

The initial encounter when the diagnosis of cancer is confirmed should be a forthright discussion between the physician and the patient (and family). It is during this moment that the patient and family begin to place their trust, faith, and confidence in the physician—truly, the golden moment. If a bond is not developed during this period or shortly thereafter, most subsequent clinical actions and suggestions will be subject to suspicion and concern. One wonders if those who do not develop such a bonding are the individuals who drift away from conventional therapy to unproven treatment fads and quackery.

The importance of defining the patient who is at psychosocial high risk cannot be underestimated. The presence of the disease of cancer and the selected therapy generates a host of psychosocial issues that are related to the patient and his family and require attention equal to the emphasis afforded the clinical problems. In the early stages of the disease, following the initial therapeutic efforts or between pulses of chemotherapy, many patients are symptom free. "Symptom free" time is time to arrange one's perspective, time to be depressed, time to feel vulnerable, and time to accept or reject the diagnosis, process of treatment, and potential outcomes. To the clinician as well as the family, it would be invaluable to know prospectively which patients are capable of effective coping while waiting for answers. How do we identify those patients who cannot cope and are in the process—during the remission which medical care has created—of eroding their personal emotional strength and the socioeconomic stability of their support systems? In order to improve the patient's level of wellness and to avoid the negative, energy-draining emotional complexes which so often accompany this disease, the identification would be of tremendous value to health care providers.

One of the major theses of this chapter is that wellness of the patient and family is as important as being free of cancer tissue. If this thesis is accepted, the objectives of cancer therapy should then be as follows:

1. Eradication of the tumor
2. Physical comfort of the patient
3. Willingness to implement and accept social and emotional interventions as needed and identified by the patient, the nuclear family, and the physician.
4. Negotiation and definition with the patient of a quality of life or state of wellness that can realistically be achieved and maintained.

Given the above objectives, there is need not only for biomedical knowledge and skill, but also for the ability to identify the nuclear family and the patient who are at psychosocial high risk and who will require assistance during the diagnostic as well as the post-diagnostic period.

It is true that the patient will cease to exist without the expertise provided by clinicians who are sufficiently knowledgeable and skillful in providing the patient with a multitude of traditional and newly tested therapeutic modalities. The results of these efforts do not, however, measure the quality of life or the state of wellness of the patient or the nuclear family. Five-year cure rates and long remissions are of little consequence if the patient's quality of life and state of wellness are less than optimal to him. In order to place the psychosocial needs of the cancer patient in perspective, there is a need for greater understanding of his emotional and social needs. These needs are different for patients of different ages and sex.

The disease of cancer results in three basic unalterable issues: first, possibility of death; second, need for emotional support; and third, need for quality medical care.

Death and cancer are equated by a majority of the populace. The initial diagnosis of cancer brings with it the real possibility of death—probably challenging the individual's sense of mortality for the first time. This ever-present potential of death continues throughout therapy, remissions, and even following the pronouncement of cure. Fear of death, I believe, can be divided into two separate concerns: first, actual death with its state of unknown and separation from the physical and social aspects of living; and second, fear of the process of dying with pain, disfigurement, dependency, and rejection. Once again, the identification of the patient who is at high psychological risk would allow the physician to manage the problems with knowledge rather than intuition. With such knowledge, plans could be made for appropriate counseling and other supportive therapeutic programs.

It is obvious that any individual who is under the stress of such a diagnosis will be in need of emotional and social support. The identification of such needs is critical, as is the identification of the resources that will best serve these needs. One concept of support consists of counselors, agencies, and other third-party individuals or institutions. It is indeed a valid concept. Another meaningful support system is the result of a more than commonplace level of communication and understanding between the patient and spouse, patient and nuclear family, and patient and physician. These components form the core of the patient's fundamental support system. Adding to this core group is the social support provided by extended family, friends, and neighbors, as well as community agencies and institutions. All are important aspects of the support system.

The third basic issue of cancer care is the need for quality medical care. The therapeutic modality needed and the duration and effectiveness of treatment will vary with age, tumor type, and medical judgment. The patient must have a degree of motivation and internal support which will provide him with the energy to meet the demands of modern therapy and continue to adhere to the protocol. Motivation is derived from understanding, communication, self-identification, and sharing. Support systems require health concern expertise and knowledge to identify and utilize.

The major variables related to cancer are

1. Tumor characteristics. These include its origin, natural history, degree of malignancy, sensitivity to therapeutic modalities, and stage at time of diagnosis.

2. Age of patient at time of diagnosis. For the purpose of discussing the psychosocial aspects of cancer, the human life span will be divided into child, adolescent, young adult, middle adult, and old adult. Each of these age groups are subject to different categories of disease, different emotional problems, and a different set of societal problems. The infant/child is emotionally and socially dependent on the societal world for total nourishment and support. The adoles-

cent is struggling for personal definition and escape from the bondage of dependency. The young adult is looking forward to planning and developing his/her societal relationships. The middle adult is choiceful; others depend on this age group, and middle adulthood can be identified in most instances as life at its least threatening time. The old adults are dependent emotionally and socially as is the infant/child. These individuals are venerated and frequently look forward to the end of their lives and death.

3. Strength and effectiveness of the various available support systems—medical, psychological, and social. The medical plans for prevention, treatment, and rehabilitation are not always well defined; however, the state-of-the-art at the present time is identifiable, and effective protocols are being used. In the psychological and social disciplines there are very few well-defined protocols—each individual and family requires a different format. Thus we have the need for identification of the psychosocial issues which impinge on the cancer patient and his family and appropriate research formats directed at the resolution of these issues.

If the goal of medicine is to assist patients in achieving and maintaining a state of well-being physically, emotionally, and socially despite the presence of disease, then an understanding of the psychosocial aspects of cancer becomes as important as the search for a greater understanding of the biological cellular aspects of cancer.

Why does an individual comply with medical instructions? Why not accept the inevitability of death? What is hope? What elements are contained within hope? The choice to live or die is a right of the patient, providing he/she intends to commit to the choice. To espouse living while emotionally seeking death results in incongruity and, inevitably, anger, despair, and misunderstanding among the patient, the family, and the physician. Under such circumstances medical therapy, if successful, results in a positive medical statistic while the patient remains in the state of "dis-ease" with himself and his society. How does this psychosocial imbalance affect the society in which the patient exists? How much entropy is generated within those who are responsible for emotional support? What is the societal and economic impact of an emotionally dis-eased person within the family? We in the health profession must impact on the total person and thereby on society, concerning ourselves with the maintenance of wellness through emotional and social support as well as the cellular cure or remission. If the health professionals are to anticipate a degree of wellness in patients despite the presence of cancer, answers to the psychosocial issues are necessary to provide guidelines for the future management of patients, utilizing psychological interventions as well as community resources.

TREATMENT

As noted previously, with the intial pronouncement of the diagnosis of cancer, the patient and family immediately seek advice and counsel related to survival.

First, they ask about the medical modes; second, at some later time, they become concerned about ability to tolerate the prescribed course of therapy, economic strength, and role in society.

At some point in the primary reaction period the patient confronts himself with the question of death—not with the possibility dependent on therapy, but with the thought that death is very realistic. The patient may wish to die for a multitude of reasons, or the patient might have an overwhelming sense of wishing to live. The medical profession should be able to allow patients to contemplate or to make such decisions. The contemplation of death is frightening to most, reflecting potential physical pain and the emotional trauma of separation, loss, and termination of worldly activities. To others death is peace and tranquility, a just reward for their productive lives. Whether it be the frightened individual or the person who has accepted termination of mortality, there should be either a verbalized or silent decision of acceptance of death or the challenge of the battle for life from this disease. Those patients who are not allowed to arrive at their individual conclusions, whatever their reasons might be, are possibly those who wish to die but are fearful of even considering, much less verbalizing, the thought of death. Those who wish to live but are frightened may have little strength to cope with the battle. Are these the patients who have difficulty accepting and coping with therapy?

If the multiple support systems in the core health-concern unit cannot provide adequate basic support (such as communicating, verbalizing, listening, understanding, sharing, and loving to produce a level of wellness acceptable to the patient), then the patient should have the privilege of accepting or denying therapy.

If the will to live is related to an acceptable degree of wellness under the circumstances of a life-threatening disease, what emotional behavioral dynamics result in the "hope" to achieve an acceptable degree of wellness? What are the guideposts that allow the family and the physician to identify those individuals who can attain and maintain a degree of hope? In short, how do we identify who is at emotional high risk and who is not?

It would appear to this observer that those who are willing to accept the challenge of living must have a penetrating understanding of themselves as individuals. They must have a commitment to their own self-worth and their self-identity in a social framework in which they are participants. In addition, their nuclear and extended families must have a high level of communication and understanding, as well as a well-defined and agreed upon value system. Are these the individuals who commit to accepting a state of good health or degree of wellness commensurate with their disease willing to accept the challenge of the battle? What other factors are present but yet undefined—interrelationships with family or spouse or orientation to the medical mode? How do we synthesize the existing data and develop new data related to patient acceptance and compliance?

From the foregoing discussion, three fundamental systems to which almost all medical and psychosocial issues relate can be identified. The first is time, the second is the interdependent milieu in which the cancer patient and family exist, and the third is the psychological and sociological environment that impacts on the patient and his family.

The "time systems" that are related to the psychosocial issues of cancer are the age of the patient and the age of the cancer. The physical and psychosocial health care of the various age groups noted previously (child, adolescent, young adult, middle adult, and old adult) varies in relation to the patient's age and to the history of the disease. A simplistic definition of the natural psychosocial history of cancer would contain four major time periods:

1. Risk. From the time at which the patient has become at risk of cancer until the clinical appearance of the disease.

2. Active Disease. From the time of clinical awareness until the onset of the stage of terminal illness. This stage may be altered by therapy, resulting in the fourth time period.

3. Remission.

4. Terminal Illness. From the identification of the stage of terminal illness until death.

There are then two dynamic time systems. The first, ever changing, is related to the patient's chronological age; the second is related to the history of the disease within that specific patient. The psychosocial inference related to the two time systems and their relationship with each other is that both medical and psychosocial needs and interventions change with age. Speaking specifically of the psychosocial interventions, changing tumor characteristics and chronological age results in increasing difficulty and complexity in defining both process and outcome related to such interventions.

The second fundamental system is the interdependent milieu in which cancer patient, nuclear family, and physician exist. Most psychosocial issues are generated by the interrelationships and interdependency of the various component health-concern units involved in the process of living with cancer. The resolution of these issues and sometimes the generation of increased complexities is the outcome of the level and quality of the transactions that occur among component parts of the total system and the patient.

The "core health care unit" consists of the patient, the nuclear family, and the physician. The strength of the bonds among these three components is directly related to the potential of success or failure of behavioral or attitudinal changes on the part of any or all of these three. The patient brings the disease into the unit, causing the interaction and all of the medical, psychological, and sociological problems pertaining to cancer.

The nuclear family can be both positive and negative. It can be positive through love and sharing, the ability to communicate, supportive acceptance of the disease process, knowledge of the disease and acceptable health habits, ethnic cultural mores, variable definitions of symptomatology, pain, disease, and cure, and most important, understanding. On the negative side the family can reject or deny or be passive, uncaring, unsharing, and unloving.

The physician can also bring to this interaction positive and negative forces. Positive forces include specific knowledge of the disease process and appropriate therapy or the ability to identify quality consultants who can provide the patient with appropriate medical care; an insight and understanding of his, the physician's, personal feelings regarding cancer and his degree of comfort with hope or hopelessness; and the ability to recognize and intervene in the psychosocial issues of his patients. The negatives are rather obvious. The physician can deny a lack of knowledge and treat the patient inadequately or inappropriately. He can subconsciously deny cancer as a disease, which potentially will deny the patient of objective evaluations and an understanding of the problems; and if there is not a psychosocial recognition and intervention, the patient and the family will be denied the opportunity of understanding and the advantages of multiple support systems.

The "peripheral health-concern units" which encircle the core unit consist of all other resources which are available for support, as well as all other impacting psychosical systems that are involved in the care of the cancer patient. It becomes obvious that psychosocial issues of cancer consist of an infinite number of such modules, each with an unlimited number of potential transactions and interactions with other peripheral modules reinforcing each other or detracting from each other. The outcome of these interactions is the impact they make on the core unit as a whole or on the individual members of that unit.

Is it any wonder that there is a blatant need for a greater reservoir of knowledge regarding the psychosocial issues of cancer?

In my own experience there has been a clearly defined need for the interactions which have occurred within the core health concern unit, and the impact of the peripheral health concern unit has been powerful and extremely supportive. How do the multitude of others who do not have the advantage of professional knowledge and insight manage with their communication problems within the core unit, as well as with the peripheral units? How do patients perceive the state of wellness? What is the family response to their fears and concerns? How is the family educated in the problems of this disease and the psychological care and the need for sociological support? How do we determine who can cope and who will accept the therapeutic regimen?

SUMMARY

The author has shared some thoughts regarding the need for more knowledge in providing cancer patients with a sound support program in the psychological and sociological aspects of the disease. Some of the behavioral aspects have been discussed and related to the clinical problems. A theoretical framework was described, defining the core health-concern unit as comprised of the patient, the nuclear family, and the physician and the peripheral health-concern unit as consisting of all other health units which may have positive or negative impact on the care of the patient.

Psychosocial Aspects of Cancer,
edited by Jerome Cohen et al.
Raven Press, New York © 1982.

Chapter 2

Scope and Magnitude of the Cancer Problem in Psychosocial Research

*Patricia Fobair and **Catherine S. Cordoba

*Lawrence Berkeley Laboratory, Berkeley, California 94720 and **American Cancer
Society, California Division, San Francisco, California 94102*

When one examines the scope and magnitude of the problem of cancer and what is known about its costs and causes, the urgent need for psychosocial behavioral research in cancer prevention becomes clear. Numerous cancers are preventable, but action on the part of both society and individuals is necessary in order to accomplish the task. A review of the current state of knowledge can indicate behavioral research needed for effective prevention programs.

OVERVIEW

There are both macro and micro aspects to describing the scope and magnitude of cancer. The number of those afflicted is enormous; yet cancer seems to affect people at random, appearing as a surprise and as a personal tragedy to each individual.

One in four persons living today will eventually have cancer. Over the years it will strike approximately two out of three families. In the United States, approximately 765,000 were diagnosed in 1979 as having cancer while about 395,000 people died of this disease (17). In 1976, 19.8% of all deaths in this country were due to cancer. Throughout the world cancer is an important cause of death. In industrial countries it is the second leading cause of death, whereas in less developed countries cancer may be the fifth of sixth cause of death (47).

It is estimated that during this decade 6,500,000 new cases of cancer will be diagnosed, 3,500,000 people will die of cancer, and more than 10,000,000 people will be under medical care for cancer (17). When family members and those close to the cancer patient are considered, the numbers of people whose lives will be touched by cancer are enormous.

The sheer weight of these numbers is impressive, but what about the people

9

they represent? We know a great deal about the physiological assault that cancer makes on the body and the physical impact of treatment. Yet we know relatively little about the impact of cancer on a person's capacity to function effectively, to experience enjoyment, and to find fulfillment in life. What happens to the family who survives the dying cancer patient? What does society lose when so many people are affected?

Cancer can seldom be viewed as an incident or "spell of illness" in a person's life; it more appropriately is considered a "chronic illness." It is treated by one or more of a combination of methods: surgical resection, radiation, and chemicals or homones. Patients may undergo repeated surgeries and several courses of radiation and chemotherapy stretching over months and years. Each of these treatment methods has varying degrees of severity and consequences. Over the years the patient and family may undergo a great deal of stress in the process of developing ways of coping with the medical, physical, psychological, economic, and social issues involved.

Those working in the clinical sphere know that the impact of cancer can be tremendous. It can disrupt personal functioning, ability to continue working, marital and family relationships, educational plans, vocational advancement, financial stability, social relationships, life style, and value systems. The human cost in suffering and deterioration of quality of life has been evident anecdotally, but has yet to be fully studied. At this point we do not have enough knowledge based on research to assist in alleviating the psychosocial pain and damage cancer may cause. There is much to be learned about the ways people cope with the problems cancer brings. More importantly, we need to learn more about how to motivate people to avoid behavior, such as cigarette smoking, which can lead to cancer; and how to motivate the general public to use available cancer detection methods. The importance of studying these issues becomes clear when one examines the incidence, mortality, and survival rates of cancer patients, the costs to society as well as to the individual, and the causes of cancer as we know them today.

> Time shall unfold what plighted cunning hides.
> *King Lear*

CANCER TRENDS

Cancer incidence and mortality rates are increasing while aggregated death rates from all causes are declining (54). While cancer mortality is going down in younger persons, overall mortality is increasing (55). An encouraging trend is that survival rates for cancer patients in certain disease sites are improving and indicate progress in both treatment and prevention (49). Although there is no nationwide system in the United States for reporting cancer incidence as there is for recording mortality, there are population-based tumor registries supported by the National Cancer Insitute in a number of cities and regions. "Cancer incidence is still increasing and the increases are not all accounted for by cigarette smoking nor by the increased detection of breast cancer resulting from the fears of the 1970s" (49). Current estimates reflect that even when smoking-related lung cancers were removed from the incidence data, there were still increases in incidence from 1969 through 1976. For white men the rate of increase was about 0.5% per year and for white women, nearer 1% per year (9). A recent study of cancer rates over the last 25 years shows that the cancer incidence rate for blacks is higher than for whites. Figures from the National Cancer Surveys of 1947 and 1969 show that the overall cancer incidence rate for blacks went up 8% while for whites it dropped 3% (5,18).

Cancer sites with the highest incidence rates, accounting for the largest percentage of all malignancies, are lung and bronchus, colon–rectum, breast, and prostate (4). Incidence rates in some cancer sites are increasing faster than others as shown in a study of time trends from 1969 to 1976 (49). Melanoma and bladder cancer incidences are increasing for whites of both sexes. White females are showing large increases in cancers of the lung and corpus uteri. Blacks of both sexes are showing increases in the incidence of lung and kidney cancers. Black males show an increasing change in the incidence of colon cancer while black females are presenting increases in the number of cases diagnosed with bladder, pancreas, and corpus uteri cancers. With our present knowledge of cancer causation, some experts believe that prevention of some of these cancers is possible (e.g., smoking cessation to prevent lung cancers and more judicious use of estrogens to prevent cancer of the corpus uteri).

It should be noted that although overall incidence is going up, there are incidence declines for stomach and cervical cancers. At this time one can only speculate about the cause(s). Perhaps stomach cancer is declining because of dietary changes evidenced by the consumption of more fresh or frozen fruits and vegetables. Improved personal hygiene and earlier diagnosis through cervical cytology may account for the decline in cancer of the cervix.

> Mortality reflects both incidence and treatment. There are some forms of cancer for which incidence has gone up but where mortality has not. While this says something about the success of earlier diagnosis and improved treatment, it also tells us to look harder for the causes and, if we succeed in identifying them, try to eliminate them. (49)

Mortality rates for colon, bladder, and pancreas cancers and for melanoma are also increasing. When race and sex differences are examined, black males and females have higher rates than whites while rates for white females went down (22,54). The cancer death rate increased 26% among black Americans while it rose only 5% for white Americans (18). It has been suggested that the differences in black and white cancer rates are attributable to environmental and social factors rather than to inherent biological characteristics (16).

> . . . the differences between blacks and whites cannot be all genetic. We do not know why black men have more prostate cancer or more lung cancer; on the average they appear to smoke less. Nor do we know why they may have more cancer of the esophagus or less bladder cancer than white men, but they do. . . . (49)

One approach has been to examine geographical distribution of mortality rates in the United States. When such rates are examined, one finds the death rates are lower in states with less industrial development (such as Utah, Idaho, and North Carolina) and higher in states where industry is concentrated (New Jersey, New York, and Rhode Island) (39).

The length of time a cancer patient lives or is free of new cancer after the initial diagnosis is a useful indicator of the success of treatment. Trends in survival indicate the progress made in treating particular types of cancer. But caution is required in interpreting total survival rates without reference to incidence or mortality data. Enstrom and Austin (24) point out that cancer survival rates vary as a function of several factors: age, sex, race, social class, degree of histological confirmation, type of treatment, cancer site, stage of disease, and host resistance. Therefore, it is most useful to look at survival rates by individual cancer sites. Perhaps as many as 41% of all patients with cancer can be expected to survive 5 years without evidence of disease. This is in contrast to a survival rate of 20% in 1930. Much of the recent improvement is due to improved approaches to chemotherapy and combined treatment programs involving surgery, radiation, and chemotherapy (23).

Survival trends in the 1970s indicate that 78% of white patients in this country with breast cancer experience an overall survival of 5 years or more. Patients with cancer of the colon have not been as fortunate. Although over 50% of these individuals survive 5 years more, the rate of improvement has been less dramatic (4). Similarly, more than 50% of patients with cancer of the bladder now achieve 5 years' survival, with white patients showing a 61% relative survival. Black patients experience 30% survival (5).

An important site for examining survival trends is lung cancer. In the 1940s the survival rate for lung cancer was 6%; in the 1960s it rose to 11% (35). In a recent study, 16% of the female lung cancer patients were surviving in the 1970s. For patients with small cell and epidermoid carcinomas of the lung, 25% were living longer than 2 years as a result of combined chemotherapy and radiation (23).

Many cancer sites which affect smaller numbers of patients are now counted in the "curable" category of survival statistics. At least 60% of osteosarcoma patients are expected to survive 5 years or more. Even more optimistic are the possibilities for cure in nonseminomatous testicular cancer where patients in early stages of disease are expected to achieve 100% curability rates and 80% of all cases are expected to survive. Among the pediatric malignancies, similarly high rates of survival have been achieved for acute lymphatic leukemia (80%), Wilms' tumor (90%), and Ewing's sarcoma (60 to 70%). Other adult cancers with improved survival rates include adult leukemia (60%), soft tissue sarcomas (over 50%), Hodgkin's disease (70%), and the non-Hodgkin's lymphomas with 70 to 80% cure rate possibilities (23).

Credit for these improvements in survival from cancer must go to better medical detection and treatment. However, how many more people might survive if treatment were instituted earlier or more successful? One estimate indicates that 17% of those diagnosed with cancer in 1978 might be saved from death had they received earlier treatment (16). If mortality from cancer were eliminated, the average length of life of the general population would be increased by more than 2 years (35).

In sum, studies of time trends show that cancer incidence and mortality rates have continued to increase in the 1970s—incidence somewhat more rapidly than mortality—probably reflecting improvement in treatment and earlier diagnosis. Survival rates in certain disease sites have been strengthened by the use of new and improved anti-cancer drugs. Although 41% of all cancer patients may now survive 5 years or more, the grim fact is that 59% of the patients who have cancer will die at some point because of the disease. We are not yet in control of the causes of the disease nor have we accounted for the differential between black and white patients in mortality and survival rates. "If we had perfect prevention, we would not need treatment" (49).

Geographical patterns of cancer distribution suggest that areas with industrial concentrations have higher mortality rates than other areas; but even states with less industrial activity are experiencing a larger number of deaths over time. Some patient groups and some areas of the country may survive better than others, but no one is really free from the risk of cancer in today's world.

Accepting that in this country approximately 400,000 people die from cancer each year and that 765,000 new cases are diagnosed, what are the costs of cancer and what financial losses do we suffer as a result of this disease?

CANCER COSTS

The costs of any illness include the direct costs connected to prevention, diagnosis, and treatment; indirect costs related to losses of productivity and earning power; and the noneconomic, intangible costs in the diminution of the quality of life for both patients and families. Just as incidence and mortality rates for cancer have increased, so have the costs and economic losses. Neoplasms accounted for 1% of the total costs of all disease in 1900, 4% in 1930, and 9% in 1975 (47). It has been estimated that direct and indirect costs combined in 1978 equaled $30 billion (17,61).

Direct economic costs include expenditures for care in acute hospitals and extended care facilities, physician and nursing services, drugs, medical research, training of medical personnel, construction of facilities, and other expenditures such as for public health activities (47). Direct costs for cancer in this country totaled $5.3 billion in 1975; this represented 5.3% of the total direct expenditures for medical care. Hospital care alone accounted for 78% of the total direct costs for cancer, a much higher rate than for other diseases. Another 13% went for physicians' services (47).

In a study by Cancer Care, Inc., carried out in 1972, three-fourths of the families studied incurred direct costs between $10,000 and $35,000. The median cost was $19,054, twice as much as the median family income of $8,000 (31). Since then, medical care costs, along with other costs, have risen rapidly making the situation worse. In 1972, families in the study spent $2,382,620. Based on cost of living statistics from the United States Department of Labor, these families would now (1979) spend $3,335,668—another million dollars (46). This reflects a 40.4% increase.

An important study of direct costs of inpatient admissions was reported in 1976. Based on a sample from the Third National Cancer Survey, the report provides hospitalization expenditure data for specific cancers from the time of first admission through a 2-year follow-up period. For the 6,332 patients sampled, hospital stay and payments averaged 15.6 days and $1,399 per admission (about $90 per day). First admissions usually were longer and costlier than subsequent admissions. Nonsurvivors averaged more admissions and longer admissions than survivors. Most admissions were paid for by two sources, with Medicare accounting for 43.7% of the total payments, followed by Blue Cross (22.9%), and other private insurance (19.3%). Out-of-pocket payments by the patient accounted for 6.5% of all payments to hospitals (52,53).

McCall (Chapter 9) points out that health insurance actuaries define the type of care provided and that the physicians, not the consumers, are the central decision makers concerning the use of services. This combination has contributed substantially to the rising costs of medical care. This mix also creates finanical dilemmas for cancer patients and families. Reimbursement of costs is geared toward treatment in acute care settings, although cancer is generally a long-term chronic illness requiring treatment in an episodic fashion that is being provided more and more on an outpatient basis. Many of the costs such at transportation to and from treatment centers and assistance in the home are not reimbursed. Many patients with advanced cancer can be cared for at home and most would prefer to be, yet the necessary supportive services are not available except to the very well-to-do.

Schweitzer (51), in considering decisions regarding reimbursement for new medical technology and in studying the social costs in relation to the effectiveness of the bone marrow transplant therapy which has taken place at UCLA Medical Center between 1974 and 1978, found that the average direct treatment cost for a single patient was $64,887, with indirect costs of $1,440 for a total cost of $66,327. He calculated the mean cost per life saved to be $473,764 and the mean cost of what was called "quality adjusted life saved" as $1,029,922. (A proxy measure used for quality of survival was a simple "degree of dependence versus independence" measure.) This program is still highly experimental, requiring enormous clinical effort, and thus far the results have been disappointing (51).

Indirect costs of an illness include the loss of productivity because of mortality, morbidity, and disability. Cancer can prevent people from leading their usual productive lives in terms of working and maintaining households. The life expectancy of persons with cancer is reduced on the average approximately 16 years,

pected 40 years ago (57). Today many scientists believe that environ-
rs interact with hereditary information in cells to produce a complex
events leading to the development of cancer (58).

of viruses in the development of cancer has been actively examined
'50s. Scientists have found that a variety of viruses are capable of
imors in almost every species of animal except humans. The emphasis
rch has recently moved from the search for cancer-causing viruses
/ of ways in which the virus affects the growth and regulation of
irus appears to act as a cofactor (59). There are some indications
genic agents as different as viruses and chemicals share a common
process of cancer development. It seems likely that viruses will be
iy a role in some forms of cancer in man (59).

radiation is perhaps the most extensively studied carcinogen'' (9).
icer associated with high doses (in excess of 50 rads) of irradiation
ibstantiated by studies from many sources. The issue of risk from
 diagnostic levels of irradiation remains uncertain (56). There is
xposure entirely without some risk. A recent study of men exposed
liagnostic radiation found that previous estimates of safety obtained
tion from high-dose levels to low-dose levels may have underesti-
ictual hazards by a factor of ten (12). Although this outcome is
uted, most scientists agree that diagnostic X-rays should not be
ted in their potential relationship to cancers (9).

 consideration for primary prevention involves the investigation of
 the workplace and environment. Since workers in many industries
to chemicals for longer periods and in higher concentrations than
ers of society, industrial exposures have been the primary means
ig chemical carcinogens in man. According to Higginson (30), "Stud-
 in the workplace have historically led to the successful identification
iicals carcinogenic to man and subsequent control."

 and lively debate concerns the degree of importance given toxic
i a cause of cancer in occupational settings. Estimates of the fraction
cidence attributed to occupational exposure are difficult to make
several problems. Many industries have not been investigated ade-
workers change jobs during their work life, they also change their
terns to carcinogens. Even the nature of cancer as a "disease of
creates difficulties for teasing out the responsibility of each agent.
ese problems is the delay of 10 or more years between the initial
i chemical and the clinical appearance of a tumor. What is needed
in chemical causation is continued examination of the temporal
rends of cancer incidence around the heavily industrialized areas
y in order to determine excess risk to workers. Collecting worker
ccupational exposure to chemicals where excess mortality has been
 along with material on the life style of workers such as smoking
he next important step.

with patients under 45 years of age losing up to 43 years and those over 65 losing approximately 9 years of life (47). The losses in manpower have been estimated at 1.8 million work years due to cancer mortality with an estimated $43,000 lost per death (47).

Mortality has direct consequences for the family, affecting work life, duration of marriage, and age at bereavement. In the long run, large reductions through mortality can influence behavioral patterns (1).

According to Feldman (25), an individual's adequacy is frequently equated with independence and measured by such criteria as work, thrift, and health. "Our society places a high premium on independence, both financial and psychological, generally blurring the two." In her two recent studies involving the work life of cancer patients, she reported that some patients felt that their condition limited their ability to carry out their occupation, whereas other patients described problems in continuing to work.

A recent study of the non-medical, out-of-pocket expenses of childhood cancer revealed that they represent a significant percentage of total family income. These expenses include transportation, special food for the patient, food eaten out, lodging for parents while the child is hospitalized, baby sitters, clothes, and so on. Out-of-pocket costs plus loss of pay averaged over 25% of the yearly gross income of half the families studied—a devastating consequence with many ramifications (34).

The financial burden of cancer contributes to psychosocial deterioration or the social cost brought about by the disease. The economic impact of cancer is a major source of stress and increases the overall distress of patient and family. Treatment decisions may have to be made on the basis of finances, and many families face the possibility of bankruptcy by seeking the best care available. Depletion of resources over extended periods has long-lasting deleterious effects on all family members who may be deprived of basic needs (34).

In sum, the social and economic implications of cancer for patients and families and for society at large involve many losses; for patients, the possibility of disability or loss of life; for the family, role disruptions and losses in economic status; for society, large sums spent on patient care, much of it for the terminally ill. To eliminate such losses in society, we must increase preventive efforts; we must deal with elements that cause the disease.

> The Cause is hidden, but the Result is well known.
> Ovid

CANCER CAUSES

It is important for behavioral scientists to grasp what is known about the causes of cancer so that they can focus their preventive efforts on human behaviors which place people at risk for this disease. Determining causal relationships in cancer is complex because it involves a process which is time-dependent and multicausal, a process in which there appear to be agents which initiate, agents which promote, and a synergistic relationship between the two stages (40).

Thoughts about the causes of cancer have evolved over the centuries because cancer has existed in animals and humans since early time. Examination of a dinosaur fossil revealed a blood vessel tumor on a vertebra. Traces of cancer have been found in bone remains of Java man and in Egyptian mummies. From this we realize that the processes causing cancer have been part of life since the earliest days. Early physicians knew of cancer; Hippocrates (400 B.C.) coined the term "carcinoma" and believed that it was due to an excess of black bile from the spleen. Galen (200 A.D.) agreed with Hippocrates, but added another idea persisting in today's research, that melancholic women, as opposed to sanguine women, had a tendency toward breast cancer. The first cancer hospital was founded in Reims, France, in the early eighteenth century at a time when cancer was thought contagious and patients were treated like lepers.

Current research evolving from the earlier work has led to our present understanding of the importance of environmental factors. For a good many years the biological role of aging was considered a major factor in causing cancer. As animal research and bioassay tests became more sophisticated and as national and international epidemiological data have continued to be analyzed, the roles of environment and of human behavior have become more important. "Cancer no longer can be assumed to occur 'spontaneously' as an inevitable accompaniment of aging; instead most cancers are now generally thought to arise through the influence of environmental factors" (59).

A carcinogen is an agent or process which substantially increases the yield of malignant neoplasms in a population (20). The number of known carcinogenic agents includes several groups of viruses, various physical factors, such as radiation and sunlight, and a number of chemicals (45,54).

Leading health planners consider four basic determinants of health in the life of an individual: biological factors (including heredity), environment, life style and personal behavior, and quality of health care. An examination of each area suggests many possibilities for interacting factors (8).

Biological Issues

Both heredity and aging processes play a role in the causation of cancer. Certain cancers tend to run in families. When there is a familial background, the causes may be from a genetic (or DNA change in the cell), congenital (present at birth), or familial trait (combination of genetic and environmental source) (42). Virtually all cancers developing in man have been identified as occuring in a heritable and nonheritable form (2).

Some genetically related cancers occur because entire lengths of genetic material are absent or present in excess in the chromosomes. For example, among

the leukemias, chronic myelocytic leukemia in the chromosomes. In acute leukemia pa were discovered along with unneeded addit

The presence of congenital defects appear defects and cancer. Wilms' tumor has been defects involving urogenital malformations with Down's syndrome is at least 11 times syndrome the coexistence of birth defects a mechanism perhaps in early gestation (42) component tend to occur at earlier ages ar than do nonheritable cancers (2).

Familial patterns of cancer incidence hav teenth century. These cancers may be refe many genes may interact with environmen one factor or gene playing a major role (4 spective studies have shown a two- to fourfe ing that a family history of cancer can inc cancer. Higher incidence was found in stuc breast, large intestine, uterus, and lung. In childhood brain tumors and sarcoma (2).

Aging may be a biological marker which exposure in the individual. During a lifetim from diet, smoking, occupation, and othe immunological defenses may decrease, ho Throughout a lifetime, there is an ever-in agent early in life will change the immu In addition, there may be a nonspecific, g wearing out of the human organism, mak all diseases including cancer (36). In ani examining the role of inherited and chemic systems which will lead to better underst (40).

The malignancies associated with hered system and are often histologically identica Some scientists believe that more such c as collaborative efforts are able to differ manifestations of disease (42).

Environmenta

Within the human environment there ruses, radiation, and chemicals may pla outcome. The degree to which environm

scarcely s
mental fac
sequence

The rol
since the
producing
in this re
to the stu
cells. The
that carci
step in th
found to

"Ionizir
Risks of
have been
low-dose
no level o
to ordinar
by extrap
mated the
already d
underestir

A secor
chemicals
are expos
other mer
for identif
ies on can
of new ch

A curre
substance
of cancer
and involv
quately. A
exposure
interaction
Added to
exposure
for resear
and spatia
in the cou
histories c
document
histories,

with patients under 45 years of age losing up to 43 years and those over 65 losing approximately 9 years of life (47). The losses in manpower have been estimated at 1.8 million work years due to cancer mortality with an estimated $43,000 lost per death (47).

Mortality has direct consequences for the family, affecting work life, duration of marriage, and age at bereavement. In the long run, large reductions through mortality can influence behavioral patterns (1).

According to Feldman (25), an individual's adequacy is frequently equated with independence and measured by such criteria as work, thrift, and health. "Our society places a high premium on independence, both financial and psychological, generally blurring the two." In her two recent studies involving the work life of cancer patients, she reported that some patients felt that their condition limited their ability to carry out their occupation, whereas other patients described problems in continuing to work.

A recent study of the non-medical, out-of-pocket expenses of childhood cancer revealed that they represent a significant percentage of total family income. These expenses include transportation, special food for the patient, food eaten out, lodging for parents while the child is hospitalized, baby sitters, clothes, and so on. Out-of-pocket costs plus loss of pay averaged over 25% of the yearly gross income of half the families studied—a devastating consequence with many ramifications (34).

The financial burden of cancer contributes to psychosocial deterioration or the social cost brought about by the disease. The economic impact of cancer is a major source of stress and increases the overall distress of patient and family. Treatment decisions may have to be made on the basis of finances, and many families face the possibility of bankruptcy by seeking the best care available. Depletion of resources over extended periods has long-lasting deleterious effects on all family members who may be deprived of basic needs (34).

In sum, the social and economic implications of cancer for patients and families and for society at large involve many losses; for patients, the possibility of disability or loss of life; for the family, role disruptions and losses in economic status; for society, large sums spent on patient care, much of it for the terminally ill. To eliminate such losses in society, we must increase preventive efforts; we must deal with elements that cause the disease.

The Cause is hidden, but the Result is well known.
Ovid

CANCER CAUSES

It is important for behavioral scientists to grasp what is known about the causes of cancer so that they can focus their preventive efforts on human behaviors which place people at risk for this disease. Determining causal relationships in cancer is complex because it involves a process which is time-dependent and multicausal, a process in which there appear to be agents which initiate, agents which promote, and a synergistic relationship between the two stages (40).

Thoughts about the causes of cancer have evolved over the centuries because cancer has existed in animals and humans since early time. Examination of a dinosaur fossil revealed a blood vessel tumor on a vertebra. Traces of cancer have been found in bone remains of Java man and in Egyptian mummies. From this we realize that the processes causing cancer have been part of life since the earliest days. Early physicians knew of cancer; Hippocrates (400 B.C.) coined the term "carcinoma" and believed that it was due to an excess of black bile from the spleen. Galen (200 A.D.) agreed with Hippocrates, but added another idea persisting in today's research, that melancholic women, as opposed to sanguine women, had a tendency toward breast cancer. The first cancer hospital was founded in Reims, France, in the early eighteenth century at a time when cancer was thought contagious and patients were treated like lepers.

Current research evolving from the earlier work has led to our present understanding of the importance of environmental factors. For a good many years the biological role of aging was considered a major factor in causing cancer. As animal research and bioassay tests became more sophisticated and as national and international epidemiological data have continued to be analyzed, the roles of environment and of human behavior have become more important. "Cancer no longer can be assumed to occur 'spontaneously' as an inevitable accompaniment of aging; instead most cancers are now generally thought to arise through the influence of environmental factors" (59).

A carcinogen is an agent or process which substantially increases the yield of malignant neoplasms in a population (20). The number of known carcinogenic agents includes several groups of viruses, various physical factors, such as radiation and sunlight, and a number of chemicals (45,54).

Leading health planners consider four basic determinants of health in the life of an individual: biological factors (including heredity), environment, life style and personal behavior, and quality of health care. An examination of each area suggests many possibilities for interacting factors (8).

Biological Issues

Both heredity and aging processes play a role in the causation of cancer. Certain cancers tend to run in families. When there is a familial background, the causes may be from a genetic (or DNA change in the cell), congenital (present at birth), or familial trait (combination of genetic and environmental source) (42). Virtually all cancers developing in man have been identified as occuring in a heritable and nonheritable form (2).

Some genetically related cancers occur because entire lengths of genetic material are absent or present in excess in the chromosomes. For example, among the leukemias, chronic myelocytic leukemia patients have been found with losses in the chromosomes. In acute leukemia patients, losses in some chromosomes were discovered along with unneeded additions in others (42).

The presence of congenital defects appears to be associated with chromosomal defects and cancer. Wilms' tumor has been known to occur with certain birth defects involving urogenital malformations. The rate of leukemia in patients with Down's syndrome is at least 11 times normal and may be higher. In each syndrome the coexistence of birth defects and cancer suggests a common causal mechanism perhaps in early gestation (42). The tumors involving a heritable component tend to occur at earlier ages and at multiple sites more frequently than do nonheritable cancers (2).

Familial patterns of cancer incidence have been documented since the seventeenth century. These cancers may be referred to as polygenic, implying that many genes may interact with environmental factors to cause disease, with no one factor or gene playing a major role (42). Disease sites examined in retrospective studies have shown a two- to fourfold excess in certain families, indicating that a family history of cancer can increase a person's risk for developing cancer. Higher incidence was found in studies involving cancer of the stomach, breast, large intestine, uterus, and lung. Increased risks were also observed for childhood brain tumors and sarcoma (2).

Aging may be a biological marker which heralds the possibility of cumulative exposure in the individual. During a lifetime, there may be environmental insults from diet, smoking, occupation, and other factors (36). As a person ages, the immunological defenses may decrease, hormonal changes take place, or both. Throughout a lifetime, there is an ever-increasing chance that exposure to an agent early in life will change the immunological status of the aging person. In addition, there may be a nonspecific, genetically determined time clock, or wearing out of the human organism, making one more vulnerable with age to all diseases including cancer (36). In animal research there is ongoing work examining the role of inherited and chemically induced DNA damage and repair systems which will lead to better understanding of biological inputs to cancer (40).

The malignancies associated with hereditary disease, then, affect every organ system and are often histologically identical to the most frequent human cancers. Some scientists believe that more such conditions are likely to be discovered as collaborative efforts are able to differentiate between clinical and genetic manifestations of disease (42).

Environmental Factors

Within the human environment there are many vulnerable places where viruses, radiation, and chemicals may play a role in contributing to a cancer outcome. The degree to which environmental factors contribute to cancer was scarcely suspected 40 years ago (57). Today many scientists believe that environmental factors interact with hereditary information in cells to produce a complex sequence of events leading to the development of cancer (58).

The role of viruses in the development of cancer has been actively examined since the 1950s. Scientists have found that a variety of viruses are capable of producing tumors in almost every species of animal except humans. The emphasis in this research has recently moved from the search for cancer-causing viruses to the study of ways in which the virus affects the growth and regulation of cells. The virus appears to act as a cofactor (59). There are some indications that carcinogenic agents as different as viruses and chemicals share a common step in the process of cancer development. It seems likely that viruses will be found to play a role in some forms of cancer in man (59).

"*Ionizing radiation* is perhaps the most extensively studied carcinogen" (9). Risks of cancer associated with high doses (in excess of 50 rads) of irradiation have been substantiated by studies from many sources. The issue of risk from low-dose or diagnostic levels of irradiation remains uncertain (56). There is no level of exposure entirely without some risk. A recent study of men exposed to ordinary diagnostic radiation found that previous estimates of safety obtained by extrapolation from high-dose levels to low-dose levels may have underestimated the actual hazards by a factor of ten (12). Although this outcome is already disputed, most scientists agree that diagnostic X-rays should not be underestimated in their potential relationship to cancers (9).

A second consideration for primary prevention involves the investigation of chemicals in the workplace and environment. Since workers in many industries are exposed to chemicals for longer periods and in higher concentrations than other members of society, industrial exposures have been the primary means for identifying chemical carcinogens in man. According to Higginson (30), "Studies on cancer in the workplace have historically led to the successful identification of new chemicals carcinogenic to man and subsequent control."

A current and lively debate concerns the degree of importance given toxic substances as a cause of cancer in occupational settings. Estimates of the fraction of cancer incidence attributed to occupational exposure are difficult to make and involve several problems. Many industries have not been investigated adequately. As workers change jobs during their work life, they also change their exposure patterns to carcinogens. Even the nature of cancer as a "disease of interactions" creates difficulties for teasing out the responsibility of each agent. Added to these problems is the delay of 10 or more years between the initial exposure to a chemical and the clinical appearance of a tumor. What is needed for research in chemical causation is continued examination of the temporal and spatial trends of cancer incidence around the heavily industrialized areas in the country in order to determine excess risk to workers. Collecting worker histories of occupational exposure to chemicals where excess mortality has been documented, along with material on the life style of workers such as smoking histories, is the next important step.

approved oral contraceptive pills, estrogens have been used by millions of women as birth control measures or for the treatment of symptoms.

Now several studies point to associations of estrogens with cancers of the breast and corpus uteri. A San Francisco–Oakland study noted a significant rise in the incidence of carcinoma of the endometrium during a 6-year period between 1969 and 1975. The rise was greatest in the most affluent areas. The data suggested that the rate of increase was due to the recent introduction of replacement hormones among postmenopausal women (3). In Seattle, physicians in a large prepaid group practice substantially reduced the number of prescriptions for replacement estrogens between July 1975 and July 1977 and then reported a sharp downward trend in the endometrial cancer incidence. The drop in overall incidence soon after estrogen discontinuance also suggests that the increased risk associated with the estrogens reverses rather quickly (19). Although estrogens have a legitimate place in the medical world, they may have been oversold to the American public without enough consideration for their potential side effects. Research will continue to help define the advantages and limits in using estrogens. Prevention efforts would appear to follow easily upon the results by minimizing or eliminating the product.

Personality Factors and Stress

The fourth area of life style, the role of personality factors and stress, has often been proposed as a factor in carcinogenesis. One view holds that the brain controls the body's susceptibility to illness and that an emotional state can alter the body's hormonal and immune systems.

Following his review of the literature, Fox (26) states that personality factors may play a small role in cancer etiology, but the research to date is entirely equivocal and unconvincing. A number of methodological problems prevent us from positing a valid and reliable connection between premorbid personality factors and cancer etiology. In the retrospective studies examined, accuracy of recall, interpretation of stress by the study subjects, and contradictory findings were three of the more compelling constraints of these studies. In the sparse and more recent prospective work, similar limitations obtain.

Morrison and Paffenbarger (41) recently reviewed the research of psychosocial variables and cancer against epidemiologic principles generally applied to research on human subjects. Among the discrepancies found was that most investigators did not consider the time lag between initiation of tumor growth and recognition of tumor presence. While ignoring the dynamic history of the disease process as it pertained to cell kinetics and tumor growth, behavioral scientists have continued to assume that past and current behaviors were equivalent or static. Other discrepancies in the research include the lack of evidence relating strength of association between catastrophic events or personality traits and cancer; the fact that associations found have not been shown to be reproducible; the fact that associations were not persistent when variables known to be risk factors for cancer were controlled; and the limitation that no dose–effect relationship has been demonstrated between personality factors, stress, and cancer. Believing there is no evidence to support the view that behavioral expression of personality traits remains constant over long periods of time, Morrison and Paffenbarger suggests that the disease itself is responsible for the behavior observed: "The disease, its progression, and its associated symptomatology account for the personality characteristics found in patients with cancer" (41).

If personality factors and stress do play a role in causing cancer, Fox (26) believes that it is a small percentage factor most likely affecting the lives of those about 35 to 55 years of age. Cancers appearing among the younger age group seem to have causes closer to genetic mutation processes, such as radiation to the unborn fetus. Patients over 70 years old are probably more affected by the body's accumulation of agents over a lifetime interacting with the aging processes (26).

The subject of personality factors and stress has not been exhausted. New research is currently in progress, which perhaps with more carefully executed methodologies will give us new clues to the personality-cancer puzzle. As Bahnson (26) wrote some years ago, "Each generation has to re-explore the relationship and reformulate it in terms of its own framework and vocabulary."

Quality of Health Care

A fourth input to health concerns the quality of health care available. Although improvements in survival statistics for cancer are due partly to improvements in treatment methodologies and their availability throughout the country, treatment progress has led to new iatrogenic problems, such as induction of second cancers by drugs or radiation. Immunosuppressive drugs used for renal transplantation have the capacity to cause reticulum cell sarcomas. Radioisotopes can cause leukemia. Cytotoxic drugs are known to induce solid tumors. An androgenic–anabolic steroid used for treatment of aplastic anemia can be associated with development of liver cancer (27). More recently, low-dose irradiation has become suspect in leukemia (12). More research efforts in iatrogenesis are needed and alternative diagnostic procedures and therapies found. And more attention will have to be given to the patients' "right to know" as they are examined or treated with these agents. While it is hoped that prevention efforts will follow research results and that iatrogenic problems will lessen in the future, it is probably more realistic to anticipate that with increasing sophistication of medical technology and therapy, new side effects will emerge with new treatments and procedures.

The causes of cancer penetrate every facet of the health care system. There are processes involved in one's biological or hereditary make-up which may enhance one's chances of having cancer. One's personal behavior or life style may add to this risk. Throughout the environment, continuingly modified by man himself, there are dangerous substances which may lead to a cancer. Even with the judicious and most often necessary application of medical technology today, there are toxic substances and numerous agents which endanger patients. The very nature of cancer, acting over time with multipotential causes coupled with the breadth and depth of the possibilities for exposure, leads one to the conclusion that prevention must be always the first line of defense.

THE NEED FOR PREVENTION

According to two important indicators—incidence and mortality rates—cancer is becoming more of a problem disease while most other health problems are declining in severity. Although survival rates are improving, the percentage of people saved does not approach the number lost. The costs of cancer to society are high, with a large portion of direct expenses going to treatment and care of dying patients rather than toward prevention of the disease. The premature losses of so many lives, especially among the productive middle-aged, disrupts family life and the economy. The underestimation of prevention as both a philosophy and a technique stands out as the missing link in the all-out war against the disease.

PREVENTION DEFINED

The approach to cancer prevention by behavioral scientists involves mobilizing action based on what is known about causes. It involves reaching attainable goals through personal and coordinated efforts in society. Since every disease entity has its own natural history, one may look at the events that determine causation and identify the weak links that might be exploited on behalf of prevention (37).

One can discuss three levels of cancer prevention:

1. *Primary prevention*—taking actions to prevent initial disease development.

2. *Secondary prevention*—taking actions to detect disease in its early asymptomatic stages and through appropriate intervention strategies arrest/reverse the progress of disease.

3. *Tertiary prevention*—taking actions to maintain a maximum level of independence and activity in the chronically ill and to improve quality of life; to continuously apply measures that will restrain the progress of disease once the disease has manifested itself (10).

All forms of prevention involve strategies which help individuals change life styles and regulate the environment.

Resistance to Prevention

There are historical sources of prevention resistance in our society. Although prevention efforts have been responsible for many improvements in health status in the United States, these efforts have seldom been endorsed as a high priority (63). As Kegeles discusses in Chapter 7, the primary health care providers during medical school training are inundated with techniques for curative procedures with little attention paid to preventative issues. Although historical evidence shows that improvements in nutrition, sanitation, infectious disease control, housing, and working conditions rather than medical care have been the major determinants of mortality reduction during the past two centuries, the public tends to equate the quality of their health with the availability of physicians and elaborate treatment procedures (13).

It is difficult to interest healthy people in preventing any chronic disease that cannot be managed with minimal effort and inconvenience, and that may not occur for decades (6). This may be a legacy from past experience with infectious disease prevention where the public has not been required to take an active role (36).

Other discrepancies confuse the picture. Americans are pluralistic and tend to be optimistic and proud of being "dominant over nature." They organize themselves to eliminate sources of fear and anger while professing a strong allegiance to the individual. They often cater more to capitalistic interests than to health care, ignoring the prevention of disease, which has limited apparent and immediate financial rewards. As McCall states in Chapter 9, "Primary prevention often costs a powerful interest group something." If prevention is seen as actions taken by society, part of its success will have to come from achieving emotional consensus with target populations (43).

What Is Not Known, What Is Needed?

Prevention is something people do; it involves actions taken by individuals and society (43). Behavioral scientists are interested in focusing research in primary prevention because of its importance in reducing the incidence of disease. Identifying high-risk persons in the population and reducing their exposures is an important field of study and application.

As Schweitzer points out in Chapter 8, environment and behavior must be dealt with together. More research is needed to examine the cause and effect relationship of agents and economics. The public needs to be better informed on hazards and major institutions (e.g., the insurance industry), and incentives for health need to be developed and marketed. He predicts that successful primary prevention will come as an interaction of medical analysis with behavioral and economic relationships.

Felton also, in Chapter 5, supports the need for research into methods of behavior modification and hazard control, but he notes that we know little about behavioral change. "No definitive research has been carried out to determine the most successful means of motivating behavioral change which will lower the pulmonary carcinoma risk level." Although the usual modalities of health education have been exercised (with shipyard workers), what is needed,

Felton believes, is a program to test all of the methods available for use in the work setting.

The lack of a supportive milieu can work against the success of behavioral change among people from lower economic groups. According to MacCalla (Chapter 10), "Individuals who find themselves in a lower socioeconomic level in society spend more of each day trying to provide self and family with the basic life needs of food, clothing, and shelter." Response to what may be viewed as an inevitable fate may be futility, passivism, and resignation. There is a need for health educators to work with low-income groups and a need for research that will examine race and ethnicity as significant variables in relation to cancer prevention compliance.

Outcome data from smoking cessation programs tend to support these points. In an analysis of successful abstainers, Gritz (29) tells us that the "successful" had (a) superior knowledge of the health hazards of smoking, (b) a more comprehensive set of reasons for stopping, including greater prior respiratory problems and serious illness, and (c) more non-smoking behavior in their families, all points being elements in the health belief model. And as Gritz points out (Chapter 4), demographic analysis of smoking cessation data from surveys also confirms MacCalla's concerns about successful efforts among the poor. The greatest proportion of ex-smokers is found among professionals, followed by white collar workers and then factory workers. When one looks at educational categories, fewer of those who have completed a college education continue to smoke than in other (lower) educational categories. Upton (59) noted in a recent publication, "It is tragic that it has taken our society two decades to react to the evidence incriminating tobacco as a major source of our cancer burden." Success among middle-class persons is a beginning, but behavioral scientists have additional work to do in developing methods which are successful with lower socioeconomic groups.

Behavioral scientists are concerned about research in many of the issues related to secondary prevention. In Chapter 6 D'Onofrio asserts that preventing the occurrence of all cancer is beyond present capabilities. Consequently, early diagnosis and treatment of the disease provides a critically important second line of defense. Progress in survival statistics is partially due to earlier diagnosis among certain cancer sites, such as cervical and breast cancers (24). Secondary prevention efforts are often located in or closely connected with the medical world, which employs the tools of detection, education, and protection of the individual.

Some factors appear to stimulate or retard the use of medical care at early stages of disease. Schweitzer speculates in Chapter 8 that the price system plays a role, as does the lack of widely available primary care. Further, the separation of health education from health services reduces the ability of the health system to intervene in the early stage of disease. He believes that the insurance sector should be encouraged to provide patient education and screening activities as a means of improving access and utilization.

A San Francisco Bay area study supports the point that people are responsive to incentives or constraints in the medical care insurance system. McCall (Chapter 9) reports on the effect of an insurance deductible on physician utilization in a prepaid plan. Over 50% of the adult males in the lowest socioeconomic group reduced their utilization of annual physical exams after the introduction of this co-insurance. Therefore, a general health screening was essentially eliminated for many people in the plan, especially the "working poor." This finding indicates that financial constraints do have an effect on medical usage.

Screening for disease became widely accepted in the late 1950s in the hope that earlier intervention would provide more successful results. The effectiveness of individual screening programs and the place of screening in the medical system are currently being evaluated by medical and behavioral scientists alike. Some have suggested (as does Kegeles in Chapter 7) that the question of who is screened needs to be tailored to the attributes of each test and the vulnerabilities of various age group populations. D'Onofrio states in her chapter that there is a critical need for research on psychosocial problems related to cancer screening and its linkages in the medical system. She calls for a disaggregation in the evaluation of the behavior of the consumer and the provider groups involved in the screening, a point supported by others. Health care personnel frequently are not representative of the populations they serve. The social distance between client and health professional, their separate priority systems, and other cultural differences may act as barriers to the effective utilization of services (7,21).

What is needed is a combination of cancer prevention and cancer screening processes. High-risk groups must be targets of both primary prevention campaigns and screening efforts to detect cancer at its earliest stages. Education and information are necessary to advise the exposed population of the risks, the effective means of minimizing the risks, and the benefits of screening and detection so that the public can make its own choice. Cancer prevention and screening activities could be developed as a multidisciplinary approach, forged as a team effort. Combining these activities could help to focus attention on specific subgroups at high risk or on groups not usually exposed to screening and educational services.

Reducing risk factors related to cancer among the population is one area where cancer prevention and cancer screening processes work together. Factors such as cigarette smoking, excessive consumption of alcohol, and exposure to certain chemicals—known to be related to the onset of cancer—are being systematically identified, opening the way for initiation of prevention projects. At the same time, new means of detecting physiological, anatomical, chemical, and genetic precursors of disease are found. The prospects for improving health through reducing risk factors have reached the point where, Breslow (11) believes, it is possible to project a systematic approach—a lifetime health monitoring program or surveillance system. Multiphasic health testing and health hazard appraisal, which are two forms of surveillance, combine the expertise of the medical world and the involvement of the consumer, thereby bridging an old gap in health education and creating an opportunity for a new thrust in preventive medicine.

An excellent source of screening for cancer is the potential patient himself. As Morrison and Paffenbarger (41) point out, "Most malignant disease is diagnosed because patients seek medical care for symptoms which are either immediately recognizable as dangerous or which persist over a long time without improvement. For breast cancer, evidence indicates that 69 per cent or more of breast lumps are found by women themselves." This reveals a need for improving effectiveness in health education in reaching the public, groups at high risk, and diagnosed patients. The time may be right for doing so; the public today appears to be interested in prevention activities, as seen in their adoption of jogging on a large scale. Although patients have traditionally failed to exercise their rights as consumers about their disease course, there are signs today of increasing patient participation in illness management, such as in the development of the Patients' Bill of Rights (38). Finding the public you want to address and getting their attention seem part of the unfinished task of behavioral scientists in secondary prevention. Another part may be to restructure the content and flow of health education ideas to the various publics and subgroups in our culture, so that greater personal options in life style have a chance to be realized (38).

Tertiary prevention involves clinically oriented behavioral scientists. This group, operating from a value-based belief in the dignity and worth of each person's life, is concerned with efforts to maintain a maximum of independence and activity in the life of the chronically ill person. Areas of research covered in this book include employment histories, psychosocial morbidity, the importance of the social support system, psychological traits, and the issue of coping patterns.

As the number of patients surviving their diagnoses for 2, 5, or more years has been increasing, greater attention has been focused on tertiary prevention. The need for this attention is prompted by the observation that traditional medical care has focused on the disease while the needs of the whole patient and family have not been considered. Where support services are lacking, there is evidence that emotional complications may take place which can be devastating to the patient.

Results from a study at Mt. Zion Hospital in San Francisco illustrate the need for support services as tertiary prevention on behalf of the cancer patient. The study was directed towards gathering first-hand material from patients and their family members who described the natural history of the disease over time. Sixty-six patients were interviewed in-depth over a 2½-year period. Thirty-five of these were 3- and 6-year survivors, and thirty-one were newly diagnosed and had been followed for 6 to 12 months. Some of the pertinent findings included the fact that, for all members of the prospective sample, the discovery and initial treatment of cancer produced considerable distress, emotional turmoil, and disruption of customary roles and activities. Six to twelve months later those with recurrent disease or crippling aftereffects continued to have serious problems in resuming the continuity of their lives, while patients who had no further problems returned to customary activities (19).

Other significant findings included the importance of body damage as a predictor of long-term distress. At all three time periods of cancer experience, the intensity of physical symptomatology and interference with bodily function was strongly associated with the degree of psychological distress. Two other factors correlating with this finding were the patient's psychological stability prior to cancer and the strength of the social support network surrounding the patient.

Sex and age factors were examined. As a group, male patients of all ages seemed more affected by the disease process than female patients. The men tended to suffer more anxiety, depression, and were more affected by negative body changes. They lost their sense of well-being and confidence in their bodies. In comparing coping styles, it was found that the men had more difficulty in "turning to others" for help. The women on the whole were more successful in maintaining a sense of emotional equilibrium, experienced fewer negative changes in self-image, and were more willing to maintain their social relationships and responsibilities.

On the other hand, age was not a predictor of psychosocial outcome; each age group studied dealt with the cancer experience from their own perspective. Although age influenced the manner in which cancer was experienced, and the style and pattern of response to the disease, "age" produced the filter through which a cancer patient viewed his experience rather than contributing to the difficulties experienced (19).

Some implications for services were concluded from the study. First, it may be possible to identify vulnerable patients from biographical factors and from characteristics of the illness itself. The three basic factors which correlated with unfavorable outcome—severity of illness (including body damage), previous psychological difficulties, and social isolation—can be evaluated on an in-service unit from a medical chart and a talk with a nurse. Making services available to the patient in distress rather than waiting for the patient to seek the services was a second recommendation. Many patients, especially men, were not able to seek help but were willing to respond to help when it was offered. A third finding involved recognition of the importance of the long-term nature of psychosocial change. The person with cancer is confronted with a series of crises and remissions and must deal with different problems at successive points in the illness. The experience of what it means to have cancer changes as the disease progresses and the patient finds that the social, vocational, and economic context in which he or she lives varies greatly.

This study confirms conclusions drawn by Koenig (33) from his study of fatally ill cancer patients. That is, social problems must be anticipated in persons with a chronic, fatal disease as a part of the natural history of the disease, and clinicians must be prepared to deal with them. A recent American Cancer

Society study verified that patients reported the time of diagnosis as the most stressful but that supportive services in general were lacking (28).

The importance of interest and research in tertiary prevention has been well stated by Schain (48), a psychologist who has had cancer:

> If one is committed to rehabilitiation of the total person and not just concerned with increasing longevity, then the issue of quality survival must be addressed.
>
> Humanistic treatment tactics demand that one acknowledge disruption not only in bodily function but also a self-esteem, and the insult to one's sense of well-being is a known consequence of a cancer diagnosis and radical surgery.
>
> Longevity is not just living; it involves loving, and rehabilitation experts must develop skills to provide assistance to preserve, enhance and liberate that energy in cancer patients (8).

In sum, there is much to be done by behavioral scientists in all aspects of prevention. In primary efforts, new energy is needed for smoking cessation with groups at high risk for disease. In secondary prevention, new directions are being sought for health education. And, in tertiary prevention, the needs of the surviving cancer patient and their families have only begun to be uncovered. When one considers how much of cancer could be prevented, or the cancer experience ameliorated through the work of behavioral scientists, the challenge becomes clear.

REFERENCES

1. Abt, C. (1975): The social costs of cancer. *Soc. Indicators Res.*, 2:175–190.
2. Anderson, A. (1975): Familial susceptibility. In: *Persons at High Risk of Cancer,* edited by J. F. Fraumeni, Jr., pp. 39–54. Academic Press, New York.
3. Austin, D., and Roe, K. (1979): Increase in cancer of the corpus uteri in the San Francisco–Oakland standard metropolitan statistical area, 1960–1975. *J. Natl. Cancer Inst.,* 62:13–16.
4. Axtell, L., Asire, A., and Meyers, M. (eds.) (1976): *Cancer Patient Survival Report Number 5,* U.S. Department of Health, Education and Welfare, National Cancer Institute, DHEW No. (NIH) 77–992.
5. Axtell, L., Meyers, M., and Shambaugh, E. (1975): *Treatment and Survival Patterns for Black and White Cancer Patients Diagnosed 1955 Through 1964.* U.S. Department of Health, Education and Welfare, DHEW No. (NIH) 75–712.
6. Bailar, J. (1979): The case for cancer prevention. *J. Natl. Cancer Inst.,* 62:727–729.
7. Berkanovic, E., and Reeder, L. (1974): Can money buy the appropriate use of services? Some notes on the meaning of utilization data. *J. Health Soc. Behav.,* 2:93–99.
8. Blum, H. (1974): *Planning for Health.* New Sciences Press, New York.
9. Boice, J., and Land, C. (1979): Adult leukemia following diagnostic X-rays? *Am. J. Public Health,* 69:137–145.
10. Breslow, L. (1976): *Theory, Practice and Application of Prevention in Personal Health Services.* Task Force Reports of the National Conference on Preventive Medicine. Prodist, New York.
11. Breslow, L. (1978): Prospects for improving health through reducing risk factors. *Prev. Med.,* 7:449–458.
12. Bross, I., Ball, M., and Fales, S. (1979): A dosage response curve for the one rad range: Adults risks from diagnostic radiation. *Am. J. Public Health,* 69:130–136.
13. Brown, E. R., and Margo, G. (1978): Health education: Can the reformers be reformed? *Int. J. Health Serv.,* 8:3–26.

14. Califano, J. (1979): Remarks to the Youth Conference National Inter-Agency Council on Smoking and Health. San Francisco, April 26, 1979. HEW News. U.S. Department of Health, Education and Welfare.
15. *Cancer in California* (1979): California Division, American Cancer Society, 25:1–19.
16. *Cancer Facts and Figures, 1978* (1977): American Cancer Society, New York, pp. 1–31.
17. *Cancer Facts and Figures, 1979* (1978): American Cancer Society, New York, pp. 1–31.
18. *Cancer Facts and Figures for Black Americans, 1979* (1978): American Cancer Society, New York, pp. 1–28.
19. Castro, J., Mages, N., Fobair, P., Mendelsohn, G., and Wolfson, A. (1978): *Exploratory Studies for Cancer Patient Rehabilitation: Final Report to National Cancer Institute.* For Grant No. 1R18–CA 16873.
20. Clayson, D. (1978): Overview, fact, myth, and speculation. *J. Environ. Pathol. Toxicol.,* 2:1–8.
21. Cohen, J. (1970): Availability and useability of social services in the south central area. In: *Los Angeles Riot: Social Psychological Study,* edited by N. Cohen. Praeger, New York.
22. Devesa, S. and Silverman, D. (1978): Cancer incidence and mortality trends in the United States: 1935–1974. *J. Natl. Cancer Inst.,* 60:545–571.
23. Devita, V. (1979): *Statement to the U.S. Congress,* Senate, Health Subcommittee from the Director, Division of Cancer Treatment, National Cancer Institute, March.
24. Enstrom, J., and Austin, D. (1977): Interpreting cancer survival rates. *Science,* 195:847–851.
25. Feldman, F. (1978): *Work and Cancer Health Histories: A Study of the Experiences of Recovered Blue Collar Workers.* California Division, American Cancer Society, San Francisco.
26. Fox, B. (1978): Premorbid psychological factors as related to cancer incidence. *J. Behav. Med.,* 1:45–133.
27. Fraumeni, J. (1975): *Persons at High Risk of Cancer.* Academic Press, New York.
28. Greenleigh Associates (1979): *Report on the Social, Economic and Psychological Needs of Cancer Patients in California.* California Division, American Cancer Society, San Francisco.
29. Gritz, E. (1977): Smoking: The prevention of onset. In: *Research on Smoking Behavior,* edited by M. Jarvik, J. Cullen, and E. Gritz, pp. 290–307. NIDA Research Monograph 17, December.
30. Higginson, J. (1979): Environmental carcinogenesis: Some misconceptions and their influence on cancer control. *AACI Newsletter,* April.
31. *Impact Costs and Consequences of Catastrophic Illness on Patients and Families* (1973): Cancer Care and the National Cancer Foundation, New York, March.
32. Johns-Manville's No Smoking Program (1978): *Johns-Manville News,* Denver, Colorado.
33. Koenig, R. (1968): Fatal illness—A survey of social service needs. *Soc. Work,* 13:71–78.
34. Lansky, S., Cairns, N., Clark, G., Loman, J., Miller, L., and Trueworthy, R. (1979): Childhood cancer: Nonmedical costs of the illness. *Cancer,* 43:403–408.
35. Levin, D., Devesa, S., Godwin, J. D., and Silverman, D. (1974): *Cancer Rates and Risks.* U.S. Dept. of Health, Education and Welfare, DHEW No. (NIH) 76–691.
36. Lilienfeld, A. (1976): *Foundations of Epidemiology.* Oxford University Press, New York.
37. McDermott, W. (1977): Medicine: The public good and one's own. *Cornell Univ. Med. Coll. Alumni Q.,* 40:15–24.
38. Mantell, J., and Cordoba, C. (1978): *An Ounce of Prevention: Social Work's Contribution to Patient Education.* Paper presented to the Council on Social Work Education, New Orleans, February.
39. Mason, T., and McKay, F. (1973): *U.S. Cancer Mortality by County, 1950–1969,* U.S. Department of Health, Education and Welfare, National Cancer Institute, DHEW No. (NIH) 74–615.
40. Miller, E. C. (1978): Some current perspectives on chemical carcinogenesis in humans and experimental animals: Presidential address. *Cancer Res.,* 38:1479–1496.
41. Morrison, F., and Paffenbarger, R. (1979): *Epidemiologic Aspects of Biobehavior in the Etiology of Cancer.* Paper presented at the Academy of Behavior Medicine Conference, Snowbird, Utah, June 5.
42. Mulvihill, J. (1975): Congenital and genetic diseases. In: *Persons at High Risk of Cancer: An Approach to Cancer Etiology and Control,* edited by J. F. Fraumeni, Jr., pp. 3–37. Academic Press, New York.
43. Mulvihill, J. (1978): *Medical and Internal Factors: Familial and Genetic Factors.* Paper presented at the Conference on Cancer Prevention—Quantitative Aspects, Reston, Va., September.
44. *A National Dilemma: Cigarette Smoking or the Health of Americans (1978):* Report of the

National Commission on Smoking and Public Policy, American Cancer Society, New York, January.

45. Nelson, N. (1976): Theory, practice and application of prevention in personal health services. *Task Force Reports of the National Conference on Preventive Medicine.* Prodist, New York.

46. Overton, M. (1977): *Costs of Cancer Care.* Testimony by Exec. Dir., Cancer Care, Inc., to Dept. of Health, Education and Welfare Hearings on National Health Insurance and Long-Term or Catastrophic Illness, October.

47. Rice, D., and Hodgson, T. (1978): *Social and Economic Implications of Cancer in the United States.* Paper presented to the Expert Committee on Cancer Statistics of the World Health Organization and International Agency for Research on Cancer, Madrid, June.

48. Schain, W. S. (1979): *Self-Esteem, Sexuality, and Cancer Care.* Paper presented at 14th Annual San Francisco Cancer Symposium, San Francisco, March.

49. Schneiderman, M. (1979): *Trends in Cancer Incidence and Mortality in the United States.* Statement before the Subcommittee on Health and Scientific Research, U.S. Congress, Senate, Committee on Human Resources, March.

50. Schwartz, J., and Rider, G. (1978): *Review and Evaluation of Smoking Control Methods: the United States and Canada, 1969–1977.* U.S. Department of Health Education and Welfare, Center for Disease Control, DHEW Pub. No. (CDC) 79–8369.

51. Schweitzer, S. (1979): Social cost versus effectiveness of bone marrow transplant therapy. *Bull. UCLA Cancer Center,* 6:3.

52. Scotto, J., and Chiazze, L. (1976): *Hospitalization and Payments to Hospitals: Third National Cancer Survey.* U.S. Department of Health Education and Welfare. National Cancer Institute, DHEW Pub. No. (NIH) 76–1094, March.

53. Scotto, J., and Chiazze, L. (1977): Cancer prevalence and hospital payments. *J. Natl. Cancer Inst.,* 59:345–349.

54. U.S. Department of Health, Education and Welfare, National Cancer Institute. SEER Report on Cancer Incidence and Mortality in the United States, 1973–1976. DHEW Pub. No. (NIH) 78–1837.

55. U.S. National Center for Health Statistics. *Vital Statistics Report, Final Mortality Statistics, 1976.* U.S. Department of Health, Education and Welfare, Public Health Service, DHEW No. 78–1120.

56. Upton, A. (1978): *Statement on Diagnostic Low-Level Radiation, July 14.* Before the Subcommittee on Health and the Environment, House Committee on Interstate and Foreign Commerce. Office of Communication, National Cancer Institute.

57. Upton, A. (1978): Important Progress Logged by NCI. *U.S. Medicine.* Office of Communication, National Cancer Institute.

58. Upton, A. (1978): The National Cancer Institute and Its Redefined Mission. *Grants Magazine,* 1:113–128. Office of Communication, National Cancer Institute.

59. Upton, A. (1978): Progress in the prevention of cancer. *Prev. Med.,* 7:476–485.

60. Upton, A. (1978): *Statement on the Role of Nutrition Research in Cancer.* Before the Subcommittee on Nutrition, Senate Committee on Agriculture, Nutrition, and Forestry. Office of Communication, National Cancer Institute, June.

61. Upton, A. (1979): *Statement on the National Cancer Institute Budget for 1980.* Office of Communication, National Cancer Institute.

62. Weisburger, J. (1978): Environmental cancer. *Tex. Rep. Biol. Med.,* 37:2–18.

63. Winkelstein, W. (1972): Epidemiological considerations underlying the allocation of health and disease care resources. *Int. J. Epidemiol.,* 1:69–74.

64. Wynder, E. (1978): A corner of history. *Prev. Med.,* 7:28–30.

65. Wynder, E. (1978): *Dietary Habits in Cancer (Epidemiology).* Paper presented to the American Cancer Society's and the National Cancer Institute's National Conference on Nutrition in Cancer, New York, June.

Psychosocial Aspects of Cancer,
edited by Jerome Cohen et al.
Raven Press, New York © 1982.

Chapter 3

Role of the Social and Behavioral Sciences in Cancer Prevention

Joseph W. Cullen

Jonsson Comprehensive Cancer Center, Division of Cancer Control, University of California, Los Angeles, Los Angeles, California 90024

Too often when the psychosocial dimensions of cancer are referred to, what is meant are those dimensions related to cancer treatment, rehabilitation, and continuing care. What is not included, or unfortunately often forgotten, is that there are other dimensions in the cancer management spectrum which have profound psychosocial implications, particularly those relating to primary prevention and early detection. Indeed, there is a number of psychosocial dimensions related to primary prevention and early detection that demands systematic investigation. This is one justification for a section on prevention in a book dedicated to psychosocial research issues in cancer.

If one thinks of the cancer management spectrum as a horizontal vector in time, proceeding chronologically from prevention through detection, diagnosis, treatment, rehabilitation, and continuing care (see Fig. 1), the latter interventions are vertical vectors intersecting the time continuum, where the health care system and public interface, subtending a complex of psychosocial considerations, issues, needs, implications, and so forth. They are interventions which the health care system chooses to consider in planning for and implementing health care under normal circumstances. Yet the amount of attention or interest and the allocation of resources both human and financial have been scanty for the study and application of these interventions. That is not to say that there have not been preventive medicine advocates, but such individuals are often seen as idealists, or even extremists. *A fortori,* psychosocial issues associated with preventive medicine are regarded as even more orthogonal and consequently are even more neglected.

It would be far too ambitious a task to attempt a correction of this imbalance in a single monograph. To begin with, there are disagreements among scientists and health care experts as to whether and what cancers are preventable. There are those who take the position that much of cancer is environmental, man-made, and therefore ought to be preventable. Such proponents point to cigarette

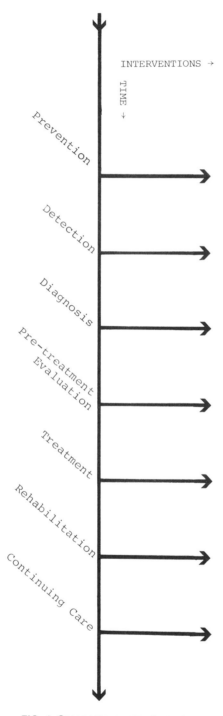

FIG. 1. Cancer management spectrum.

smoking, diet, alcohol consumption, ultraviolet radiation, and occupational carcinogens as major sources of carcinogenesis. Others offer compelling arguments for reducing cancer mortality by preventing its noninevitable growth through early detection and effective treatment. While the majority of these prevention attributions needs no reexamination, it should at least be noted that, when mortality ratios from current cigarette-only smokers are analyzed by cause of death, as has been done in several major epidemiologic studies (1,2,6), individuals in the age brackets 45 to 64 and 65 to 69 years (males and females alike) have a considerably elevated rate of cancer of the lung, bronchus, larynx, oral cavity, pharynx, and esophagus. There is an even higher than expected cancer rate for the bladder, pancreas, kidney, and stomach. The fact is that of all the deaths from cancer occurring among men in the United States in the period 1967 to 1971, as much as 34.5% were mainly or partly due to smoking (3). When one adds to this impressive statistic that as much as 3% of all cancers in the United States in 1974 were attributable to alcohol consumption (7), and that approximately 5% are now attributable to occupational exposures (4), one has already accounted for a large portion of cancer incidence without invoking neoplasms related, albeit speculatively, to diet or to the other suspected agents including food additives, drugs, radiation, and biorefractories in drinking water.

The role of the environment in cancer causation, according to Higginson and Muir (5), "has been recognized for many years, and the criticism that the scientific community has failed to study these problems has little justification." Nevertheless, man continues to search for a "silver bullet," a cancer cure or some other biomedical *Deus ex machina.* Man resorts to the tradition of treating the disease with robust enthusiasm and unfailing devotion.

The dialogue continues to grow louder, and justifiably so, in relation to carcinogenesis and lifestyle. Indeed, many believe that the 1980s will witness a dramatic modification in some of the more traditional biomedical models to include the nostrum of cancer prevention. The time truly has come, then, to consolidate whatever gains have already been made by social and behavioral scientists, relating to health issues and to prioritize prospective research activities that are necessary to guarantee that the war on cancer does not continue "on one wing."

So as not to appear excessively glib about the promise to reduce cancer incidence by modifying life styles or by any other behavioral/social means, it should be noted that resistance to these gains and even failures will probably precede or parallel any successes. There is already evidence that behavioral and social scientists are found wanting in providing society with answers to health care solutions in general. But as a rejoinder to that unfortunately true allegation, it is documentable that the resources historically allocated to these scientists have not been adequate. That fact, together with the long history of attention that such scientists have given to other fields of endeavor, specifically mental health, alcoholism, and psychosomatic diseases, accounts for the gaps in the theoretical models required for sound psychosocial research in cancer and the ensuing paucity of research data which would have issued from such models and studies. This situation will not change unless these scientists are encouraged to join the fray and are supported accordingly.

In the chapters that follow in this section, important behavioral and social research considerations in cancer prevention are addressed across several fronts. Because of the limitation of space, the specific topics selected are to a degree arbitrary; nonetheless, they stand out as critical points for the development of a comprehensive cancer plan for the 1980s.

Smoking behavior among females is foremost in this category. The discussion by Gritz relating to the situational factors influencing female smoking behavior and intervention strategies to change it are of utmost concern for society to confront and the scientific research world to consider. In fact, in this particular instance, there is no arbitrariness in pointing to smoking behavior as an issue to be considered for research promulgation. It is one of the most destructive forms of human behavior today engaged in by a civilized society.

The malignant diseases induced in industrial settings where thousands of Americans are captive throughout their working years are highlighted by Felton. Although there is no categorical definition about the number of cancers caused in the workplace, the potential health impact of industrial exposure since the massive industrialization in this country in the past half century could be ominous. While some of the diseases caused in these settings may be difficult or even impossible to eradicate because of considerations beyond reasonable or available technology, it is not an empty postulate to examine systematically where behavioral issues are causal or correlative in these processes. Where they are either of these there must be a better means to manipulate them. Embarrassingly, we know of very few of these means in a society that can perform virtually any technological feat.

Much has been written about the relationships of early screening and detection to reduction in mortality from cancer. However, D'Onofrio and Kegeles meticulously outline that there are numerous gaps in our informational base relating to the human element in this process, including how to motivate the public to respond to health education exhortations or even to perceive symptomotology with responsibility and alacrity thereby guarding against the progression of unnecessary life-threatening disease.

The economic aspects of all of these issues are focal points for the nation's health leaders and policy makers. The Congress and the people continue to ask questions that imply concern with or confront the cost of health care, and rightly so. Our country has come to a decision point. Either the choice is made to provide the necessary technologies required to manage the diseases of the populace (this strategy, of course, implies a diminution of expenditures in other categories of national priority), or we mount carefully designed realistic programs in disease prevention, where the prospects are promising. Both Schweitzer and McCall deal with such issues and with the research strategies to be considered in a program to deal with them.

Finally, as MacCalla points out, there are the broad and complex social and cultural dimensions related to the prevention of cancer. America, as the proverbial melting pot, subtends a plethora of ethnic and cultural differences that rule out monolithic intervention strategies for virtually any societal program, including health and cancer prevention. At this point in time little is known about the groups and their differences as they relate to education, attitude, and behavior change. Indeed, not even enough is known about the epidemiologic characteristics of the various subpopulations. The challenge, then, is to examine what is known, even from other fields of endeavor besides health and/or cancer, and to match that knowledge base with the target audiences, their needs, and the prospects of a future payoff given an expenditure of funds and energy.

Promises have been made in the past across all aspects of health care. In the case of cancer the National Cancer Program optimistically and incredulously capitulated to the mandate to develop a "silver bullet" in order to treat cancer more effectively. It seems that the charisma of being able to cure disease (allowed in some instances to have occurred through excessive or inappropriate consummatory behavior) exceeds the pride or recognition that comes when the disease is prevented from onset. But prevention has now become the nostrum for the future. Society cannot afford to ignore it. Where treatment is still necessary, prevention truly does not apply. But where treatment would not be necessary if prevention were applied, it does not speak well of our national system to perpetuate such a delusion. If we have the knowledge, we must learn how to use it more effectively. Where we do not have such knowledge, we must learn systematically to investigate ways of gaining it. That is the nature of science.

REFERENCES

1. Doll, R., and Peto, R. (1976): Mortality in relation to smoking: 20 years' observation on male British doctors. *Br. Med. J.,* 2:1525–1536.
2. Hammond, E. C. (1966): Smoking in relation to the death rates of one million men and women. In: *Epidemiological Approaches to the Study of Cancer and Other Chronic Diseases,* edited by W. Haensael, pp. 127–204. U.S. Public Health Service, National Cancer Institute Monogr. 19.
3. Hammond, E. C., and Seidman, H. (1980): Smoking and cancer in the United States. *Prev. Med.,* 9:169–173.
4. Higginson, J. (1980): Proportion of cancers due to occupation. *Prev. Med.,* 9:180–188.
5. Higginson, J., and Muir, C. S. (1979): Environmental carcinogenesis: Misconceptions and limitations to cancer control. *J. Natl. Cancer Inst.,* 6:1291–1298.
6. Hirayama, T. (1972): Smoking in relation to the death rates of 265,118 men and women in Japan. A report on 5 years of follow-up. Presented at the American Cancer Society's 14th Science Writer's Seminar, Clearwater Beach, Florida, pp. 24–29.
7. Rothman, K. J. (1980): The proportion of cancer attributable to alcohol consumption. *Prev. Med.,* 9:174–179.

Psychosocial Aspects of Cancer,
edited by Jerome Cohen et al.
Raven Press, New York © 1982.

Chapter 4

The Female Smoker: Research and Intervention Targets

Ellen R. Gritz

Veterans Administration Medical Center, Brentwood, Los Angeles, California 90073; and Department of Psychiatry, The Neuropsychiatric Institute, School of Medicine, University of California, Los Angeles, Los Angeles, California 90024

Smoking is not a harmless habit. Its potential lethality is recognized by the medical community, health professionals in related fields, and a majority of the lay public.

In the early 1960s evidence was clearly set forth causally linking cigarette smoking and lung cancer (34,49). Since that time this relationship has been further defined and the connection confirmed between smoking and increased risk of developing cancer at several other sites. These include larynx, pharynx, oral cavity, esophagus, and bladder (18,35,51). Other serious disorders linked to smoking include coronary heart disease and other vascular diseases, chronic obstructive lung disease, and peptic ulcer.

Through education, legislation, and publicity, a tremendous effort is being made to promote a reduction in tobacco consumption and in the number of smokers and to prevent the initiation of smoking in teen-agers. The success of this campaign is measurable (50). The proportion of the United States population that smokes is on the decline. Unfortunately, men seem more responsive to this campaign than do women. Not only do males seem to quit smoking more readily than do females, but the pattern of initiation of smoking among teen-age females shows increases in smoking while males maintain stable rates.

People begin to smoke for social reasons. The influence and models provided by friends, siblings, and parents are extremely important (5,38,44). The following relationships were found consistently in the National Clearinghouse for Smoking and Health (NCSH) surveys: in two-parent homes the likelihood of a teen-ager smoking was directly related to the number of parents who smoked. Even more teen-agers who lived in one-parent homes were likely to be smokers than in two-parent homes. Teen-agers, especially girls, were more likely to become smokers if their mother was a smoker than if their father was. Having an older sibling who smoked increased the likelihood of a teen-ager's becoming a smoker over having a nonsmoking sibling. With both older sibling and parental smoking in the home, there was a fourfold greater probability that a teen-ager would smoke than if neither parent nor older sibling smoked. This information clearly supports the critical role of the family as a modeling structure.

In a parallel vein, the interview data concerning the smoking behavior of "four best friends" revealed that teen-agers congregate with others with similar habits. Among teen-age girls who were regular smokers, 88.6% had at least one friend who was also a current regular smoker, whereas only 30.2% of teen-agers who were never-smokers or experimenters had at least one friend who was a regular smoker. In this latter group of nonsmokers/experimenters, therefore, 69.8% reported friends with the same nonsmoking patterns.

A variety of studies have reported that smoking prevalence was inversely associated with socioeconomic status and academic performance/aspirations, and directly associated with alcohol use (27,36,37,44). Students who worked were more likely to be smokers than those who did not hold jobs (44), but this finding may be linked to socioeconomic status and the need to contribute to family income or earn one's own spending money.

The dynamics of teen-age smoking were further explored in the 1974 NCSH survey (44). Eight factors were identified which describe teen-agers' attitudes toward smoking: health effects, nonsmokers' rights, positive aspects of smoking, rationalizations supporting smoking in the face of medical evidence, stereotypes surrounding the initiation of smoking, stereotypes of the personality of smokers, feelings toward authority, and individual control over the future. The factor scores of teen-age boys and girls did not differ substantially on any factor, but smokers did differ from nonsmokers in both sexes. It is relevant to this discussion that education regarding the health hazards of smoking is effective, being accepted by smoking and nonsmoking teen-agers alike. Smokers assert that cigarettes can make one feel good; nonsmokers rarely agree to this statement. Smokers rationalize their behavior by maintaining more strongly than nonsmokers that smoking is "okay" if quitting occurs before habituation. On the other hand, smokers are also much more willing to become "hooked" on something, including cigarettes, than nonsmokers. Nonsmokers seem more inclined to think that smoking makes one more popular with the opposite sex and that it is associated with precocious maturation and showing off ("bad" tendencies) than do smokers. Finally, teen-age smokers appear to have more conflictual feelings toward adult authority than nonsmokers.

The most recent and extensive survey of smoking behavior among teen-age girls and young women in the United States was carried out in 1975 under the auspices of the American Cancer Society (ACS) by a survey opinion corporation (48). The report confirms and extends the NCSH findings. The smoking habits of women 18 to 35 years of age are similar to those of teen-age girls. Both groups show a marked increase in the proportion of heavy smokers (at least a pack a day), while teen-age boys have not made similar increases. The respective proportions of teen-age boy, teen-age girl, and young women smokers smoking at least 30 cigarettes per day in 1975 were 31%, 39%, and 61%.

Changing social norms are gradually blurring gender-specific roles in large segments of our society. These changes have affected females more than males. Summarizing an extensive body of interview data, the authors state:

> In general, the teenage girls have been more influenced by the new youth values than the boys. These "New Values," originally generated by college youth in the sixties and now permeating the majority of all young people, represent the breakdown of previous moral norms and are characterized by the rejection of authority, emphasis on the emotional rather than the rational, freer sexual morality, a strong accent on self and self-fulfillment, the acceptance of illegal drugs and a more informal life style (48, p. 9)

The pervasiveness of the "smoking environment" is reinforced by the influence of the media portraying smokers as attractive, popular, affluent, and healthy; by the reduction in televised antismoking commercials; and by the provision of "smoker" rooms in high schools. Furthermore, a full 70% of the teen-age girl smokers and 73% of young women claimed their physicians had not counseled them against smoking, although knowledge of the health risks is widespread and well accepted in their groups.

For most of the teen-agers, however, the anti-smoking education came too late, in the 7th to 10th grades, after they had already begun to smoke. Timing appears to be critical as an intervention strategy when a child is exposed to the smoking behavior of parents from birth and to the smoking behavior of siblings and friends at ever earlier ages. With this factual background, research and intervention strategies become apparent.

PREVENTING THE ONSET OF SMOKING

The first test intervention that comes to mind is to expose children to anti-smoking education in the elementary schools, before much experimentation has taken place. At least three such projects have been undertaken, with two still in progress (6,13,47). The Houston (13) and Los Angeles (6) studies are primarily peer-teaching interventions, aimed at providing techniques of recognizing peer, parental, and media influences promoting smoking and of successfully resisting them. No special approaches were designed for girls as opposed to boys. The concept of dealing with present behaviors and pressures instead of future health risks seems to be a sound one, since the health knowledge is apparently widely disseminated through a variety of sources. The limitations on these intervention studies involve the amount of exposure to counterproductive (pro-smoking) influences, selective attrition of volunteer subjects, and uncontrollable events such as student transfers.

We need more simultaneous interventions to affect a wider sphere of the teen-ager's life, and we need to coordinate these efforts. Such a test intervention would be best carried out in a small community or cohesive suburb. In a large urban environment, the teen-ager may be exposed to a multiplicity of physical settings with differing smoking-related stimulus patterns, such that the effect of an anti-smoking campaign does not "transfer" into very different physical sectors of life.

Suggested avenues for target interventions could be provided by the media, social clubs of various forms (for example, Scouts), religious organizations, athletic organizations, health professionals, and parent-teacher organizations. A campaign of this type is being carried out in North Karelia Province, Finland, to reduce the rate of cardiovascular disease in the entire populace (30); the local food and dairy industries are simultaneously involved.

Interventions of this magnitude, if successful, fail to differentiate the effectiveness of the various components. It is therefore critical to evaluate separately each aspect of an intervention. In every case, a sample group of teen-agers exposed to a particular experimental technique should be matched as closely as possible with a control group which remains unexposed.

Another suggestion involves designing gender-specific interventions and testing them against coeducational interventions. Although the survey data cited here show that teen-age girls have caught up with teen-age boys in smoking prevalence, there are suggestions of different social dynamics at work. Teen-age girl smokers appear to be self-confident, socially sophisticated, and extroverted, whereas teen-age boy smokers are described as socially unsure and using cigarettes as a demonstration of masculinity and male assertiveness (48). In both sexes, smoking seems to be associated with an attitude of rebellion against adult authority, but one of more recent and drastic form among girls. Specific approaches dealing with these dynamics could be developed and presented to single-sex audiences, to be compared to a mixed audience. Research by sociologists and psychologists is needed to confirm and delineate further these findings.

THE YOUNG WOMAN SMOKER: AGES 18 TO 35

In the 18- to 35-year age range, interventions involving the place of work become appropriate. The American Cancer Society study (48) reported that 39% of young women smokers are employed full or part time, and 61% fall into the category of housewife, unemployed, or student. Within these subgroups of smokers, 66% of the housewives, unemployed, and students are heavy smokers, compared to only 53% of the working women. Anti-smoking programs located in the place of employment provide a specific focus for women in a place where stress is likely to be encountered. The work environment also provides a locus where a supportive environment can be formally organized and utilized to sustain cessation and abstinence efforts. The importance of social support will be elaborated on when discussing cessation methodology.

Anti-smoking campaigns should be organized to reach the housewife via the daytime media, perhaps outside of supermarkets and in large shopping malls, and even through preschool and elementary school parent contact programs. We can be much more active in this realm.

The young woman smoker is also the target for anti-smoking interventions related to fertility and childbearing status. Although oral contraceptive use alone does not increase the risk for developing coronary heart disease (CHD), women who both smoke and use oral contraceptives are subject to higher risk (21,22,26). Compared to those who neither smoke nor take oral contraceptives, the relative risk for CHD is about $12:1$, and rises to $15:1$ in heavy smokers (21). Furthermore, a report of an association between smoking and current oral contraceptive use in increasing the risk for subarachnoid hemorrhage has recently been made (31). There may be a range of vascular diseases which occur with increased frequency in female smokers who use oral contraceptives.

These well-documented findings could be used to spearhead interventions in target populations through gynecologists and other sources of birth control information. The teen-ager who is simultaneously beginning to use birth control and to smoke is an especially important candidate for such anti-smoking campaigns. Women have traditionally been more concerned with health and health care in our society than have men (24), and this age may be an optimal time to introduce such information. Rap groups and feminist centers provide other locales in which to reach the target population.

SMOKING DURING PREGNANCY

The prime childbearing period falls between 18 and 35 years of age. In this time span the smoking status of women is of special importance because of potential harmful effects during pregnancy. Since 1957, when the first report of fetal growth retardation appeared in the literature (42), the connection between maternal smoking and the birth of small-for-date infants has been repeatedly confirmed (2,19,28,29,35,43). On the average, full-term babies born to smokers are 200 g lighter than those born to women who do not smoke. If a woman quits smoking by the end of the fourth month of pregnancy, this effect on the fetus does not occur. However, if she continues to smoke throughout her pregnancy, she has a nearly twofold risk compared to a nonsmoker of delivering a low birth weight baby, one weighing less than 2,500 g. This relationship between smoking and low birth weight holds when other influences, such as socioeconomic status, have been controlled and has been demonstrated in a variety of races, cultures, and geographical settings (43).

Higher fetal and infant mortality among smokers' infants is another finding of serious consequence (28,43). Increased risks associated with both low birth weight and premature delivery of infants of women who smoke have been related to the excess perinatal mortality observed. A number of complications of pregnancy leading to early fetal loss have also been reported to occur more frequently among smokers. These include spontaneous abortion and miscarriage, abruptio placentae, placenta previa, and premature and prolonged rupture of the membranes (19,23,28). When making such comparative analyses, it is important to rule out potentially confounding variables such as maternal age, health status, parity, attitude toward pregnancy, and medication use (43).

The one finding reflecting a potentially protective influence of smoking during pregnancy is that of reduced incidence of toxemia and pre-eclamptic toxemia in smokers. These are conditions associated with hypertension, clinical edema, and proteinurea. The published reports have controlled for other risk factors, and present as a possible explanation the muscle capillary dilation action of nicotine or the hypotensive effects of thiocyanate, the detoxification product of cyanide (1,2,11,43). An alternate explanation is provided by the suggestion that pregnant women at risk for these disorders may abort, resulting in lower incidence rates. In fact, when one sums the incidence rates for spontaneous abortion, pre-eclampsia, and toxemia, it is observed that smoking and nonsmoking pregnant women do not differ (35).

Despite this accumulation of evidence warning against smoking in pregnancy, there is little medical and public health activity to assist women in quitting during this specific time period. There are only three published reports of systematic smoking deterral and cessation programs, and these did not achieve marked success (3,7,8). It is estimated that one-third of pregnant women smokers spontaneously quit for the course of their pregnancy, one-third cut down, and one-third continue to smoke at their previous rate (3,48).

A number of strategies must be employed to convey the urgency and the benefits of abstinence during pregnancy to smoking women. Obstetricians must be persuaded to take a far more active role in this regard than they have up to the present. The report of a positive pregnancy test and the early prenatal visits are ideal times to deliver printed materials, make nurse-patient and physician-patient contacts, and perhaps even suggest a local smoking cessation group just for pregnant women. Although women in higher socioeconomic classes who have been exposed to advanced education tend to be more receptive to educational materials, the working class woman may rely more on lay referral systems, such as family and friends (3,14). Furthermore, the studies which concentrated on the working class women (in Great Britain) pointed out the salience of personal experience: primiparous women showed greater acceptance of educational materials than women who had already borne a child (3,9). Ordered by frequency, sources of information were television, posters and leaflets, husbands, family and friends, books or magazines, a doctor, and a nurse (3).

Personalized approaches for smoking cessation during pregnancy and continued abstinence after childbirth must be developed carefully. Ethically, there are issues to consider regarding the woman who cannot or will not stop smoking; the provision of information must always be delivered in a non-guilt-inducing fashion. In the past, an extreme of this point of view—that the pregnant woman is so delicately emotionally balanced that she cannot be disturbed with "unpleasant" information—has been used as an excuse to avoid any intervention whatsoever. The positive viewpoint involves the concept that this 9-month period in a woman's life is a unique one in which she is responsible for the care of two individuals. With high motivation, it can become an especially good and perhaps easy time to initiate a major life change in health habits.

SMOKING CESSATION

Information regarding smoking cessation in women is gathered from two sources: the population surveys conducted by the NCSH and the treatment literature. Concentrating on the most recent data, the surveys conducted by the NCSH between 1964 and 1975 show that there has been a gradual increase in the percentages of former smokers in both sexes, although the patterns of incidence and prevalence differed (39,45). In general, males were giving up smoking in greater proportions than females. The 1975 survey reported that 42.6% of males who had ever smoked were now ex-smokers, compared with 33.5% of females (45). Males may also remain abstinent for longer time periods than women: a 2-year follow-up of more than 500 ex-smokers identified in the 1964 survey showed significantly greater success among males on this measure (12).

Demographic analyses of the smoking cessation data from these surveys reveal that in every occupational category a greater proportion of males than females who had ever smoked had quit (45). The greatest proportion of ex-smokers is found among professionals, followed by white-collar workers, and then factory workers. Quitting rates for male and female professionals are closest; however, among male health professionals (physicians, dentists, and pharmacists), 55 to 64% were former smokers in 1975, compared to only 36% of nurses (46).

As in the case of occupation, fewer of those who have completed a college education continue to smoke than in other educational categories; 52% of males and 48% of females who fall into the former category who had ever smoked were ex-smokers in 1975 (45). Combining all other categories, 40.5% of males and 31.3% of females were ex-smokers in this survey.

The treatment literature for smoking cessation includes a wide variety of interventions. These span a range from educational approaches, such at those offered by the American Cancer Society, to experimental evaluations of aversive conditioning techniques performed in university settings to pharmacotherapy with a variety of drugs, offered in a formal medical clinic. Treatment populations also range—from college students to middle-aged individuals with a 20-year history of smoking two packs of cigarettes a day. It is not always easy to tease out effects of demographic and smoking history-related variables on treatment success rates. For detailed consideration of the problems and results of research in this area, the reader is referred to a number of sources (16,25,32,40). The overall finding is that initial end-of-treatment success rates tend to be rather high, but that recidivism rates are equally high. If one examines maintenance rates for abstinence among those who have successfully quit smoking, only 35% are still abstinent at 3 months, and only about 20% remain abstinent at 1 year (20,32).

Examining the treatment literature for evidence of gender differences in cessation success rates is difficult, since only a tiny fraction of published reports include the relevant information. In a recent examination of the literature, only 30 reports of differential quitting rates for male and female smokers were located, and an additional 9 which treated only female subjects (see ref. 15 for a more extensive treatment of this subject). These studies covered the full variety of treatments: education, psychotherapy, behavior modification, and pharmacotherapy.

Both at end-of-treatment and long-term (1 year or greater) follow-up, the majority of studies showed no significant difference between male and female quitting rates. Approximately half of the studies contained reports of data which were inadequate for comparison purposes at either evaluation period. In the remaining studies, a significantly greater proportion of men were abstinent at end-of-treatment in 30% of the reports (6 of 20), and at long-term follow-up in 44% of the reports (7 of 16). There were only isolated incidences of women showing higher abstinence rates than men, none of which reached statistical significance. Thus, when a significant difference was found, it was in the direction of greater male success in smoking cessation and long-term abstinence. This result must be considered suggestive in this light. It points to the critical importance of including gender-specific data in future treatment studies and to specifying gender as a systematic independent variable in the research design wherever possible.

Only on the most tentative ground may one draw conclusions regarding the origin of gender differences in quitting success from this small sample of treatment reports. However, a social-support hypothesis is often cited and seems to deserve credence and further exploration. According to this hypothesis, women are more successful in programs which provide social support and therapist-client contact, and less successful in programs in which such support is absent or when external environment supports are lacking. In general, women do more poorly in treatments characterized by educational and pharmacotherapeutic regimes, which are apt to be less individualistically oriented. They seem to do better in programs which fall into the general categories of psychotherapy and behavior modification, where there tends to be a greater frequency of individual or small-group contact.

Several examples of studies supporting the social-support hypothesis can be mentioned. Guilford (17) was one of the first to demonstate that women were significantly more successful in quitting in a group (Aided Treatment) than on their own (Unaided Treatment), whereas men were equally successful across treatments. Within each treatment, Aided and Unaided, male and female success rates did not differ; the women simply did much more poorly on their own. In a study of group-plus-medication treatment, women who scored higher on the Social Introversion Scale of the Minnesota Multiphasic Personality Inventory achieved lower quitting rates than those who scored lower on this scale (33). This scale measures degree of discomfort in social situations; those with outgoing tendencies score lower than shyer, more introverted people. Interestingly, scores on this scale did not differentiate successful from unsuccessful quitters among males, pointing again to a lesser need for social support. One must be careful in drawing such a generalization as findings to the contrary have been reported; spousal support was important for successful cessation in a large male subject population (41). Similarly, the number of nonsmokers versus smokers in the environment was critically related to the success of quitting efforts of women but not of men (4). Media-conducted stop-smoking campaigns can be considered on the extreme low end of a continuum measuring within-program social support. Although twice as many women as men participated in a recently televised smoking cessation campaign, fewer women were able to achieve abstinence, perhaps because of lack of clinic or personal contact (10).

These suggestive findings certainly provide a spur to experiments designed to test the hypothesis that increasing social support improves female success in giving up smoking. They may also serve as a key to designing interventions for those programs already in action.

We are desperately in need of both good research designs and better intervention strategies to decrease the proportion of women who presently smoke and to prevent the initiation of smoking in our teen-age girl population. Both the lay public and health professionals are more aware than ever of the deleterious day-to-day health effects of smoking, of the increased risk of potentially fatal illnesses such as cardiovascular disease and lung cancer, and of the negative complications of smoking during pregnancy. As women carry a major responsibility for the health care of the family in our society and are more somatically oriented than men, our research and intervention strategies must capitalize on these orientations before the mortality risks for major smoking-related diseases reach unity.

ACKNOWLEDGMENTS

The author gratefully acknowledges the support of the Medical Research Service of the Veterans Administration and of the American Cancer Society, Inc., Grant No. PDT 2K.

REFERENCES

1. Andrews, J. (1973): Thiocyanate and smoking in pregnancy. *J. Obstet. Gynecol.*, 80:810–814.
2. Andrews, J., and McGarry, J. M. (1972): A community study of smoking in pregnancy. *J. Obstet. Gynaecol. Br. Commonw.*, 79(12):1057–1073.
3. Baric, L., MacArthur, C., and Sherwood, M. (1976): A study of health education aspects of smoking in pregnancy. *Int. J. Health Educ.* [*Suppl.*], 19:1–17.
4. Berglund, E. (1969): Tobacco withdrawal clinics: The five-day plan. In: *The Final Report.* Norwegian Cancer Society, Oslo.

5. Bewley, B. R., Bland, J. M., and Harris, R. (1974): Factors associated with the starting of cigarette smoking by primary school children. *Br. J. Prev. Soc. Med.,* 28:37–44.
6. Community Cancer Control/Los Angeles (1976): A proposal to implement a community based cancer control program in Los Angeles, California, pp. 108–110.
7. Danaher, B. G., Shisslak, C. M., Thompson, C. B., and Ford, J. D. (1978): A smoking cessation program for pregnant women: Exploratory study. *Am. J. Public Health,* 68(9):896–898.
8. Donovan, J. W. (1977): Randomised controlled trial of antismoking advice in pregnancy. *Br. J. Prev. Soc. Med.,* 31:6–12.
9. Donovan, J. W., Burgess, P. L., Hossack, C. M., and Yudkin, G. D. (1975): Routine advice against smoking in pregnancy. *J. R. Coll. Gen. Pract.,* 25:264–268.
10. Dubren, R. (1977): Evaluation of a televised stop-smoking clinic. *Public Health Rep.,* 92:81–84.
11. Duffus, G. M., and MacGillivray, I. (1968): The incidence of pre-eclamptic toxemia in smokers and nonsmokers. *Lancet,* 2:994–995.
12. Eisinger, R. A. (1971): Psychosocial predictors of smoking recidivism. *J. Health Soc. Behav.,* 12:355–362.
13. Evans, R. I., Rozelle, R. M., Mittelmark, M. B., Hansen, W. B., Bane, A. L., and Mavis, J. (1978): Deterring the onset of smoking in children: Knowledge of immediate physiological effects and coping with peer pressure, media pressure, and parent modeling. *J. Appl. Soc. Psychol.,* 8:126–135.
14. Graham, H. (1976): Smoking in pregnancy: The attitudes of expectant mothers. *Soc. Sci. Med.,* 10:399–405.
15. Gritz, E. R. (1980): Problems related to the use of tobacco by women. In: *Research Advances in Alcohol and Drug Abuse, Vol. 5,* edited by O. Kalant. Plenum Press, New York.
16. Gritz, E. R., and Jarvik, M. E. (1978): Nicotine and smoking. In: *Handbook of Psychopharmacology, Vol. 11,* edited by L. L. Iverson, S. D. Iversen, and S. H. Snyder, pp. 426–464. Plenum Press, New York.
17. Guilford, J. S. (1967): Sex differences between successful and unsuccessful abstainers from smoking. In: *Studies and Issues in Smoking Behavior,* edited by S. V. Zagona, pp. 95–102. University of Arizona Press, Tucson.
18. Holbrook, J. H. (1977): Tobacco and health. *CA,* 27:344–353.
19. Hollingsworth, D. R., Moser, R. S., Carlson, J. W., and Thompson, K. T. (1976): Abnormal adolescent primiparous pregnancy: Association of race, human chorionic somatomammotropin production, and smoking. *Am. J. Obstet. Gynecol.,* 126(2):230–237.
20. Hunt, W. A., Barnett, L. W., and Branch, L. G. (1971): Relapse rates in addiction programs. *J. Clin. Psychol.,* 22:455–456.
21. Jain, A. R. (1976): Cigarette smoking, use of oral contraceptives, and myocardial infarction. *Am. J. Obstet. Gynecol.,* 126(3):301–307.
22. Jick, H., Dinan, B., and Rothman, K. J. (1978): Oral contraceptives and non-fatal myocardial infarction. *J.A.M.A.,* 239(14):1403–1408.
23. Kline, J., Stein, Z. A., Susser, M., and Warburton, D. (1977): Smoking: A risk factor for spontaneous abortion. *N. Engl. J. Med.,* 297:793–796.
24. Lewis, C. E., and Lewis, M. A. (1977): The potential impact of sexual equality on health. *N. Engl. J. Med.,* 297:863–869.
25. Lichtenstein, E., and Danaher, B. G. (1976): Modification of smoking behavior: A critical analysis of theory, research and practice. In: *Progress in Behavior Modification Vol. 3,* edited by M. Herson, R. M., Eisler, and P. M. Miller, pp. 79–132. Academic Press, New York.
26. Mann, J. I., Doll, R., Thorogood, M., Vessey, M. P., and Waters, W. E. (1976): Risk factors for myocardial infarction in young women. *Br. J. Prev. Soc. Med.,* 30:94–100.
27. McKennell, A. C., and Thomas, R. K. (1967): *Adults' and Adolescents' Smoking Habits and Attitudes* (Government Social Survey). Her Majesty's Stationery Office, London.
28. Meyer, M. B., and Tonascia, J. A. (1977): Maternal smoking, pregnancy complications and perinatal mortality. *Am. J. Obstet. Gynecol.,* 128(5):494–502.
29. Miller, H. C., Hassanein, K., and Hensleigh, P. A. (1976): Fetal growth retardation in relation to maternal smoking and weight gain in pregnancy. *Am. J. Obstet. Gynecol.,* 125(1):55–60.
30. Pallonen, U., Puska, P., and Koskela, K. (1978): A community anti-smoking program as part of a comprehensive CUD control program. In: *Progress in Smoking Cessation,* edited by J. L. Schwartz, pp. 199–204. American Cancer Society.

31. Petitti, D. B., and Wingerd, J. (1978): Use of oral contraceptives, cigarette smoking, and risk of subarachnoid hemorrhage. *Lancet,* 2(8083):234–236.
32. Raw, M. (1978): The treatment of cigarette dependence. In: *Research Advances in Alcohol and Drug Problems, Vol. 4,* edited by Y. Israel, H. Kalant, R. E. Popham, W. Schmidt, and R. G. Smart, pp. 441–485. John Wiley & Sons, New York.
33. Resnikoff, A., Schauble, P. G., and Woody, R. H. (1968): Personality correlates of withdrawal from smoking. *J. Psychol.,* 68:117–120.
34. Royal College of Physicians of London (1962): *Smoking and Health.* Pitman, London.
35. Royal College of Physicians of London (1977): *Smoking or Health.* Pitman, London.
36. Russell, M. A. H. (1971): Cigarette smoking: Natural history of a dependence disorder. *Br. J. Med. Psychol.,* 44:1–16.
37. Salber, E. J., and Abelin, T. (1967): Smoking behavior of Newton school children—5-year follow-up. *Pediatrics,* 40:363–372.
38. Salber, E. J., Welsh, B., and Taylor, S. V. (1963): Reasons for smoking given by secondary school children. *J. Health Hum. Behav.,* 4:118–129.
39. Schuman, L. M. (1978): Patterns of smoking behavior. In: *Research on Smoking Behavior,* edited by M. E. Jarvik, J. W. Cullen, E. R. Gritz, T. M. Vogt, and L. J. West, pp. 36–66. National Institute on Drug Abuse Monograph No. 17, Rockville, Md.
40. Schwartz, J. L. (1978): Smoking cures: Ways to kick an unhealthy habit. In: *Research on Smoking Behavior,* edited by M. E. Jarvik, J. W. Cullen, E. R. Gritz, T. M. Vogt, and L. J. West, pp. 308–338. National Institute on Drug Abuse Monograph No. 17, Rockville, Md.
41. Schwartz, J. L., and Dubitsky, M. (1968): One-year follow-up results of a smoking cessation program. *Can. J. Public Health,* 59:161–165.
42. Simpson, W. J. (1957): A preliminary report on cigarette smoking and the incidence of prematurity. *Am. J. Obstet. Gynecol.,* 73:808–815.
43. U.S. Department of Health, Education, and Welfare, Public Health Service (1973): *The Health Consequences of Smoking,* DHEW Publication No. (HSM) 73–8704, Washington, D.C.
44. U.S. Department of Health, Education and Welfare, Public Health Service (1976): *Teen-age Smoking: National Patterns of Cigarette Smoking, Ages 12 Through 18, in 1972 and 1974.* DHEW Publication No. (NIH) 76–931, Washington, D.C.
45. U.S. Department of Health, Education and Welfare, Public Health Service (1976): *Adult Use of Tobacco.* Center for Disease Control, Atlanta, and National Cancer Institute, Washington, D.C.
46. U.S. Department of Health, Education and Welfare (1976): *Survey of Health Professionals, 1975,* pp. 1–9. NCSH, Bureau of Health Education, Center for Disease Control, Public Health Service, Washington, D.C.
47. U.S. Department of Health, Education and Welfare (1976): *San Diego Smoking Research Project: Five Year Status.* Health Education Project, pp. 1–7. NCSH, DHEW Project No. 200–75–0516, Washington, D.C.
48. U.S. Department of Health, Education and Welfare, Public Health Service (1977): *Cigarette Smoking Among Teen-agers and Young Women.* DHEW Publication No. (NIH) 77–1203, Washington, D.C.
49. U.S. Public Health Service (1964): *Smoking and Health.* Report of the Advisory Committee to the Surgeon General of the Public Health Service, Publication No. 1103, Washington, D.C.
50. Warner, K. E. (1977): The effects of the anti-smoking campaign on cigarette consumption. *Am. J. Public Health,* 67:645–650.
51. Williams, R. R., and Horm, J. (1977): Association of cancer sites with tobacco and alcohol consumption and socioeconomic status of patients: Interview study from the Third National Cancer Survey. *J. Natl. Cancer Inst.,* 58(3):525–547.

Psychosocial Aspects of Cancer,
edited by Jerome Cohen et al.
Raven Press, New York © 1982.

Chapter 5

Contemporary Problems and Needed Research Related to Industrially Induced Malignant Disease

Jean S. Felton*

Naval Regional Medical Center Branch Clinic, Long Beach, California 90822

The presence of a known carcinogen as a work contactant in the industrial setting presents many problems demanding a highly specialized body of medical and health care knowledge. With the increasing evidence provided by epidemiologic studies of the relationship of asbestos to (a) fibrogenic lung disease, (b) cancer of the lung, (c) mesothelioma, and (d) other forms of malignant disease, asbestos-using industries, in compliance with federal and state mandates, have initiated rather intensive medical surveillance programs in an effort to detect the early presence of disease among their workers.

ASBESTOS AND HEALTH BEHAVIOR

It has been shown by Selikoff and other investigators (1–3) that the individual who uses asbestos as a work material in an uncontrolled environment places himself at risk for asbestosis, carcinoma of the lung, or both. In addition, it has been demonstrated by several writers (4–6) that persons who either were in contact with asbestos products or were children in the homes of asbestos workers years ago absorbed sufficient asbestos fiber through contact with industrial materials or soiled work clothing to develop disease at a later age. Revealed by these epidemiologic investigations has been the close correlation of cigarette smoking and the increased risk of the development of pulmonary carcinoma (7). In essence, a considerable portion of any medical surveillance program must consist of changes in life style, reversal of self-polluting practices, and motivation of the population at risk toward a more appropriate health behavior. Although the diseases created by such a fibrogenic material are physical and

* Present address: Departments of Community Medicine, University of Southern California School of Medicine, Los Angeles, California 90033; and University of California, Irvine, Irvine, California 92717.

demonstrate pathophysiologic tissue alteration, the prevention, in great part, lies in efforts aimed at behavioral modification.

It has been common experience in large industrial groups that even though the presence of a carcinogenic work substance is known, the employees will not undertake spontaneously the cessation of any practice which will further impair their already damaged health status. Actions to have such personnel cease smoking, limit the intake of beverage alcohol, assume an exercise program, or lose weight meet with little compliance. In many heavy industry areas, such efforts at health improvement do not always match the macho self-image of workers. Further, habits of the nature of cigarette smoking are of such long duration as to make workers feel that fracture of such a habit would be impossible. It is understood also that there are few other means perceived by such personnel to handle the periods of inactivity present in the course of the normal work day. Smoking is resorted to, as is the excessive intake of high carbohydrate food, refined sugar products, and the like.

These findings point to the need for an intensive dual program of research into the methods of behavioral modification and hazard control. One example of a work population for which such a project could be developed is a West Coast shipyard with some of the following characteristics: There are approximately 7,500 employees, nearly 7% of whom are women. The mission of the shipyard engaging these workers consists of the repair, overhaul, and modification of ships from the Pacific Fleet. Many of the vessels are recycled at periodic intervals and are brought back to the shipyard for stays of 8 to 12 months. The civilian work force, in joint effort with the forces afloat (the ships' crews), then carry out the repairs or modifications indicated by diagnostic studies conducted prior to the return of the ships to the Pacific Coast. Since the elimination of asbestos as an insulating material was mandated only in the last several years, much of the current heat-repressing material found in piping systems aboard is asbestos. Newer installations involve the use of fiberglass, and only in rare situations, when the fiberglass has been destroyed by high levels of heat and pressure, is asbestos still used.

The development of asbestos-related disease takes years, and the long latent period has been demonstrated by numerous investigators. It has been pointed out that asbestosis can develop in about 10 years, cancer of the lung possibly after 20 years of work exposure, and mesothelioma 20 to 40 years after first contact (3). It has been shown clearly that among asbestos workers there is a close correlation between cigarette smoking and the development of cancer of the lung. When we compare smoking asbestos workers with other nonsmoking workers, we find an increased risk in the former of 92 times for the potential development of cancer of the lung. Were we to compare smoking asbestos workers with nonsmoking asbestos workers, the risk would be a difference of over 8 times. The objective, therefore, is the cessation of smoking in a group for which smoking has been nearly a lifelong practice.

RESEARCH PROGRAM RESOURCES

Although the usual modalities of health education have been utilized with such work populations (8), no definitive research has been carried out to determine which has been most successful in motivating behavioral change so as to lower the pulmonary carcinoma risk level. What is needed is a program that would test all of the methods, techniques, and media available for use in the work setting. Are one-to-one interviews more productive of change than group sessions with accepted and recognized peers? Are visual media such as filmstrips, motion pictures, or videotape shows more likely to produce change than printed materials which might be distributed to the workers? Would involvement of family members be helpful in behavioral alteration? Are the safety devices that workers currently are being asked to wear the most comfortable and the most effective that could be designed? Does the practice of giving such workers so-called hazard pay attenuate efforts to improve health behavior?

Exposure to a work material involves more than the immediate interface between employee and the hazardous substance. There are many issues, arising from a variety of courses, to be resolved. These include considerations of physical safety; disease prevention; acceptance and obeying of regulations; possible pay differentials; alterations of work time, including odd-shifting; careful placement of handicapped persons in relationship to work constraints; introduction and inclusion of pertinent material into management-labor contract negotiations; submission of grievances based on alleged unfair labor practices or Equal Employment Opportunity infractions as they might relate to work with a carcinogen; lost time because of occupationally incurred illness, with its attendant workers' compensation administrative and costing activities; communication between in-plant health service personnel and physicians and hospitals in the community; and the establishment and maintenance of effective relationships between the occupational health authority and both management and labor.

Most of these issues are resolved by the promulgation of consensus documents, all too often produced unilaterally (a labor council distributes a seething diatribe to its membership; management develops a regulatory document without review by the union; plant medicine establishes a new operational procedure, not discussed previously with the target consumers, and on, and on, and on). Other problem areas are explored through the meet-and-confer system of joint consultation. In managerially sound enterprises a document is distributed in draft form so that affected parties may have the opportunity to comment before possible adverse impacts result. In some settings there is constant warring among certain organizational components, or there is a chronic flight of memoranda back and forth with no oral communication, or there is the attitude that if the other source produced or suggested something, it is, by definition, unacceptable. In many institutions, if a worker files a claim following an injury, or enters into litigation regarding such a trauma, the company immediately fights the claim even though the plaintiff may be completely right in his allegation and have absolute proof of the correctness of his contention.

These interpersonal, interdepartmental, and interfactional difficulties are mentioned because for any program to succeed there must be agreement on objectives, procedural methods, and anticipated risks or benefits. Research necessitates agreement and community knowledge, and can be executed only in a climate where labor–management, medicine–management, and medicine–labor relationships have been carefully cultivated and constantly refined to meet new needs. To work effectively with executive and union leaders requires full faith and credibility in the medical leadership, and these elements are not always readily attained; they arrive only with persistently hard work on the part of all medical staff members (9). Once obtained, they can never be taken for granted but must be recast, rehoned, and valued as the most important commodities in any potential research milieu.

In attempting a reconfiguration of workers' life styles, it is particularly important to remain aware of the tenuous planking of these relationships. The introduction of alternatives in behavior will always be questioned for motivation, particularly if the entities suggested provide some benefits. Workers are consistently highly suspicious of change, and many remain so even when their trade union leaders request support. If a research project is to be introduced, a great deal of planning is required so that total support will be obtained. Only in a company where valued work relationships exist can an investigative effort succeed.

Resources for health services often are in short supply because industry has yet to realize the full impact of federal and state occupational safety and health legislation. Only with heavy fines and with significant increases in workers' compensation premiums have some companies grudgingly conceded the need for control of an occupationally encountered carcinogen. Nearly every organization has a training branch that could help arrange educational inputs. The trade unions have indicated willingness to aid in programs of worth to their membership. Most physicians and nurses have done some teaching and could be utilized in the retraining activity. And in most instances management is willing to allow time for training if the program does not require an excessive amount of down time and it can see a positive cost-benefit relationship.

A PROJECT PROPOSAL

A population of the type described previously offers certain enclaves of personnel that might present different challenges to the educator. For example, of the 7,500 employees in this particular shipyard there are approximately 125 American Samoans, nearly 100 Guamanians, and possibly double this number of persons from the Philippine Islands, in addition to the usual representation of Caucasians, Blacks, Chicanos, and Asians. In any kind of surveillance program consisting of physical examinations, chest radiography, pulmonary function measurement, environmental sampling, and sputum cytology, these ethnic groups could present differences in anthropometry that might influence the acquisition of, or immunity to, industrially created disease.

A surveillance program requires a computerized system of records, a call-in system, and an epidemiologic treatment of the data resulting from the diagnostic procedures carried out. A research effort of the type envisioned would require a physician director, an epidemiologist and/or a biostatistician, a creative specialist in patient education, and a facility for the development of teaching media.

In the course of obtaining the medical histories of asbestos workers, it was learned that several of such personnel had already ceased smoking. When investigators questioned the motivating force behind such action, many reasons were given. Hence a research investigation should be able to identify what factors in the lives of these successful workers produced habit conversion—whether, as happens many times, change results from the pressure of family members, from peer group influence, from altered image of a group, and so on.

L'ENVOI

In substance, at this point in the development of knowledge of occupational disease, we need a research program at an installation where the population has been and continues to be at risk because of respiratory contact with free asbestos fiber. The research activity should include not only all the elements of medical surveillance, but a trial of a variety of methods aimed at life style changes which will lead to a new health behavior, and ultimately in the lowering in the prevalence of asbestos-related disease (as seen in pleural and pulmonary fibrosis, carcinoma of the lung, mesothelioma, carcinoma of the digestive tract, and carcinoma of the oral cavity). Only through environmental control and behavioral change can a work population be protected from the ill effects of an industrially needed material—at least until an adequate substitute is discovered which can replace asbestos in all of its more than 3,000 uses.

REFERENCES

1. Anderson, H. A., Lilis, R., Iaum, S. M., Fischbein, A. S., and Selikoff, I. J. (1976): Household contact asbestos neoplastic risk. *Ann. N.Y. Acad. Sci.,* 271:311–323.
2. Felton, J. S. (1979): A comprehensive program in asbestos hazard surveillance and education. *Am. Ind. Hyg. Assoc. J.,* 40:11–18.
3. Felton, J. S. (1977): Occupational health relates to management and labor. *Navy Lifeline,* 6:18–21.
4. Harries, P. G., Mackenzie, F. A. F., Sheers, G., Kemp, J. H., Oliver, T. P., and Wright, D. S. (1972): Radiological survey of men exposed to asbestos in naval dockyards. *Br. J. Ind. Med.,* 29:274–279.
5. Lillington, B. A., Jamplis, R. W., and Differding, J. R. (1974): Conjugal malignant mesothelioma. *N. Engl. J. Med.,* 291:583–584.
6. Navratil, M., and Trippe, F. (1971): Epidemiological study of pleural calcifications in persons living in the area close to an asbestos factory. In: *IVth International Pneumoconiosis Conference,* Bucharest, 27 September–2 October. Apimodia, Bucharest.

7. Selikoff, I. J., Churg, J., and Hammond, E. C. (1965): The occurrence of asbestosis among insulation workers in the United States. *Ann. N.Y. Acad. Sci.,* 132:139–155.
8. Selikoff, I. J., and Hammond, E. C. (1978): Asbestos-associated disease in United States shipyards. *CA,* 28:87–99.
9. Selikoff, I. J., Hammond, E. C., and Churg, J. (1968): Asbestos exposure, smoking, and neoplasia. *J.A.M.A.,* 204:106–112.

Psychosocial Aspects of Cancer,
edited by Jerome Cohen et al.
Raven Press, New York © 1982.

Chapter 6

Psychosocial Research Needed to Improve the Use and Evaluation of Cancer Screening Techniques

Carol N. D'Onofrio

School of Public Health, University of California, Berkeley, California 94720

Since completely preventing the occurrence of all cancer is beyond present capabilities, earlier diagnosis and treatment of the disease provides a critically important second line of defense. Although data relating earliness of cancer care to greater length of survival are far from definitive (4,12,58), medical authorities widely agree that cancers which are localized or restricted to a limited site are more amenable to control than those which have metastasized (1,5,126,133). The detection and treatment of cancer in its early stages therefore aptly has been termed secondary prevention—a challenging arena for psychosocial research.

The timely discovery of cancer depends upon the development of accurate detection methods, their effective application to at-risk populations, and prompt action to assure definitive diagnosis of suspicious signs and symptoms. Once the diagnosis is confirmed, promptness in initiating treatment obviously is essential. The secondary prevention of cancer thus involves a complex process, the efficacy and efficiency of which are affected both by biomedical knowledge and technique, and by the behavior of consumers, providers, and larger systems in applying these tools.

This chapter is particularly concerned with identifying priorities for research into behavioral problems related to the earlier detection of cancer in apparently healthy people through the appropriate utilization of screening methods. Problems of delay in diagnosis and treatment once signs or symptoms are discovered have received much more research attention (e.g., 4,10,14,26,63,64,68,70,74, 76,77,84,88,89,91,122,123,131) and therefore will be only minimally considered here. The fact that two recent reviews of the literature on delay (4,68) concluded with recommendations for more effective screening programs further justifies a closer examination of psychosocial research needs in this area.

As defined by the National Commission on Chronic Illness (29), screening is "the presumptive identification of unrecognized disease or defect by the application of tests, examinations, or other procedures which can be applied rapidly." Screening is not diagnostic, but rather identifies asymptomatic persons in selected populations who may be harboring incipient disease and who therefore should undergo diagnostic procedures. Since many cancers develop slowly over a period of years before symptoms appear on the clinical horizon, the development and application of effective screening techniques promise to contribute importantly to improved cancer control through earlier case finding (127).

Whether conducted on a mass basis, as in community programs, or individually through periodic physical examinations and health appraisals, cancer screening must rest upon a solid foundation of biomedical research. The cumulative results of this research at any point in time determine the cancer sites subject to earlier detection through screening, the sensitivity and specificity of available screening methods, and the range of human behaviors, material resources, and other conditions essential to their effective application. Taken together, these factors define the technological potential and limitations of screening for improved cancer control.

Since the ultimate purpose of behavioral research in cancer screening is to discover ways in which more people may be benefited by technological advances in earlier cancer detection, psychosocial investigations require a close relationship with the biomedical sciences. Scientific knowledge about the cancer each screening procedure is designed to detect and the technical requirements for applying the screen delimit the broad parameters of relevant behavioral problems. Epidemiologic data on risk factors define the consumers whose behavior is of particular concern, while the nature of the screening test determines the specific actions which must be performed by members of this target population and by health professionals, as well as the systems conditions which must be present to achieve screening objectives. The performance standards by which observed actions and conditions are judged also are based upon the goals of the screening effort and their underlying scientific rationale. For these reasons, a consideration of priorities for psychosocial research in cancer screening must begin with a brief review of present screening technology.

SCIENTIFIC FOUNDATIONS FOR CANCER SCREENING

Papanicolaou and Traut (105) made a landmark contribution to the development of modern cancer screening when, in 1943, they demonstrated the potential of the cervical smear for earlier cancer detection. This accomplishment precipitated an "explosive evaluation of diagnostic cytology" (39,66), which, accompanied by other technological advances, led to the development of additional screening methods. Of the screening techniques currently available, the most widely known and applied are the "Pap" test for cervical cancer, the chest X-ray for lung cancer, mammography and breast self-examination for breast cancer, the guaiac test and proctosigmiodoscopy for colorectal cancers, observation of "danger signals" for skin cancers, and visualization of the oral cavity and oral exfoliative cytology for cancers of the mouth and larynx. Other screening tests have been developed, such as thermography for breast cancer (59,90,128), the vaginal irrigation smear (VIS) for cervical cancer (40,41,72,99), the cytosputum test for lung cancer (6,7,94), testicular self-examination (111), and self-examination for oro-facial cancer (114). However, these as yet have been less generally accepted. New cancer screening methods continue to appear (e.g., 46,102,103).

The incidence of the various cancers toward which these screening procedures are directed, related mortality data, and 5-year survival rates for localized and regionalized disease have been widely publicized. Major risk factors for each of these cancers also have been identified and estimates made of the impact which earlier detection would have on cancer control (e.g., 1,2,50,55,75,135). Nevertheless, it must be stressed that the scientific community by no means has reached consensus on these matters. To the contrary, they are issues at the heart of much intensive biomedical research.

On the basis of existing evidence, the American Cancer Society (ACS) (1) and others (e.g., 7,15–17,19,21,23–25,33,38,43,45,51,53,60,61,71,73,78,87,93, 96,100,108,110,117,115,119,129) project that numerous lives could be saved by the application of current screening techniques and other early detection measures to at-risk populations. The ACS figures are dramatic: one out of every four cancer deaths might be averted by earlier diagnosis and prompt treatment— an estimate which in 1981 translated into approximately 134,000 preventable deaths. The ACS further points out that the high costs of cancer could be reduced through earlier detection, noting, for example, that, "the cost of a fatal cancer of the uterus can amount to $25,000 or more, while the same cancer, when found early and cured, may cost only a few hundred dollars" (1). Other benefits which have been attributed to cancer screening include longer survival times, less drastic treatment, increased patient productivity, and a better quality of life (42,101).

On the other hand, screening programs in general have been criticized as too expensive, too comprehensive, and poorly evaluated (e.g., 27,36,37,49,65,-80,85,106,116), while a number of criticisms have been leveled at specific cancer screening tests. Thus benefits which have been claimed for cervical cytology have been discounted by others who point out that a beginning decline in morbidity and mortality rates for invasive cancer of the cervix was observable prior to the development of the Papanicolaou smear (33,57). Evidence is lacking that earlier detection of lung cancer leads to improved survival rates (18,52,79,95). The encouragement of breast self-examination also has been attacked on the grounds that its efficacy has not been proved (e.g., 120). As Moore (97) recently editorialized:

we must insist on some sort of evidence, before we set millions of women nervously palpating their breasts in front of a mirror every month in response to subway advertisements, Cancer Society commercials, television and books published for the lay public.

While the ability of mammography to detect breast cancer earlier had been demonstrated (11), numerous issues surround mammography screening for women under 50 years of age (62,98,119,121). Concern especially has been expressed that irradiation from repeated tests over time might induce the disease iatrogenically (8,9,34,35,48,69). The difficulty of pathological interpretation of minimal lesions presents another problem—that of false positive findings. In the National Cancer Institute (NCI) field trials of mammography screening, 66 (13%) of the 506 lesions originally classified as malignant were later reclassified as benign and a further 22 (4%) as borderline or uncertain. Notwithstanding, 58 of the 66 women had been treated by some form of breast surgery, 27 of them by a radical procedure. Of the 22 cases reclassified as borderline, 20 also had been treated with breast surgery (35,104).

The relatively high rate of false positive slides from the guaiac test for colorectal cancers is not associated with unnecessary surgery but does require expensive and time-consuming diagnostic workups, consequently reducing the cost-effectiveness of this approach (30). In addition, variability in the performance of guaiac screening makes it difficult to judge the usefulness of this procedure (47). Proctosigmoidoscopy also has been criticized as expensive, as well as distasteful to consumers and potentially dangerous in inexperienced provider hands (125). Most important, it has not yet been definitively demonstrated that either of these screening methods can produce a reduction in mortality for colorectal cancer (67,82,113,118).

Oral cytology is another screening procedure found lacking in cost-effectiveness, for although the rate of false positive readings is acceptable, the relatively low incidence of oral cancer in the population means that a great many slides must be read to find one case (124,130). This problem, of course, is exacerbated when screening is applied too broadly, rather than selectively to those most at risk—a count upon which both oral and cervical cancer screening programs have been negatively judged (e.g., 44,75).

Finally, the psychosocial consequences of screening have been a concern, particularly as false positive results may arouse needless anxiety and as false negative findings may produce an unwarranted sense of security (3,22,83). Thus with the exception of mammography for women over 50 years of age (104), the scientific rationale for cancer screening is presently in dispute (112).

In view of these problems, the NCI currently recommends only three cancer screening procedures: mammography for women over age 50 and those at special risk, breast self-examination for other women, and the Papanicolaou smear for cervical cancer. At the same time, the NCI is working to develop the scientific basis for additional recommendations by rigorously reviewing available data on screening procedures (e.g., 30,52,104), by supporting major demonstrations on selected screening techniques, and by mounting further basic research (127).

Clearly, the scientific foundations for secondary cancer prevention need to be strengthened through continuing biomedical investigations. Technical limitations in the accuracy of current cancer screening procedures, ambiguities about the risk factors which should indicate their use, doubts about their impact on cancer control, and related issues of cost-effectiveness all underscore the need for further biological, clinical, and epidemiological research (12,20,28,31,36,

37,80,106,113,116,118,124,134,135). In addition, new and improved screening techniques must be developed for the earlier detection of cancers of the lung (95) and other sites, now typically discovered only in advanced stages less subject to treatment and control.

Nevertheless, even the most technically perfect detection method cannot reduce the ravages of cancer unless it is effectively applied (12,13,32). Thus there is an equally critical need for psychosocial research on problems related to the utilization of cancer screening techniques. This need was recognized nearly two decades ago by an Expert Committee of the World Health Organization, which stated in its report on the *Prevention of Cancer* (132) that "There are wide gaps in our knowledge of social, psychological, and educational factors that inhibit the utilization of preventive knowledge." Unfortunately, research support for the systematic investigation of the behavioral aspects of cancer prevention and control has been minimal, for as Frei and Frechette (56a) have observed, there has been a tendency "to assume that the problems of application are relatively uncomplicated in comparison with the thorny scientific questions the disease presents." As these authors conclude, however, and as the following discussion demonstrates, much still remains to be understood about how research findings are converted into better service.

Psychosocial research is imperative not only to further the full application of the screening technology presently available, but also to acquire insights which will facilitate the effective application of improved screening methods as these are developed. In addition, such research can contribute importantly to answering fundamental questions about the adequacy of present and future cancer detection techniques.

In 1951, the National Conference on Chronic Disease (29) established five criteria for screening tests. Although subsequently augmented and refined by others (3,20,50,130,133,134), these criteria remain central concerns in evaluating cancer screening procedures today. Determining the extent to which a given screening method meets the first two of these criteria, *reliability* and *validity* of test results, is primarily a task for biomedical investigation. Nevertheless, as Grant (65) has pointed out, sensitivity and specificity as measures of the internal validity of a screening test may vary significantly with the skill of the operator, an observation which had implications for behavioral as well as bench research.

Judging the merits of a screening procedure according to the criteria of yield, cost, and acceptance clearly requires both psychosocial and biomedical data. *Yield,* for example, is measured by "the number of previously unknown verified cases of disease among the total population surveyed, the number of persons with previously unknown verified disease benefited by referral to medical care, and the number of previously known cases not under medical care benefited by return to it" (29). These outcomes are affected not only by the technical accuracy of a screening test, the incidence of cancer in the population, and the precision with which epidemiological risk factors are defined, but also by variables in human behavior which determine who is tested and how often, the competency with which tests are performed and interpreted, and the appropriateness of follow-up actions which are taken (32). Data on these behavioral factors therefore must be obtained in order to evaluate both the actual and potential yield of screening methods.

Weighing the *costs* of screening against the benefits also involves complex psychosocial as well as biomedical issues. The effectiveness and efficiency of alternative methods for recruiting at-risk populations and delivering screening services must be fully explored before accurate cost estimates can be made. The psychosocial consequences of screening also must be better understood if both the costs and benefits of screening are to be well measured (81). Finally, since determining cost-benefit ratios inevitably involves making value judgments (11,54), psychosocial research is needed to clarify the values which scientific experts, public policy makers, individual consumers and health providers, and society as a whole place on cancer screening in terms of the investments anticipated, the outcomes which may be expected, and competing goals to which available resources might be directed (80,134). Some of these same issues, of course, are involved in estimating the cost-effectiveness of cancer screening as compared to other alternatives for cancer control.

Since the reliability, validity, yield, and cost of screening tests all affect the *acceptability* of screening procedures to physicians, allied health professionals, individual laypeople, and the community, it follows that the degree to which a screening method meets this last criterion will be affected by both biomedical and psychosocial considerations. On the other hand, the acceptability of a test also will affect its use and therefore will influence its performance on the criteria of yield and cost. Accordingly, psychosocial research to assess the acceptability of various screening procedures among at-risk populations, health providers, and community institutions is needed to evaluate the potential of these tests for improved cancer control. As Knox (86) points out, data on levels of test acceptability in each age group additionally are necessary to formulate the best ages and frequencies for conducting screening. A better understanding of the factors affecting the acceptability of screening methods to those who must apply them also may prove useful to biomedical investigators in setting priorities among promising laboratory leads for the development of new and improved screening procedures.

Psychosocial research in cancer screening therefore need not—and indeed must not—await perfection of the biomedical basis for earlier cancer detection. If the full benefits of present screening technology, as well as those of future technological progress, are to impact upon the control of cancer with minimum delay, investigations into behavioral factors affecting the utilization of screening procedures must proceed apace with biomedical studies. Likewise, if present and future screening techniques are to be evaluated adequately, relevant behavioral data must be made available. Assuring a sound foundation for secondary cancer prevention, therefore, necessitates the advancement of knowledge through research in both the biomedical and behavioral sciences.

SCOPE AND FOCUS OF PSYCHOSOCIAL RESEARCH IN CANCER SCREENING

Psychosocial research is concerned with the description, understanding, prediction, and modification of human behavior. A consideration of psychosocial research needs in cancer screening therefore appropriately begins by identifying those specific behaviors required for the successful conduct of the screening process. Since applying each of the cancer detection techniques currently available requires different actions by different agents, the behavioral dimensions of screening are exceedingly complex.

To underscore this critical point, Table 1 outlines behaviors involved in applying a common screening test. Although more detail is needed about precisely

TABLE 1. *Summary of behaviors required for the effective application of Papanicolaou screening for cervical cytology*

CONSUMER BEHAVIORS

Women aged _____ to _____ years, and other women at risk, make and keep an appointment for a Pap test every _____ years.

Women with suspicious or positive Pap test results make and keep one or more medical appointments for additional tests and evaluation.

Women with a confirmed diagnosis of cervical cancer consult with health personnel about available options for treatment, decide on the preferred course of action, and take all steps necessary to implement this course.

PROVIDER BEHAVIORS

Health personnel advise women aged _____ years and older of the need for a Pap test every _____ years, as well as when and where the test can be obtained.

Health care providers take Pap tests on women who seek screening and as a routine part of health care in other situations as appropriate, e.g., periodic health checkups, family planning clinics, and gynecological care.

Health personnel assure that women receiving a Pap test understand its purpose, how it is performed, the range of possible results, and how results should be interpreted, including indications of the need for repeat screening.

Laboratories process Pap smears and return accurate reports of the findings to the physician or clinic which submitted the smear.

Health personnel inform women who have had a Pap test of the findings and their interpretation and assure that these women understand additional actions they should take, as well as when and how to take them.

Health personnel follow up women with suspicious or positive test results to assure that additional diagnostic, referral, and treatment procedures are completed as appropriate.

Health personnel maintain appropriate records and tickler systems to notify women who should be rescreened and to follow up positive and suspicious screening test results.

SYSTEM BEHAVIORS

Health agencies and other qualified organizations organize, conduct, and evaluate screening programs, including outreach and education, to encourage women at risk for cervical cancer to obtain Pap tests at appropriate intervals.

Health planning agencies and other organizations as appropriate assure that trained personnel, clinical and laboratory services, and supportive educational programs are available for the conduct of cervical screening and that efforts and resources are coordinated.

who should do what, where, when, and how, making such determinations necessitates balancing a range of information, some of which is not available or in dispute (86). Consequently, actual and recommended screening practices vary, while decision making about screening represents another aspect of behavior meriting psychosocial investigations (109,112). In general, however, screening requires the cooperative action of many different people behaving in various roles and settings as consumers, health professionals, and members of larger social systems. These realities carry important implications for the scope and focus of psychosocial research.

First, a great many varieties of human behavior must be investigated. It cannot be assumed that participation in cancer screening is a single phenomenon for consumers, for providers, or for the systems in which they interact. Thus, for example, conducting monthly breast self-examination is not behaviorally equivalent to requesting proctosigmoidoscopy from a private practitioner nor even to seeking a professional breast exam (107). Not only are different skills and resources, frequencies and sequences of action, behavioral settings, and time frames involved in each of these screening procedures, but so are different body parts. Moreover, one type of screening can be performed independently whereas the others require patient and physician cooperation. Different knowledge, beliefs, attitudes, values, social relationships, and other determinants of behavior therefore undoubtedly are associated with each of these actions. Accordingly, they must be studied independently.

Second, while the particular actions and persons who must take them vary with the screening method, it is clear that consumer, provider, and system behaviors in some unique mix are essential to the application of each procedure. Therefore, psychosocial research must be concerned with the extent to which *all* of these actions are performed, as well as with more detailed studies of each of them. Only through a focus on the entire behavioral system of the screening process can relationships and interactions between essential factors be examined, and it is here, rather than with the isolated behaviors of consumers or providers that the most critical behavioral problems may exist. Moreover, a focus on only one part of the system may result in failure to identify weak links elsewhere in the chain of behaviors essential to the successful application of the screening method.

Thus, for example, if psychosocial research is to discover ways in which breast self-examination can be more effectively used as a screening tool, the extent to which women practice BSE obviously will be a variable of central concern. In addition, however, research also must examine the behavior of physicians, nurses, and outreach workers in teaching and encouraging women to practice BSE. At another level, the amount of training these providers themselves have had in BSE *and* in effective techniques for teaching it to others should be assessed. To complete the picture, the behavior of women who discover a breast abnormality and of the professionals and laypeople they consult should be explored to determine the extent to which their actions support the earlier detection and treatment of breast cancer (70). In this regard, the availability and use of diagnostic facilities and other resources in the community also should be examined.

With the collection of these data, however, only the descriptive phase of psychosocial research will have been accomplished. At this point, theoretical and empirical understanding of human behavior must be combined to develop potential explanations for the actions observed. Usually this requires gathering additional descriptive data about factors which intentionally or unintentionally may influence the behaviors of primary interest. Thus formal and informal communications about BSE and breast cancer within the community and its relevant subsystems may be studied, and a broad range of other possible influences on behavior may be explored (e.g., 92). Further research must then be undertaken to test the validity and reliability of the most likely explanatory hypotheses, ideally through prospective studies designed to examine their predictive power. From the fruits of such research, possible interventions to improve BSE practices may be suggested, and these, of course, should be subjected to experimental field testing in the context of action research.

As discussed thus far, the scope of psychosocial research in cancer screening is already very large, involving the investigation of consumer, provider, and systems behaviors, both singly and in interaction as these are unique to each screening method. In addition, however, psychosocial research is also concerned with searching for possible similarities and differences in the utilization of various screening tests.

Clearly the identification of valid generalizations about screening behavior would permit a more parsimonious approach to understand how to improve the effective application of any given screening technique. Such generalizations also would assist in evaluating the degree to which a cancer screening test meets the criteria of yield, cost, and acceptability. Accordingly, research might explore patterns of individual acceptance of both BSE and cervical cytology, and possibly also screening for diabetes and hypertension. Participation in different types of screening programs might be compared and contrasted within and among different classes and subclasses of at-risk populations, as well as among various health agencies and community groups. The extent to which physicians routinely screen patients for a range of diseases could be examined, and referral relationships among private practitioners and medical institutions could be traced in following up the results of different cancer screening procedures, as well as referrals for other reasons.

Similarly, research might investigate the extent to which determinants of the behaviors involved in screening are common from one test to another and the extent to which they are specific to each screening method. More generally, the relationship of participation in screening to other preventive health actions could be probed. Quite possibly, additional understanding in this area would suggest new interventions to improve earliness of cancer detection. Likewise, cross-cutting studies of consumer and provider behaviors when confronted with symptoms may lend new insights into problems of following up positive or suspicious screening results (70). Numerous other linkages between cancer screening and various dimensions of human behavior also might productively be explored.

The scope of psychosocial research in cancer screening therefore spans a very wide range of human behavior and potentially involves an enormous number of variables. The focus, however, must remain firmly fixed on the paramount objective of improving the appropriate utilization of cancer screening techniques, which in turn will contribute to the fuller evaluation of these procedures.

REFERENCES

1. American Cancer Society (1978): *Cancer Facts and Figures.* The American Cancer Society, New York.
2. American Cancer Society (1980): *Cancer Facts and Figures.* The American Cancer Society, New York.
3. American Medical Association (1955): *A Study of Multiple Screening.* Council on Medical Service, The American Medical Association, Chicago.
4. Antonovsky, A., and Hartman H. (1974): Delay in the detection of cancer: a review of the literature. *Health Educ. Monogr.,* 2:98–128.
5. Axtell, L. M., and Meyers, M. H., editors (1974): *Recent Trends in the Survival of Cancer Patients.* DHEW Pub. No. (NIH) 75–767, U.S. Govt. Printing Office, Washington, D.C.
6. Ayre, J. E. (1963): You *can* do more about lung cancer! *Consultant.*
7. Ayre, J. E., Snyder, A. J., and Fegeri, H. E. (1970): The impact of modern cytology upon cancer detection and prevention in industry. *Indust. Med.,* 39:33.
8. Bailar, J. C. III (1976): Mammography: a contrary view. *Ann. Intern. Med.,* 84:77–84.
9. Bailar, J. C. III (1977): Screening for early breast cancer: pros and cons. *Cancer,* 39:2783–2795.
10. Battistella, R. M. (1971): Factors associated with delay in the initiation of physicians' care among late adulthood persons. *Am. J. Public Health,* 61:1348–1361.
11. Bay, K. S., Flathman, D., and Nestman, L. (1976): The worth of a screening program: An application of a statistical decision model for the benefit evaluation of screening projects. *Am. J. Public Health,* 66:145–150.
12. Berlin, N. I. (1974): Early diagnosis of cancer. *Prev. Med.,* 3:185–186.
13. Biocca, S. M., and Joly D. (1960): Fighting cancer in Argentina. *Int. J. Health Educ.,* 3:174–177.
14. Blackwell, B. L. (1963): The literature of delay in seeking medical care for chronic illness. *Health Educ. Monogr.,* 16:3–31.
15. Boyes, D. A. (1969): The British Columbia screening program. *Obstet. Gynecol. Surv.,* 24:1005–1011.
16. Breslow, L. (1972): Early case-finding, treatment, and mortality from cervix and breast cancer. *Prev. Med.,* 1:141–152.
17. Butler, B. B., Erskine, E., and Godfrey A. (1970): Public health detailing: selling ideas to the private practitioner in his office. *Am. J. Public Health,* 60:1996–2002.
18. Cameron, C. S. (1974): Cancer control: challenge or chimera? *Cancer,* 33:402–413.
19. Canadian Task Force on the Periodic Health Examination (1959): The periodic health examination. *CMA J.,* 121:1–45.
20. Canadian Task Force on Cervical Cancer Screening Programs (1976): Cervical cancer screening programs. *CMA J.,* 114:1103–1033.
21. Candau, M. G. (1970): Cancer: where we stand. *World Health* (Feb.-March), p. 3.
22. Chamberlain, J. (1972): Mass screening: its use in defining populations at-risk for health education. In: *Behavioral Sciences in Health and Disease,* edited by L. Baric for the Health Education Council, London, pp. 93–99. Published by Int. J. Health Educ., Geneva.
23. Christopherson, W. M. (1966): The control of cervix cancer. *Acta Cytol.,* 10:6–10.

24. Christopherson, W. M., Parker, J. E., Mendez, W. M., and Lundin, F. E., Jr. (1970): Cervix cancer death rates and mass cytological screening. *Cancer,* 26:808–811.

25. Christopherson, W. M., Lundin, F. E., Jr., Mendez, W. M., and Parker, J. E. (1976): Cervical cancer control: a study of morbidity and mortality trends over a twenty-one period. *Cancer,* 38:1357–1366.

26. Cobb, B., Clark, R. L., McGuire, C. and Howe, C. D. (1954): Patient responsible delay in treatment of cancer. *Cancer,* 7:920–925.

27. Collen, F. B., Feldman, R., Soghikian, K., and Garfield, S. R. (1973): The educational adjunct to multiphasic health testing. *Prev. Med.,* 2:247–260.

28. Collen, M. F., Dales, L. G., Friedman, G. D., Flagle, C. D., Feldman, R., and Seigelaub, A. B. (1973): Multiphasic checkup evaluation study. 4. Preliminary cost benefit analysis for middle-aged men. *Prev. Med.,* 2:236–246.

29. Commission on Chronic Illness (1957): *Chronic Illness in the United States.* Vol. 1. Prevention of Chronic Illness. Published for the Commonwealth Fund by Harvard Univ. Press, Cambridge, Mass.

30. (1978): Consensus group does not recommend mass screening for colo-rectal cancer; mortality reduction not shown. *J.A.M.A.,* 240:2625–2626.

31. Coppleson, L. W., and Brown, B. (1976): The prevention of carcinoma of the cervix. *Am. J. Obstet. Gynecol.,* 125:153–159.

32. Coulehan, J. (1975): Screening yield in an urban low income population. *Am. J. Public Health,* 65:474–479.

33. Cramer, D. W. (1974): The role of cervical cytology in the declining morbidity and mortality of cervical cancer. *Cancer,* 34:2018–2027.

34. Culliton, B. J. (1976): Breast cancer: second thoughts about routine mammography. *Science,* 193:555–558.

35. Culliton, B. J. (1977): Mammography controversy: NIH's entree into evaluating technology. *Science,* 198:171–173.

36. Cutler, J. L., Ramcharan, S., Feldman, R., Siegelaub, A. B., Campbell, B., Friedman, G. D., Dales, L. G., and Collen, M. F. (1973): Multiphasic checkup evaluation study. I. Methods and population. *Prev. Med.,* 2:197–206.

37. Dales, L. G., Friedman, G. D., Ramcharan, S., Siegelaub, A. B., Campbell, B. A., Feldman, R., and Collen, M. F. (1973): Multiphasic checkup evaluation study. 3. Outpatient clinic utilization, hospitalization, and mortality experience after seven years. *Prev. Med.,* 2:221–235.

38. Dales, L. B., Friedman, G. D., and Collen, M. F. (1979): Evaluating periodic multiphasic health checkups: a controlled trial. *J. Chronic Dis.,* 32:385–404.

39. Davis, H. J. (1962): The irrigation smear: accuracy in detection of cervical cancer. *Acta Cytol.,* 6:459–467.

40. Davis, H. J. (1962): The irrigation smear: a cytologic method for mass population screening by mail. *Am. J. Obstet. Gynecol.,* 84:1017–1023.

41. Davis, H. J., and Jones, H. W., Jr. (1966): Population screening for cancer of the cervix with irrigation smears. *Am J. Obstet. Gynecol.,* 96:605–613.

42. Day, E. (1963): Cancer screening and detection: medical aspects. *J. Chronic Dis.,* 16:397–405.

43. Dowdy, A. H., Barker, W. F., Lagasse, L. D. Sperling, L., Zeldis, L. J. and Longmire, W. P., Jr. (1971): Mammography as a screening method for the examination of large populations. *Cancer,* 28:1558–1562.

44. Duffy, B. J. (1976): Papanicolaou testing—are we screening the wrong women? *N. Engl. J. Med.,* 294:223.

45. Dunn, J. E., Jr. (1958): Preliminary findings of the Memphis-Shelby County uterine cancer study and their interpretation. *Am. J. Public Health,* 48:861–873.

46. (1979): Early detection of uterine Ca pushed. *Med. Tribune,* 20:27.

47. (1979): Experts not yet ready to back mass guaiac testing. *Med. World News,* April 16, 1979, pp. 22–23.

48. Feig, S. A. (1979): Low-dose mammography: application to medical practice. *J.A.M.A.,* 242:2107–2109.

49. Feinlieb, M., and Zelen M. (1969): Some pitfalls in the evaluation of screening programs. *Arch. Environ. Health,* 19:412–415.

50. Ferrer, H. P. (1968): *Screening for Health: Theory and Practice.* Butterworth, London.

51. Fidler, H. K. and Boyes, D. A. (1965): The cytology program in British Columbia. *Canad. J. Public Health,* 46:109–112.
52. Fink, D. J., and Upton, A. C. (1979): Consensus conference on screening for lung cancer, Sept. 18–20, 1978: Summary. National Cancer Program, Special Communication, USDHEW, April 19, 1979.
53. Foster, R. S., Jr., Lang, S. P., Costanza, M. C., Worden, J. K., Haines, C., and Yates, J. (1978): Breast self-examination practices and breast-cancer stage. *N. Engl. J. Med.,* 299:265–270.
54. Fox, B. H. (1975): Probable payoff in primary prevention of cancer. Paper presented at Workshop on Preventing Cancer, sponsored by the New Mexico Health Education Coalition, Albuquerque, N.M., March 21, 1975.
55. Fraumeni, J. F., Jr., editor (1975): *Persons at High Risk of Cancer: An Approach to Cancer Etiology and Control.* Academic Press, New York.
56. Fulghum, J. E. (1967): *Cervical Cancer Detection Through Cytology.* Monograph Series No. 11. Florida State Board of Health, Jacksonville, Fla.
56a. Frei, E., and Frechette, A. L. (1978): The future of cancer control. Editorial. *N. Engl. J. Med.,* 298:567–568.
57. Gardner, J. W., and Lyon, J. L. (1977): Efficacy of cervical cytologic screening in the control of cervical cancer. *Prev. Med.,* 6:487–499.
58. Garwin, J. L. (1975): Survival rates calculated from date of diagnosis. Correspondence. *N. Engl. J. Med.,* 293:1045.
59. Gerson-Cohen, J., Hermeb, M. B., and Murdock, M. G. (1970): Thermography in detection of early breast cancer. *Cancer,* 26:1153–1156.
60. Gilbertsen, V. (1969): Detection of breast cancer in a specialized cancer detection center. *Cancer,* 24:1192–1195.
61. Gilbertsen, V. (1974): Proctosigmoidoscopy and polypectomy in reducing the incidence of rectal cancer. *Cancer,* 34:936–939.
62. Gold, R. H. (1979): Indications and risk-benefit of mammography. *J. Fam. Pract.,* 8:1135–1140.
63. Goldsen, R. K. (1963): Patient delay in seeking cancer diagnosis: behavioral aspects. *J. Chronic Dis.,* 16:427–436.
64. Goldsen, R. K., Gerhardt, P. R., and Handy, V. H. (1957): Some factors related to patient delay in seeking diagnosis for cancer symptoms. *Cancer,* 10:1–7.
65. Grant, J. A. (1974): Quantitative evaluation of a screening program. *Am. J. Public Health,* 64:66–71.
66. Gray, L. A. (1969): The frequency of taking cervical smears. *Obstet. Gynecol. Surv.,* 24:909–913.
67. Greegor, D. H. (1971): Occult blood testing for detection of asymptomatic colon cancer. *Cancer,* 28:131–134.
68. Green, L. W., and Roberts, B. J. (1974): The research literature on why women delay in seeking medical care for breast symptoms. *Health Educ. Monogr.,* 2:129–177.
69. Greenberg, D. S. (1977): Medicine and public affairs: X-Ray mammography, silent treatment for a troublesome report. *N. Engl. J. Med.,* 296:1015–1016.
70. Greenwald, H. P., Becker, S. W., and Nevitt, M. C. (1978): Delay and noncompliance in cancer detection: a behavioral perspective for health planners. *Milbank Mem. Fund Q.,* 56:212–230.
71. Greenwald, P., Nasca, P. C., Lawrence, C. E., Horton, J., McGarrah, R. P., Gabriele, T., and Carlton, K. (1978): Estimated effect of breast self-examination and routine physician examinations on breast cancer mortality. *N. Engl. J. Med.,* 299:271–273.
72. Gutkowski, T. J., and Loftus, J. F. (1970): Vaginal irrigation smear technique for mass screening. *CA,* 20:168–171.
73. Guzick, D. S. (1978): Efficacy of screening for cervical cancer: a review. *Am. J. Public Health,* 68:125–134.
74. Hackett, T. P., Cassem, N. H., and Raker, J. W. (1973): Patient delay in cancer. *N. Engl. J. Med.,* 289:14–20.
75. Hall, D. J., editor (1976): *Cancer Screening in Routine Primary Care.* Report of a workshop for primary care physicians and medical staff. Sidney Farber Cancer Institute and Massachusetts League of Neighborhood Health Centers, Boston.

76. Henderson, J. G. (1966): Denial and repression as factors in the delay of patients with cancer presenting themselves to the physician. *Ann. N.Y. Acad. Sci.,* 125:856–864.
77. Henderson, J. G., Wittkower, E. D., and Lougheed, M. N. (1958): A psychiatric investigation of the delay factor in patient to doctor presentation in cancer. *J. Psychosom. Res.,* 3:27–43.
78. Hicks, M. J., Davis, J. R., Layton, J. M., and Present, A. J. (1979): Sensitivity of mammography and physical examination of the breast for detecting breast cancer. *J.A.M.A.,* 242:2080–2083.
79. Holmes, E. C. (1978): State of the art: screening programs for early detection of lung cancer. *UCLA Cancer Center Bull.,* 5:12.
80. Hutchinson, G. B. (1960): Evaluation of preventive services. *J. Chronic Dis.,* 11:497–508.
81. Ibrahim, M. A. (1978): The case for cervical cancer screening. Editorial. *Am. J. Public Health,* 68:114–115.
82. Jaco, D. (1977): Colon cancer: etiological issues and prospects for early detection. *Prev. Med.,* 6:535–544.
83. Kaiser, R. F., Erickson, C. C., Everett, B. E., Gilliam, A. G., Graves, L. M., Walton, M., and Sprunt, D. H. (1960): Initial effect of community-wide cytologic screening on clinical state of cervical cancer detected in an entire community. Results of Memphis-Shelby County, Tennessee Study. *J.N.C.I.* 25:863–881.
84. Katz, J. L., Weiner, H., Gallagher, T. F., and Hellman, L. (1970): Stress, distress, and ego defenses. *Arch Gen. Psychiatry,* 23:131–142.
85. Knox, E. G. (1974): Multiphasic screening. *Lancet* (Dec. 14), pp. 1434–1436.
86. Knox, E. G., (1976): Ages and frequencies for cervical cancer screening. *Br. J. Cancer,* 34:444–452.
87. Koss, L. G., and Phillips, A. J. (1974): Summary and recommendations of the workshop on uterine-cervical cancer. *Cancer,* 33(Suppl.): 1753–1754.
88. Kutner, B., Makover, H. B. and Oppenheim, A. (1958): Delay in the diagnosis and treatment of cancer: a critical analysis of the literature. *J. Chronic Dis.,* 7:95–120.
89. Kutner, B., and Gordan, G. (1961): Seeking care for cancer. *J. Health Human Behav.,* 2:171–178.
90. Lilienfeld, A. M., Barnes, J. M., Barnes, R. B., Brasfield, R., Connell, J. F., Diamond, E., Gershon-Cohen, J., Haberman, J., Isard, H. J., Lane, W. Z., Lattes, R., Miller, J., Seaman, W., and Sherman, R. (1969): An evaluation of thermography in the detection of breast cancer. A cooperative pilot study. *Cancer,* 24:1206–1211.
91. Lynch, H. T., and Krush, A. M. (1968): Delay: A deterrent to cancer detection. *Arch. Environ. Health,* 17:204–209.
92. MacCalla, T. (1981): Socio-cultural dimensions relevant to preventing cancer. In: *Psychosocial Aspects of Cancer,* edited by J. Cohen, J. W. Cullen, and L. R. Martin, Raven Press, New York *(this volume).*
93. Marshall, C. E. (1965): Effects of cytologic screening on the incidence of invasive carcinoma of the cervix in a semi-closed community. *Cancer* 18:153–155.
94. Melamed, M., Flehinger, B., Miller, D., Osborne, R., Zamon, M., McGinnis, C., and Martini, N. (1977): Preliminary report of the lung cancer detection program in New York. *Cancer* 39:269–382.
95. Miller, A. B. (1973): Screening for lung cancer. *Can. J. Public Health,* 64(Suppl.): 832–835.
96. Miller, A. B., Lindsay, J., and Hill, G. B. (1976): Mortality from cancer of the uterus in Canada and its relationship to screening for cancer of the cervix. *Int. J. Cancer,* 17:602–612.
97. Moore, F. D. (1978): Breast self-examination. *N. Engl. J. Med.,* 299:304–305.
98. Moskowitz, M. (1978): Mammography in medical practice: a rational approach. *J.A.M.A.,* 240:1898–1899.
99. Naguib, S. M., Lundin, F. E., and Davis, H. J. (1966): Relation of various epidemiologic factors to cervical cancer as determined by a screening program. *Obstet. Gynecol.,* 28:451–459.
100. Naguib, S. M., Geiser, P. B., and Comstock, G. W. (1968): Response to a program of screening for cervical cancer. *Public Health Rep.,* 83:990–998.
101. Neuberger, M. G. (1966): Statement. In: *Detection and Prevention of Chronic Disease Utilizing Multiphasic Health Screening Techniques.* Hearings before the Subcommittee on Health of the Elderly of the Special Committee on Aging. U.S. Senate, 89th Congress, Second Session, Sept. 20–22. U.S. Govt. Printing Office, Washington, D.C.
102. (1971): New diagnostic tool for uterine cancer. *HSMHA Health Reports,* 86:597.

103. (1979): New screening test for colorectal cancer developed in Canada. *J.A.M.A.*, 242:1005–1006.
104. (1978): NIH/NCI consensus development meeting on breast cancer screening. *Prev. Med.*, 7:269–278.
105. Papanicolaou, G. N., and Traut, H. F. (1943): *Diagnosis of Uterine Cancer by the Vaginal Smear*. The Commonwealth Fund, New York.
106. Ramcharan, S., Cutler, J. L., Feldman, R., Siegelaub, A. B., Campbell, B., Friedman, G. D., Dales, L. G., and Collen, M. R. (1973): Multiphasic check-up evaluation study. 2. Disability and chronic disease after seven years of multiphasic health checkups. *Prev. Med.*, 2:207–220.
107. Reeder, S., Berkanovic, E., and Marcus, A. C. (1980): Breast cancer detection behavior among urban women. *Public Health Rep.*, 95:276–281.
108. (1975): Regular screening would reduce cancer of the colon and rectum toll. *J.A.M.A.*, 234:137.
109. Reinke, W. A. (1969): Decisions about screening programs: can we develop a rationale basis? *Arch. Environ. Health*, 19:403–411.
110. Report of the Canadian Task Force (1976): Cervical cancer screening programs. *Can. Med. Assn. J.*, 114:1003–1033.
111. Rowan, R. (1976): Self-exam of the testicles. *Penthouse Forum* (Feb. 1976).
112. Sackett, D. L., and Holland, Walter, W. (1975): Controversy in the detection of disease. *Lancet* (Aug. 23): 357–359.
113. (1979): Screening for colorectal cancer. *Lancet* (Dec. 8): 1222–1223.
114. (1976): Self-exam for orofacial cancer. *Med. World News*, May 3, 1976, p. 23.
115. Shapiro, S., Strax, P., and Venet, L. (1971): Periodic breast cancer screening in reducing mortality from breast cancer. *J.A.M.A.*, 215:1777–1785.
116. Shapiro, S., (1973): Evaluation of two contrasting types of screening programs. *Prev. Med.*, 2:266–277.
117. Shapiro, S., (1977): Evidence on screening for breast cancer from a randomized trial. *Cancer*, 39:2772–2782.
118. Sherlock, P., and Winawer, S. J. (1974): Modern approaches to early identification of large bowel cancer. *Am. J. Digest. Dis.*, 19:959–964.
119. Smart, C. R., and Beahrs, O. H. (1979): Breast cancer screening results as viewed by the clinician. *Cancer*, 43:851–856.
120. Smith, E. M., Francis, A. M., and Plissar, L. (1980): The effect of breast self-exam practices and physician examinations on extent of disease at diagnosis. *Prev. Med.*, 9:409–417.
121. Stevens, G. M., and Weigen, J. F. (1969): Survey mammography as a case finding method for routine and postmastectomized patients. *Cancer*, 24:1201–1205.
122. Sutherland, R. (1960): *Cancer: The Significance of Delay*. Butterworth, London.
123. Titchener, J. L. Zwerling, I., Gottschalk, L., Levine, M., Culbertson, W., Cohen, S., and Silver, H. (1956): Problem of delay in seeking medical care. *J.A.M.A.*, 160:1187–1193.
124. U.I.C.C. (International Union Against Cancer) (1967): *Cancer Detection*, Monograph Series, Vol. 4. Springer-Verlag, New York.
125. U.I.C.C. (1978): *Screening in Cancer: A Report of a UICC International Workshop, Toronto, Canada, April 24–27, 1978*. UICC Technical Report Series Vol. 40, Geneva.
126. U.S. Dept. Health, Education and Welfare (1976): *Cancer Questions and Answers About Rates and Risks*. DHEW Pub. No. (NIH) 76–1040. USPHS.
127. U.S. Dept. Health, Education and Welfare (1976): National Cancer Program 1976. Annual Plan for FY 1978–1982.
128. U.S. Dept. Health, Education and Welfare, (1979): *The Breast Cancer Digest: A Guide to Medical Care, Emotional Support, Educational Programs, and Resources*. NIH Pub. No. 80–1691. National Cancer Institute, Bethesda, Md.
129. Whitted, H. H. (1963): Early detection of cancer among low income groups. *Arch. Environ. Health*, 6:280–285.
130. Wilson, J. M. G., and Jungner, G. (1968): *The Principles and Practice of Screening for Disease*. World Health Organization. Public Health Papers No. 34, Geneva.
131. Worden, J. W., and Weisman, A. D. (1975): Psychosocial components of lagtime in cancer diagnosis. *J. Psychosom. Res.*, 19:69–79.
132. World Health Organization. (1964): *Prevention of Cancer*. WHO Technical Report Series No. 276, Geneva.

133. World Health Organization (1969): *Early Detection of Cancer.* WHO Technical Report Series No. 422, Geneva.
134. World Health Organization. (1971): *Mass Health Examinations,* Public Health Paper 45. WHO, Geneva.
135. Wynder, E. L. (1969): Identification of women at high risk for breast cancer. *Cancer,* 24:1235–1240.

Psychosocial Aspects of Cancer,
edited by Jerome Cohen et al.
Raven Press, New York © 1982.

Chapter 7

Psychosocial Research Issues Related to Cancer Screening: Some Additional Concerns About Research Issues in Community Cancer Research

S. Stephen Kegeles

Department of Behavioral Sciences and Community Health, University of Connecticut Health Center, Farmington, Connecticut 06032

I hope to accomplish three things in this response to Dr. D'Onofrio's chapter. First, I wish to compliment her on the issues she chose to discuss, and in the quite sophisticated manner in which she discussed them. Second, I intend to enlarge on some of the points she made. Third, I intend to discuss some matters suggested by her chapter which have concerned me in my own research and in reviewing grant and contract proposals submitted to the Division of Cancer Control and Rehabilitation of the National Cancer Institute during the last 4 years.

Initially, I wish to underline Dr. D'Onofrio's concern that the behavior on which social researchers concentrate their efforts be appropriate. For years I took the position that as social researcher I need be concerned only with formulating and carrying out legitimate scientific studies and reporting the data collected to both health practitioner and health scientist audiences. I would be guided exclusively by expert medical opinion about whether the behavior which a population was asked to follow was appropriate. Social researchers have taken this position quite frequently. Thus, for instance, there have been many aversive conditioning studies in the smoking and weight control areas without concern on the part of the social researcher about whether a sudden cessation of smoking or a sudden rapid weight loss might, in fact, create greater health risk than continuation of "inappropriate" behavior. Human experimentation committees sometimes question such endeavors, but not yet frequently enough. I now believe that social researchers must personally assess the quality of evidence themselves about the appropriateness of the behavior to be modified before an attempt is made to change the behavior, no matter what "expert opinion" holds. Such an assessment is frequently very difficult for the social researcher; however, any other position runs great risk as unethical human experimentation.

73

Let me be clear about this issue. I do not mean that social researchers have no role in socio-community research other than that of technical persuaders. Indeed, they must be full partners in all endeavors based on their level of expertise. Neither do I mean that social researchers have legal responsibility for community health endeavors. Societal demand rests this authority with physicians. Rather, social researchers have equivalent ethical and moral responsibility with physicians for actions taken. This ethical and moral responsibility can be discharged best by full knowledge of the consequences of actions which people are urged to follow.

This point relates to cancer screening in obvious ways. Although cervical cancer has decreased greatly in areas in which many women have taken Pap tests, it has also decreased greatly in areas where few or no women have taken Pap tests. Moreover, the Memphis–Shelby County data (11) show one of the few instances of a direct relationship between Pap tests by high-risk women and decreases in cervical cancer. In most other instances, we commit what sociologists have called the "demographic fallacy"; we correlate increases in cervical cytology with decreases in cervical cancer, despite the minimal data which show worldwide increases in Pap tests taken by high-risk women. Even though Cramer (5) makes a convincing case for the fact that cervical cytology reduces cervical cancer, we must attend carefully to Knox's statement (13) on the kinds of research that are needed to show the relationship clearly.

Even if there is agreement that most data suggest a need for continued and accelerated Pap testing, we must deal with the frequency with which women should be urged to take such examinations. As Dr. D'Onofrio notes, if Pap tests are needed less often than once a year, it seems clearly inappropriate, needless, and perhaps unethical to insist that women obtain yearly tests. It is certainly as inappropriate to involve social researchers in research activities which attempt to lead people to take costly and inappropriate actions. Does informed consent by the potential participant of such actions take care of this problem? Perhaps, in some cases. Unfortunately, a large number of people are willing to consent to do inappropriate things when asked to do so by a "scientist." I do not believe the informed social researcher who consents to persuade people to take inappropriate actions is absolved of his ethical responsibility. The recent article by Breslow and Somers (4) is a step in the direction of defining the appropriate timing of health actions by the population. We certainly need specific statements of the frequency with which people should take actions for health and cancer screening which match the reality of disease progression.

Such ethical considerations are directly relevant to early breast cancer screening. Ray Fink, an extremely capable sociologist, was instrumental in persuading women to take part in the large Health Information Program (HIP) effort on which most of the evidence on early breast cancer screening is based (7,8). These women were examined by thermography and mammography. Prior to the HIP studies, little was known about either the dangers of such technology or their benefits; thus such studies were needed in order to determine the value of early breast examination. However, the recent National Cancer Institute Con-census Report (15) suggests that thermography is inefficient and that the cancer risk of mammography for women under age 50 may be greater than its benefits. Hence Fink inadvertently contributed to placing some women in a dangerous situation. It is obvious in this case, however, that his behavior was ethical at the time of the study; he did communicate what was known at the time the studies were carried out.

If there is to be continued social research in breast self-examination, one must take into consideration the evidence for the effectiveness and timing of such screening rather than providing false assurance for behavior which might be inadequately done. Such concern must be even greater in efforts to get people to take cancer screening actions for which evidence is even less impressive than in breast and cervical cancer. Thus I suggest great concern not only for program efforts, but for involving social researchers in situations in which the medical evidence is, at best, fuzzy.

The second of Dr. D'Onofrio's points on which I wish to expand concerns the behavioral unit to be assessed. Too often, "compliance" has been treated frequently as if it were a unitary concept. Thus, for instance, the original Health Belief Model (17) and the revised Health Belief Model (1) have been used to attempt to explain all of health behavior by many health educators and social researchers. The model has been useful in explaining behavior, and most recently in predicting mothers' behavior, in regard to children's activities (2,3). However, it has been far less useful for predicting behavior or for modifying repeated instances of health behavior. A more detailed analysis of the behavior to be changed might suggest a less indiscriminate use of this model. A related point is in the general overattention to psychological theory and explanations. As I have worked with some postdoctoral social psychology fellows over the last couple of years, I have found quite sophisticated specification, elaboration, and conceptualization of the independent variable—that which is conceived of as psychological theory, and much less attention to the dependent variable. A primary stress within our post-doctoral teaching is directed toward moving fellows from such global concepts as "learned helplessness" or "psychological stress" or "fear appeals" to an analysis of the types of health behavior these notions are being used to explain or to label. Definitions need to be made in terms of the frequency, duration, and place of behavior and of the characteristics of the person who needs to carry it out.

Another reason for this type of analysis is that success in explaining health behavior will not be accomplished by dependence on what people say is in their heads or how they explain their own past behavior. Instead, success in building both a technology and a theory of health behavior will come by thinking in terms of contingent stimulus conditions and contingent reinforcement condi-tions. Without clear demarcation of the behaviors necessary for action to occur, there will be available only quite limited notions of how stimulus conditions and contingent reinforcements should be arranged. Hence Dr. D'Onofrio's expressed concern about the need for a sophisticated analysis and definition of behavioral units for cancer control programs is to be applauded.

Third, Dr. D'Onofrio's suggestion that research is needed badly on provider behavior and on health care system activities needs repetition. Medical school curricula during the "clinical years" and activity during internship and residency reinforce interests in curative medicine and in sick rather than well people. Since the medical establishment is provided societal sanction to define all health activities (9), primary and secondary prevention are less important and receive short shrift in both the learning process and the general health arena. Academic medical school departments of behavioral sciences, community health, and most recently, family practice or family medicine have all attempted to offer curricula to change this orientation. They have succeeded for a few students, for a short period of time, and in a few institutions. However, most medical students still emerge from school as physicians who are interested essentially in providing clinical services for sick people. Research is certainly needed in means for rearranging the activities of practitioners. However, it is difficult to be optimistic that the interactive feedback system of community practitioner and medical teacher, each of whom reinforces the primary of curative medicine, can be broken easily.

TECHNOLOGY TRANSFER

The next point is that of "technology transfer," the newest public relations term of the Department of Health, Education and Welfare. Cancer control—which includes some cancer screening—is to be directed toward the transfer of scientific and technological data to the community. That certainly seems appropriate; the inventions and the knowledge which have emerged in the "war on cancer" (an earlier public relations term) need to receive dissemination. However, it is mandated that federal support for "technology transfer" must serve a demonstration and not a service function. In addition, these demonstration activities must be evaluated carefully to determine which are and which are not effective so that communities throughout the country can use successful activities without additional federal funding. On this basis the cancer centers were organized, the 27 breast cancer centers were funded, and contracts were written for institutions and individuals to bid on. This is an eminently sensible orientation; the public is provided with the fruits of scientific knowledge most rapidly. However, there are problems with these notions, both in their inception and in their commission. Frequently, for instance, persons who propose to carry out these activities either are not trained or experienced in research, or are well trained and experienced in biological and/or physical science research but not in community or behavioral research.

In research grants submitted by members of both of these groups, one finds many instances of proposals to carry out community activities (including screening) in which it is impossible to determine what the potential grantee proposes to do and why. When and if such proposals are funded (and some have been over the years) and a request is then made by the investigator for refunding after 2 to 3 years, one frequently finds it almost impossible to determine what was done, why, and with what effect during the original funded period. Those investigators without prior training or experience frequently do not seem to have carried out the activities which one supposed they were intending to, or which they promised to do, nor have they evaluated the effects of these activities. Those with good training appear convinced that science means laboratory animal or molecular research; community activity can be done by anyone, especially a public relations person.

Frequently, there is little or no technology available for transfer. Thus one finds frequent statements in grant or contract proposals such as follow:

1. We will use (or have used) audio tapes from such and such institution to inform physicians of cancer problems and/or solutions.

2. We will use (or have used) 24-hr "hot line" telephones for consumers and for community practitioners.

3. We will use (or have used) a series of experts on public television to talk about cancer and/or cancer screening.

4. We will use (or have used) a series of symposia at out medical school, hospital, health center.

There is nothing inherently wrong with any of these statements; they may all be appropriate and sensible or, again, they may not be. The problem is that there are minimal data available about the kind of impact these activities have, the kinds of persons on whom they have impact, or the cost-to-benefit ratio they have as compared to using funds otherwise. Certainly, none of these is a technology which is transferable to new communities.

Let us return to screening for some instances of activity, with appropriate or nonexistent evaluation.

1. During the early meetings in Columbia, Maryland, in order to help define what should be done in cancer control, each invitee was requested to bring projects which might be promoted by the Division of Cancer Control. Individuals then met within groups to define priorities for cancer control. A proposal I brought to the meetings concerned the need to determine appropriate techniques for eliciting repeat cervical tests from among high-risk population groups. The proposal was to try a series of experimental approaches for small groups of high-risk women. It was most reasonable for state health departments to be involved in the activity since they deal frequently with low-income groups, the high-risk population in this situation. Subsequently, a Request for Proposal (RFP) was written which resembled the early proposal. The two may not have been connected, but they looked similar. However, the RFP did not require the experimental component, mandated bids only from state health departments, required obtaining many Pap tests in a short period of time, and required assessment of the reliability and validity of the tests. A number of states were provided

funds to carry out the activity; their focus was generally on numbers of tests. (The program was eventually discontinued because little or no research was carried out.) We have no greater knowledge now than we had in 1974 about how to elicit repeat Pap tests from groups at high risk for cervical cancer.

2. Each of the 27 breast cancer centers was mandated to teach breast self-examination and to evaluate the effectiveness of its teaching. Kathleen Grady, one of my colleagues, has recently conducted a mail survey of the 27 centers to find out what they have done in these regards. We received 24 responses to repeated mailings. We found that most, if not all, of the centers which responded did teach breast self-examination. It appears as if most used either American Cancer Society (ACS) pamphlets or materials built on the ACS pamphlets for teaching, and some used the Betsi Model. Only two centers, the Fox Chase Center in Philadelphia and the Houston Center, spontaneously mentioned doing any formal evaluation of its teaching activity. The Fox Chase Center utilized the Betsi Model for its teaching and used an additional non-center population for its evaluation. The evaluation resulted in an interesting report (b).

Two points should be made about the breast self-examination (BSE) activity carried out in the breast cancer centers. First, we did a simple Andie Knutson-like (14) evaluation, each lasting between 5 and 15 min, with 18 housewives who had read two separate ACS pamphlets on BSE, and we found that one-third of the women made mistakes. Such mistakes related to where they should start the examination, how often they should do the examination, or what they were looking for. Most explicitly, women were unable to define when they should do the examination after reading the pamphlet. The term "once a month, after your menstrual period" left women in limbo. Most of the women liked the pamphlet, however, and most could recite the danger signals. These pamphlets could have been evaluated in much the same way we evaluated them by any of the centers. As a result of 3 to 4 hr of evaluation, the centers would have determined whether what they were doing was having the success they desired, and modifications could have been made. Instead, the centers chose to use the pamphlets provided without determining their utility.

Secondly, as just noted, some of the centers used the Betsi Model for teaching; yet there appear to be no data which indicate that learning to determine lumps on the Betsi Model has any relation to whether, how frequently, how correctly, or how often women do BSE. Again, I do not intend to suggest that what is taught in the breast centers is wrong. There simply are no data about whether it has had impact or not. We have been able to locate about 15 studies of BSE carried out over the past 25 years, about 7 or 8 of which have been carried out in the last decade. A few of these have been intervention studies: they all indicate that women instructed in BSE state they start to examine their breasts; however, only about 20% of women state they continue to do BSE on a regular basis. The only data on accuracy and adequacy of their BSE performance is demonstrated on the Betsi Model and not on their own bodies. A more complete statement on the current status of and factors which appear to be related to breast self-examination is contained in a forthcoming publication (12). Thus instruction provided in BSE at the breast cancer centers probably does help in starting BSE, but not in continuing BSE. Moreover, despite all the money spent in the breast cancer centers, we do not know whether any of the teaching has resulted in greater accuracy in self-detection of breast cancer, how frequently breast self-examination should be done, or whether there should be increased efforts to induce women to do breast self-examination.

This response certainly should not be construed as an attack on the American Cancer Society, an organization without which much of what is done in the community would not otherwise be done. Over the years, the only organization concerned with the public side of cancer control has been the American Cancer Society. Nor should it be inferred that the Cancer Control Division of the National Cancer Institute should be discontinued. Without that Division and its sophisticated but tough-minded review process, there would be no sensible psychosocial research in community cancer activities; in fact, little community activity would be carried out at all. Instead, these statements should be construed as further emphasizing the last point from Dr. D'Onofrio's chapter I wish to discuss—the great need for research in technology transfer in cancer, including that of cancer screening. What should this research be like?

Because of the limited space available and the subsequent chapter by Dr. Spinetta (Chapter 21) this need be mentioned only briefly. Most important is that cancer control needs to be dealt with as research and not as an advertising or public relations venture. Thus whatever is done must follow the standard rules for research that we have all learned. This means, at a minimum, that expected outcomes need to be specified in sufficient and articulated detail to enable them to be tested, that potentially contaminating variables need to be controlled for, that data need to be collected and analyzed in ways which meet scientific standards and statistical assumptions, and that reports need to be made which reflect the samples studied. In addition, the research carried out must be on populations who are real for the area under consideration, and the behavior to be assessed should be appropriate to the samples to which it will be generalized. My current research interest is in attempting to build a technology and a theory of preventive health behavior. Thus, with a group of younger colleagues, all social psychologists, I am carrying out and planning a series of tightly controlled experiments on health behavior which cross disease and age characteristics of populations. All of these experiments have in common the following characteristics:

1. Repeated measures of personal characteristics of the sample;
2. Intervention activities which provide, with them, a free health service;
3. Comparison of two or more intervention methods; and
4. Assessment of the effects of the interventions on repeated measures of behavior over at least 1 year.

Each of these studies uses cognitive and/or behavioral interventions and training.
Obviously, this is not meant to suggest that everyone carry out research of

this kind, especially if we are to continue to obtain funds to do so. However, there is an essential need for systematic and integrated research which builds findings, comparable to the studies carried out by Dr. Lazarus (see Chapter 15) on stress and coping, to the studies carried out by the Michigan group on the health belief model (17), and to the research by Jenkins and others at Boston University on type A personality (10,16). We hope the era of the single social researcher who wanders into a health field, carries out a study, and then goes back to his parent discipline never to return to health research is over. Only through systematic research can we obtain a technology that is transferable to community cancer programs.

REFERENCES

1. Becker, M. H. (ed.) (1974): The health belief model and personal health behavior. *Health Educ. Monogr.,* 2:326–473.
2. Becker, M. H., Maiman, L. A., Kirscht, J. P., Haefner, D. P., and Drachman, R. H. (1977): The health belief model and prediction of dietary compliance: A field experiment. *J. Health Soc. Behav.,* 18:348–366.
3. Becker, M. H., Radius, S. M., Rosenstock, I. M., Drachman, R. C., Schuberth, K. C., and Teets, K. C. (1978): Compliance with a medical regimen for asthma: A test of the health belief model. *Public Health Rep.,* 93:263–277.
4. Breslow, L., and Somers, A. R. (1977): The lifetime health monitoring program: A practical approach to preventive medicine. *N. Engl. J. Med.,* 296:601–817.
5. Cramer, D. W. (1974): The role of cervical cytology in the declining morbidity and mortality of cervical cancer. *Cancer,* 34:2018–2027.
6. Crosson, K. E., Nessel, A. E., Engstrom, P. F., and Grover, P. L. (1978): Health education in preventive oncology: A study of factors influencing practice of breast self-examination. *Proc. 2nd Annual American Society of Preventive Oncology,* New York. Preprint.
7. Fink, R., Shapiro, S., and Lewison, J. (1968): The reluctant participant in a breast cancer screening program. *Public Health Rep.,* 83:479–490.
8. Fink, R., Shapiro, S., and Roester, R. (1972): Impact of efforts to increase participation in repetitive screenings for early breast cancer detection. *Am. J. Public Health,* 62:328–336.
9. Friedson, E. (1974): *Professional Dominance: The Social Structure of Medical Care, 2nd Ed.* Aldine, Chicago.
10. Jenkins, C. D. (1976): Recent evidence supporting psychologic and social risk factors for coronary disease. *N. Engl. J. Med.,* 294:987–994, 1033–1038.
11. Kaiser, R. F., Erickson, C. C., Everett, B. E., Gillaim, A. G., Graves, L. M., Walton, M., and Sprunt, D. J. (1960): Initial effect of community-wide cytologic screening on clinical stage of cervical cancer detected in an entire community. Results of Memphis–Shelby County, Tennessee, study. *J. Natl. Cancer Inst.,* 25:863:881.
12. Kegeles, S. S., and Grady, K. E. (1980): Behavioral dimensions in cancer control. In: *Cancer Epiemiology and Prevention,* edited by D. Schottenfeld and J. F. Fraumeni, Chapter 66. Saunders, Philadelphia.
13. Knox, E. G. (1966): Cervical cytology: A scrutiny of the evidence. In: *Problems and Progress in Medical Care,* edited by G. McLachlan, pp. 277–309. Oxford University Press, London.
14. Knutson, A. L. (1953): Application of pretesting in health education. *Public Health Monograph No. 8.* U.S. Department of Health, Education and Welfare, Public Health Service, Washington, D.C.
15. NIH/NCI (1977): Background discussion and recommendations, *Consensus Development Meeting on Breast Cancer Screening,* Bethesda, Md. Sept. 14–16, Oct. 18.
16. Rosenman, R. H., Brand, R. J., Jenkins, C. D., Friedman, M., Straus, R., and Wurm, M. (1975): Coronary heart disease in the Western collaborative group study: Final follow-up experience of 8.5 years. *J.A.M.A.,* 233:872–877.
17. Rosenstock, I. M. (1974): The health belief model and preventive health behavior. *Health Educ. Monogr.,* 2:354–386.

Psychosocial Aspects of Cancer,
edited by Jerome Cohen et al.
Raven Press, New York © 1982.

Chapter 8

Concepts and Research Issues in the Economics of Cancer Prevention

Stuart O. Schweitzer

Division of Health Services, School of Public Health, University of California, Los Angeles, Los Angeles, California 90024

Neither the inception of cancer nor its progression can be viewed as isolated medical events in the life of a patient. Interactions exist among a person's life style, his environment, and his health status which are now becoming better understood (1,8). We are becoming aware, as well, of the effects which the health system itself imposes on individual health. We have understood implicitly some of these relationships for many years. When the term "Health Maintenance Organization" (HMO) was first coined, the assumption was that a group of providers organized into a coordinated system would be better able to "maintain" the health of subscribers than would a traditional clustering of independent practitioners. Today this assumption is being subjected to closer scrutiny (9). Additionally, cost containment is now a priority goal in health policy, and prepaid medical care is seen by many as a useful component within a health system. The characteristic of HMOs most appreciated at the national policy level now appears to be their potential for increased efficiency in delivering health care services. It is ironic that the original objective of improved health status has been supplanted by economic realities.

The ways in which health system characteristics induce changes in health are manifold. We shall consider in this paper some of the economic aspects of health care in an effort to understand better the role of incentives of all types in the prevention of a dread disease—cancer.

PRIMARY PREVENTION

Primary prevention of disease is the only phase which truly prevents illness, as it defines a set of actions which will reduce the incidence of disease rather than deal with its sequelae.

We are still trying to understand the biological actions which cause cancer, and until we have fully understood this process our actions in cancer control must be more inferential than we would like. With only a few cancer entities do we feel confident in stating that selected agents cause cancer. Other agents seem to exacerbate it, whereas for still other cancers we observe an association without being certain of a causal link. This distinction is extremely important, because many programs to reduce exposure to certain agents involve a realloca- tion of resources: disruption of industries, increased capital expenditures, higher use of other—often limited—productive resources, and higher consumer prices. If social benefits of some new prevention programs are uncertain because we know little about the causality, a recommendation to expend new resources is less easily justified. Given this rather important caveat, we are now able to ask what kinds of economic factors might affect the primary prevention of cancer, and how do they work? If we consider those agents whose causal role in cancer seems virtually certain—tobacco, asbestos, and certain chemicals (e.g., PPB and PVC)— we see that each exposes itself to individuals in a different setting. Tobacco products are consumed regularly by some 60 million Americans at home, at work, and during leisure activities. Exposure to this risk factor is basically a personal decision on the part of the individual (although secondary exposure from another's smoking is now recognized as harmful).

Incentives to reduce the incidence of smoking traditionally rely on access and cost variables for the smoker—restricting consumption. Use of media to educate smokers and potential smokers is advised, of course (15). Cigarette taxes are used in other countries more than they are in the United States for the direct purpose of reducing demand. One version of the cigarette tax is the flat per-cigarette tax used in the United States. Recently the suggestion has been made that a tax which is graduated according to the tar content of the cigarettes would be useful in deflecting demand toward the less harmful brands (6). One of the reasons for our reluctance to rely heavily on a cigarette tax lies in the regressive nature of the tax, as the poor will typically pay a higher percentage of their income than will the wealthy. Measures have been proposed to reduce the regressivity by returning to the tax payers the tax proceeds in some other form, such as in smoking-related research.

A second approach recently employed on behalf of nonsmokers may act as a disincentive to smokers as well—restricting smoking to fewer areas of public facilities. Regulations to this effect have been adopted in Berkeley, Los Angeles, Chicago, and the state of Utah; a statewide proposal was narrowly defeated in California in 1978. This makes smoking less convenient, of course, but it also raises the density of smoke within those ever smaller areas where smokers are segregated. It is not unlikely that we may be increasing the risk of cancer to those who choose to smoke in public places.

The health or life insurance industries have a distinct incentive to discourage smoking by policyholders, but have not generally taken up the challenge. En- forcement is cited as a problem in offering lower premiums to nonsmokers; but there is no reason why smoking could not be treated like any other previous medical condition, relying on individual response to questions only until a large claim arises, at which time the insurer would retain the right to verify the insured's statements.

For other carcinogenic agents, policies acting to reduce exposure must typically be applied to those who create the exposure to environmental pollutants at industrial sites. The control measures available in this sort of setting are different from those which influence consumers directly. Both direct regulation and taxation can be used to control emissions of industrial plants. The former has been the method of choice (3–5), but advocates of an economic incentive (taxation) scheme would rather retain flexibility for firms while avoiding the enforcement problems inherent in regulation. In the case of a new liquified natural gas plant proposed for Southern California, the suggestion has even been made that reduction in pollutant levels at other sites of the firm be used to permit the new facility to conform to area-wide clean-air standards. The major difficulty in imposing effluent regulations or taxes currently is the paucity of data justifying the action. In nearly every case, a reduction in exposure to a pollutant can be achieved only through higher production costs, which translates into reduced employment. Thus, although the benefits of the action may be widespread, the costs will be borne directly by a few—those workers whose jobs are threatened by higher production and retail costs of the product. A community sees the decision in a similar way, as the benefits are weighed against loss of local tax revenues if firms reduce employment or, in the extreme, close down altogether. [A case in point is that of Minnesota's Reserve Mining Company, found guilty of polluting Lake Superior for many years (10).]

The difficulty underlying both an individual's and a community's response to such an exposure-reducing measure is an imbalance in the nature of risks and, more importantly, a difference in the way these risks are portrayed.

How is one to weigh increased mortality or morbidity against loss of one's economic livelihood? The former is probabalistic and can be expected to occur only in the future, if at all. The latter loss, unemployment, is a more immediate threat. The costs of both illness and unemployment have differential impacts on individuals at different stages of their life cycles.

The rate of time preference of individuals tends to make people value current events more than future ones. Premature loss of life or limb occurring in later life is seen only vaguely by a younger worker but more clearly by one approaching advancing years. Thus the threat of future cancer, not viewed seriously by the young, increases as one ages. The risk of unemployment, on the other hand, is taken more seriously by the young, who are creating a family and building a career. As one's family responsibilities decline with age, along with one's productive life expectance, the seriousness of the threat of unemployment falls. This leads us to predict that a community of primarily youthful individuals would be less likely to adopt such an environmental action than would one whose proportion of elderly individuals were greater. The politics of environmental protection would seem to be consistent with this model. Our model describes, as well, the psychology of teen-age smoking if we replace the threat of unemployment with the penalty of "peer ostracism." The threat of future illness is viewed as being far less serious than this (current) social disapproval.

Further confusing this objective assessment is the way in which the loss trade-off is portrayed by those engaged in the policy debate. Here we see the typical inequality in access to information that has hampered legislative and regulatory bodies in their attempts to deal with large, well-staffed, powerful industries. At the national level we have seen the creation of the Congressional Office of Technology Assessment (OTA) as a response to the problem. Several states have created parallel research and analysis departments for the purposes of developing independent estimates of the impacts of potential industry-oriented policy for the benefit of the legislature.

With regard to the reduction of exposure to carcinogens, several questions arise where the public side of the issue is all too often deficient in pertinent information. The first question is the extent of the carcinogenic nature of the pollutant. Evidence is often more inferential, as mentioned before, and subject to different interpretations. Secondly, we know little about the "dose-response" relationship between amount of exposure to a carcinogen and the amount of disease produced. Is the relationship a linear one, implying that a 50% reduction in pollution would reduce the incidence of disease by that amount? Or is there a threshold effect, such that marginal improvements in exposure would produce no real change in morbidity? The end result of our inadequate information is that any regulatory or policy decision concerning primary prevention action is likely to be effectively opposed by pressure groups with substantial resources and an ability and motive to use the courts to improve their prospects for protection from interference.

There is little in the way that elements of our health care system presently work to counter these pressures. As evidence of this, one notes that only a short-lived anti-smoking media campaign has ever been employed to reduce the incidence of teen-age smoking. Effective campaigns to educate teen-agers, reduce media advertising, or raise cigarette taxes have not been enacted. Physicians are rarely able to provide a role model, and outside of an HMO with its defined membership, there is no mechanism to disseminate ideas about more healthful life styles. Incentives to encourage primary cancer prevention can, of course, be directed at employers, but the difficulties inherent in either the consumer or employer strategy are similar. First, a clear understanding must exist with respect to a program's objectives in terms of specific reduction in exposure to an agent in order to produce a specific improvement in health outcome. Second, a behavior model—of either the consumer on the one hand, or the employer on the other—must be created to explain the relationship between incentives and cancer-inducing behavior. How do consumers of cigarettes or hair dyes respond to increased education regarding health risks? Do market variables enter into the behavior pattern? What are the costs of alternative means of producing PVC, or of insulating steam pipes?

The interaction of the medical analysis and the behavioral and economic relationships will permit an effective primary prevention program. One might argue that in some areas the basic research has already been done, and yet we are unable to suggest policy initiatives because there has been little in the way of synthesis of these individual studies.

Other characteristics of a health care system which influences preventive care affect an individual's prospensity to seek care early in the course of the disease, and so we turn to secondary prevention.

SECONDARY PREVENTION

The early, presymptomatic detection and treatment of illness is termed secondary prevention because the serious consequences of many diseases can be prevented this way. Strictly speaking, the disease is not literally being prevented but is merely being detected and treated early.

Since secondary (and tertiary) prevention pertains to treatment of disease within the person, we look exclusively at the use of personal health services rather than the community aspects of the cases of illness discussed earlier. What factors stimulate or retard the use of medical care at an early, often presymptomatic, stage of a disease (12)?

One important class of such variables is economic, as economic incentives alter our pattern of consumption in many ways. We include in the class of economic factors those which affect time costs as well as direct money costs. Using this broader definition, we could enumerate a number of access variables which describe a health system; geographic access to physicians and waiting time are but two examples. Third-party reimbursement, determining net price of services, is of course recognized as a major determinant of patterns of use by patients. Traditional third-party reimbursement historically has covered inpatient care more fully than ambulatory care. Within the category of ambulatory services, those least often covered are those for routine diagnostic care. Although substantial empirical evidence indicates that more comprehensive insurance coverage of ambulatory care would increase the utilization of those services, there is less understanding of the nature of the increase. Is the price sensitivity equally great for all ambulatory services? The reason for the particular pattern of insurance is clear. Preservation of the independence between insurance coverage for services and use of services requires that insurance cover only those services for which demand elasticity is low; thus full coverage for hospital care assumed to be nondiscretionary, and shallow coverage for physician care assumed to be nondiscretionary, and shallow coverage for hospital care assumed to be readily overconsumed will prevail. But there is an obvious conflict between short-term efficiency in the management of an insurance program and minimizing the long-run social costs of illness.

If insurance coverage were altered to include preventive services, would use of services become less rational? Would use of less necessary services expand as much as the use of more necessary services? An answer to this question, of course, assumes an understanding of what constitutes "necessity" of services. Although agreement is easy to reach on services at either end of this "necessity" spectrum, the gray area in the middle is very wide. "Need" has both medical and mental aspects which make a service of great value to one person while being frivolous to someone else. Traditionally, we employ the price system to allocate services to those most desirous of purchasing them. However, for large segments of the population, the elderly and the poor, we have largely removed money price as an allocation mechanism, relying instead on a time price (a queue) or access barriers, such as the proportion of providers accepting assignment under Medicare or agreeing to see Medicaid patients. The price mechanism is therefore employed on a shrinking population: the non-poor, non-elderly without outpatient medical insurance coverage.

Although we have studied the determinants of the demand for medical care intensively, at least at an aggregate level (7), we have less understanding of the supply response. We know that the supply of some health services is very responsive to economic stimuli. For example, physicians tend to locate in more affluent neighborhoods (2). Secondly, as reimbursement for services improved, supply increased: access to health care for the poor and the elderly has improved markedly since the inception of Medicaid and Medicare in 1965. Also, the growth of high technology medicine generally follows third-party reimbursement, with kidney dialysis and CAT scanning being but two examples.

With respect to preventive services, the lack of widely available primary care for much of the population and the separation of health education from health services reduce the ability of the health system to intervene in an early stage of a disease. Where the incentives on the part of the providers clearly favor early detection, as in the case of HMOs, one would expect to see evidence of successful early detection. But such a comparison has not yet been done. If such a linkage could be demonstrated, one could envision a number of policy ramifications related to the structure of insurance benefits and premiums. Both patient education and a specified subsidized regimen of screening activities could be encouraged by the insurance sector, which would have the double effect of increasing demand and access as well.

TERTIARY PREVENTION

Many of the inhibiting factors affecting use of tertiary preventive services are the same as those previously discussed under the heading of secondary prevention. These relate to the way in which the medical care system, both providers and the financing mechanism, de-emphasize early detection and prompt intervention. There is one additional factor that concerns tertiary prevention specifically, however.

Tertiary preventive care utilizes to a unique degree nonmedical providers as well as physicians. The concepts involved in tertiary care are to a large extent psychological and social, as they are concerned with the way in which an individual copes with his disease, both personally and as a member of a community. We look, therefore, at the role of counseling and education for the patient and for the patient's family, colleagues, and neighbors.

Where these support services are lacking (as they typically are), there is substantial evidence that even organic, let alone nonorganic, emotional complications of illness arise which can be devastating in the case of disease as feared as cancer (11).

If we look at the health system to see how it deals with this side of the "caring" mission, we see numerous inadequacies. The first barrier to an integrated care system is that the patient's physician, who assumes the central role in treatment, neither is trained in psychosocial aspects of medicine nor is particularly interested in or appreciative of them. The practitioner therefore is both incapable of providing needed nonmedical services directly and likely to be insensitive to the patient's need for an appropriate referral to a specialist.

Were this barrier overcome and appropriate counsel sought, economic forces then become evident. Third-party health coverage rarely includes nonphysician-rendered services. If social worker or psychologist services are included at all, they are only for a brief, crisis mode of service not conducive to adequate resolution of the social correlates of cancer.

INSURANCE AND EMPLOYMENT ASPECTS

Another aggravation of the tertiary phase of prevention is the discrimination against cancer patients by insurers and employers because of heightened risk of future illness.

The fragmented insurance system prevailing throughout the country imposes severe risks on individuals who change employers or those whose employer changes insurance carriers. If one is undergoing cancer treatment, one's insurer's obligation to support the costs of care are clear. This insurance, however, is tied not to the individual but to the employer or the employee group. Only 16% of private hospital insurance policies were individual policies with the remainder arising from group coverage (13). For physician expense, the proportion of individual policies was only 7%.

A frequent scenario is that a cancer patient relocates, necessitating re-employment. The new employer finds that the patient is not eligible for the existing standard group coverage because of his pre-existing condition and often decides not to hire the individual at all, citing the policy that every employee must be covered by the group insurance plan.

If the employee stays at his former job, a variation of this scenario occurs. His insurer typically raises the group's premium because of the worsened experience rating of the group. If the employer retains the old coverage, this employee group (often very small) must bear the burden of the group's "experience." If he opts to switch insurers, the cancer patient will not be covered under the new policy, necessitating the retention of his/her old policy converted to individual rather than group status at a higher premium rate (and reduced coverage).

Thus the financial loss of cancer treatment remains a significant threat, in spite of the widespread coverage of private health insurance. The uncoordinated, fragmented nature of the insurance industry does little to assuage the fears of financial ruin that are all too often felt by cancer patients, even in the earliest phases of the disease.

PREVENTION AND ACCESS

Access to primary medical care has two dimensions: the physical availability of practitioners in numbers adequate to meet demand, and financial accessibility. The inadequacies of the distribution of primary care physicians in the United States is well documented (14). A shortage in personnel creates an undue length of time for scheduled appointments, and either directly precludes prompt medical attention to health problems or does so indirectly by discouraging use of primary care. It is easier to justify a drop-in visit to a crowded physician's office or clinic with an acute episode of illness than it is with only a vague impression of abnormality.

Many economic factors have either created or exacerbated the primary practitioner shortage, especially in inner-city and rural areas. The reimbursement system, for example, has never made medical practice in low-income areas as lucrative as it is in wealthier areas. Low Medicaid reimbursement rates combined with bureaucratic problems of collection have created a virtual absence of primary care in the style that it exists in other urban or suburban areas, and have fostered instead a style of practice that reflects the lower reimbursement levels—one that raises the "productivity" of the practice to the maximum attainable consistent with legally defensible standards of care. "High productivity" means, in this context, maximum dollar revenue per hour. This is hardly the setting that is conducive to eliciting personal information from the patient that might indicate the early stage of a major illness. The lack of coordinated care associated with the lack of a single practitioner willing to assume responsibility for the total health of a patient (or his family) similarly favors acute crisis-oriented care rather than prevention.

A RESEARCH AGENDA

In this chapter we have explored numerous economic facets of the prevention and detection phases of cancer and have noted ways in which patterns of prevention and detection, judged optimal from a medical standpoint, are often discouraged or, at best, not stimulated by the workings of the medical system, including our system of financing medical services. If ways can be found to make economic incentives more supportive of cancer prevention—primary, secondary, and tertiary—there is little doubt that our success in dealing with the disease would be greatly improved.

Our analysis of the role of economic incentives in the utilization of preventive health services has suggested areas where our ignorance of behavioral relationships precludes prompt policy-oriented intervention.

We have seen that the incentives that have stimulated our health care system to provide advanced crisis-oriented care are correspondingly absent with respect to such care for prevention or early detection. Patients and practitioners alike respond to the need for acute care more readily than the need to prevent illness. A change in these priorities necessitates a better understanding of a number of relationships that span all three stages of prevention. We shall enumerate these below, together with specific examples of research questions with significant potential impact:

1. Identification of (a) realistic objectives in terms of altered health status and (b) the requisite levels of exposure to carcinogens to accomplish these goals.

In some cases, the exposure goal should be near zero, such as for industrial exposure to carcinogens, whereas for other agents a realistic goal might be a substantial reduction—a decrease of perhaps 50% in teen-age cigarette consumption or a reduction of a similar percentage in exposure to microwave of X-ray radiation. What is the dose-response relationship in each case? Should we attempt to reduce the incidence of smoking, or alternatively, to reduce the daily cigarette consumption of smokers?

2. Identification of the role of incentives in the production or consumption process.

How responsive are consumers to altered prices of cigarettes? In the industrial setting, how do economic factors enter into the choice of production methods in various chemical processes? In the case of shipyard workers, for instance, what are the actual costs associated with providing ventilation in work spaces sufficient to reduce exposure to asbestos dust?

3. What is the demand elasticity for preventive medical services as opposed to acute services? What will be the long-run consequences of providing such insurance coverage? Are the economic and health consequences of improved patient education positive? What do such programs cost, and what are the most effective means for organizing these services? Are prepaid systems more successful in intervening earlier in cancers that are known to be responsive to early treatment, such as cancer of the breast or cervix?

4. What is the best way to stimulate preventive care in any National Health Insurance (NHI) initiative? What forecasts can we make of the impacts of NHI on access to care for population groups, and what will this altered access picture mean for the use of preventive services? If difficulties are predicted, can New Health Practitioners be instrumental in alleviating the shortage?

5. What policy initiatives can remedy the insurance and employment conse-

quences of cancer? What changes in the structure of the insurance industry will be necessary to solve these problems? What is the proper role of government in this area?

It is ironic that the American health care system is thought by many to offer the finest that medical science has created for the treatment of disease, including cancer. Although our biomedical technology is among the most advanced in the world, our ability to care for patients in a psychosocial, supportive sense is woefully lacking. For no disease is this dichotomy more apparent than for cancer, for this disease requires inordinate inputs of both dimensions of service—cure and care. Unfortunately, we are now beginning to discover that our ability to cure is seriously impaired by our reduced capacity to care.

This linkage between the psychosocial and the medical aspects of cancer has been insufficiently appreciated until recently. With the realization that the health care system itself determines to a large extent the medical course of disease comes a new mandate to create a structure that will foster prevention as well as treatment, and care along with cure.

REFERENCES

1. Belloc, N. B., and Breslow, L. (1972): Relationship of physical health status and health practices. *Prev. Med.,* 1:409–421.
2. Benham, L., Maurizi, A., and Reder, M. W. (1968): Migration, location and remuneration of medical personnel: Physicians and dentists. *Rev. Econ. Statistics,* 50:332–347.
3. Clean Air Act (1970): PL 91-604.
4. Clean Air Ammendments (1977): PL 95-95.
5. Clean Water Act (1977): PL 95-217.
6. Harris, J. E. (1980): Taxing tar and nicotine. *Am. Econ. Rev.,* 70:300–311.
7. Holtman, A. G., and Olsen, E., Jr. (1978): *The Economics of the Private Demand for Outpatient Health Care,* John E. Fogarty International Center for Advanced Study in the Health Sciences, U.S. DHEW Publication No. (NIH) 78–1262, Washington, D.C.
8. Knowles, J. H. (1977): The responsibility of the individual. In: *Doing Better and Feeling Worse—Health in the United States,* edited by J. H. Knowles, pp. 57–80. W. W. Norton, New York.
9. Luft, H. A. (1978): How do health-maintenance organizations achieve their savings? *N. Engl. J. Med.,* 298:1336–1343.
10. *New York Times* (1978): Reserve Mining is ordered to heed pollution agency, p. 10. April 15.
11. Rahe, R. H. (1972): Subjects' recent life changes and their near-future illness susceptibility. *Adv. Psychosom. Med.,* 8:2–19.
12. Schweitzer, S. O. (1974): Incentives and the consumption of preventive health care services. In: *Consumer Incentives for Health Care,* edited by S. J. Mushkin, pp. 34–60. Prodist, New York.
13. *Source Book of Health Insurance Data, 1978–1979* (1979): Health Insurance Institute, Washington, D.C.
14. Stevens, R. (1973): *American Medicine and the Public Interest.* Yale University Press, New Haven, Ct.
15. Warner, K. E. (1977): The effects of the anti-smoking campaign on cigarette consumption. *Am. J. Public Health,* 67:645–650.

Psychosocial Aspects of Cancer,
edited by Jerome Cohen et al.
Raven Press, New York © 1982.

Chapter 9

Financing and Delivery System Research Issues

Nelda McCall

Stanford Research Institute, Menlo Park, California 94025

Any discussion of the health delivery and financing system with respect to the cancer client points out the present problems in the general health delivery system. A rationalization of our present delivery system will benefit all clients, including those who have cancer. Unfortunately, expansion in federal government health programs has historically been accomplished by including successive categories of beneficiaries—merchant seamen, veterans, the aged, the poor, the disabled, those with end-stage renal disease—rather than providing coordinated health services to everyone. Thus emphasis has been placed on curing through high-technology services that are easily reimbursed by federal health programs. This orientation is not desirable. The problems in the health delivery system for the cancer client may be more acute because of the nature of their illness, but they mirror the underlying problems faced by all participants in the system.

This chapter will first comment on the current financing and delivery system; this will serve as a background for the discussion of financing and delivery system research issues for clients with cancer.

CURRENT DELIVERY AND FINANCING SYSTEM

The health care system in the United States is unique. In the medical care market, traditional demand relationships—those in which demand is a function of price of the commodity, price of alternative goods and income, tastes and preferences of the consumer—are complicated by insurance coverage and by the special role of the provider.

The price of importance in specifying the consumer demand relationship in the medical care market is the price the consumer must pay out of pocket for the additional service net of insurance, that is, the marginal user price. By establishing this net price, health insurance actuaries are defining the type of care provided. Thus they may make a useless operation "free" to a client but exclude outpatient services from coverage. The insurance companies' main interest is in the solvency of the plan, and only indirectly in the benefit to the client (27).

In addition, the role of the physician is unique among suppliers of services. The physician is the central decision maker in the health care sector. Although expenditures on physician services account for only 19% of health spending, physicians are primarily responsible for decisions concerning the use of services representing over 70% of all health care spending (8). They order all lab tests, X-rays, and drugs and are responsible for all decisions to hospitalize. Once the consumer makes an initial decision to seek the services of a physician, almost all subsequent medical care consumption decisions rest primarily with that physician.

Historically in the United States, physicians have had the luxury of expecting to use virtually whatever resources they wanted without regard to effective or efficient use. They have not been asked—either by the client or by the financing system or by their peers—to evaluate if an expenditure of resources results in long-term improvements in society's health status, or even if it promotes the individual client's survival in a life of sufficient quality.

The mix of physician decision making and third-party payment has contributed substantially to the rapidly rising cost of medical care. In fiscal 1977 the nation spent $163 billion for health care, $737 per person, an increase of 12% over the previous 12 months. This represented an 8.8% share of the GNP. Third-party payments financed 70% of personal health expenditures, with government paying 40% (20).

The government's concern with this problem of increasing cost is complicated by their parallel concern with lack of access by the near poor who are not currently eligible for government programs. These concerns will, of necessity, lead to efforts to foster increased efficiency. The creation of the Health Care Financing Administration in 1977, integrating Medicare and Medicaid responsibilities, is clearly an effort in that direction.

The government in the past has taken a relatively passive role in using its substantial economic power to promote changes in the way medical care services are delivered. However, it is clear that efforts will be made in the future in several areas to promote specific reforms in the delivery system. Some of the areas are premature implementation of technology, planning failures, unrealistic consumer expectations, defensive medicine, physician maldistribution, and physician reimbursement. In the physician reimbursement area the government has been particularly remiss. Reimbursement systems—over which the government has control—have financially rewarded surgical procedures as compared with medical visits, paid more to those in urban areas than to those in rural areas, and paid more to specialists compared to GPs for providing the same service (6,18,29,31,35).

A good example of problems inherent in government financing and what can result if systems are not developed thoughtfully is Medicare coverage of end-stage renal disease. In 1972 Medicare coverage was given to those with chronic renal failure. No hearings were held and less than half an hour of floor time was allotted to consideration. In 1977 the program cost $901 million for 37,100 beneficiaries or over $24,300 per client (13). Data available for the Colorado Medicare program for end-stage renal beneficiaries for part of 1976 and 1977 suggest that Medicare reimbursed costs of approximately $23,400 per beneficiary person year—over 400% higher reimbursement for physician services and for inpatient hospital services than for other Medicare beneficiaries (24). With the passage of the legislation the numbers receiving dialysis have grown as the increased coverage has removed the necessity for discrimination by physicians in selecting candidates for dialysis. Our dialysis rates per million population are 143% higher than those in the United Kingdom (39).

In addition, in the 5 years since the program began, there has been movement toward dialysis in centers and away from home dialysis. In 1977 only 13% were on home care compared with 40% in 1972 (15). This compares to a home dialysis rate of 66% in the United Kingdom (5). This shift has occurred even though home patients do as well as those who have facility dialysis (80% 2-year survival) and cost 40% less (19).

Why has this shift occurred? Because insurance and provider incentives are in the wrong direction. Medicare has provided less coverage for home treatment, and physicians favor center-care treatment over home care. The program, while well intentioned, was initiated with not nearly enough thought to possible consequences. There is a lesson in this for all of us who are anxious to see special disease-specific treatments covered under public programs.

Turning to a discussion of the three kinds of prevention, this chapter will change the customary order of discussion and consider secondary prevention or diagnosis first, primary prevention second, and tertiary care third.

SECONDARY PREVENTION OR DIAGNOSIS

Traditionally, health insurance plans have provided less coverage for preventive services—both clinical and ancillary—than they have for illness-related services. Medicare does not cover annual physical exams although it covers X-ray services, such as a mammogram, if these are ordered by a physician. Only Health Maintenance Organizations (HMOs) have traditionally offered coverage for nonsymptomatic visits and tests at the same level as for illness-related care.

In a study undertaken several years ago with Anne Scitovsky on the effect of the introduction of a coinsurance provision on physician utilization in a prepaid plan, we found the impact on the use of annual physical exams after the introduction of 25% coinsurance was less for the annual physical exams than for other physician visits. However, this finding did not hold true by income group. Our data showed that adult males in the lowest socioeconomic group reduced their utilization of annual physical exams quite substantially (over 50%) (34).

In a more recent study conducted with Anne Scitovsky and Lee Benham

(33), we examined annual physical examination use in two prepaid plans. We had data on family income, major medical coverage, other insurance coverage, attitude toward seeking care, satisfaction with the plan, health status, and regular source of care. We found having a regular in-plan physician was the most important determinant of use. Those who identified the plan as a regular source of care but did not identify a specific physician had a 6% lower probability of having an annual physical examination, and those with no regular source of care or those who identified a place or provider outside of the plan were 18% less likely to have had an in-plan annual physical examination. These are relatively large differences because the typical plan member had only a 31% probability of having obtained an annual physical examination.

Those with incomes less than $20,000 were less likely—but not significantly less likely—to have had an annual physical examination. However, when the data were examined by plan, the pattern was inconsistent in the case of the prepaid plan with more extensive financial coverage; in the other plan there was some evidence—again it was not significant—of a positive relationship between income and the use of annual physical examinations. Interestingly, some of those who were heavy users of all physician visits—female spouses and those who perceived their health as less than excellent—did not have a higher rate of annual physical examinations. This may have been because they were receiving preventive services as part of their illness-connected visits. Other groups with statistically significant lower use of annual physical examinations were those who were not satisfied with the plan and those who were widowed, separated, or divorced. By age, those under 5 were most likely to have had an annual physical examination, followed by those 5 to 14 and those over 55 (33).

Screening became popular in the late 1950s based on the assumption that discovering a disease in a presymptomatic stage permits favorable intervention. It is, however, not altogether clear that screening asymptomatic people results in appreciable benefit. The only randomized clinical trial of the effect of a screening program on measurable health status of a population found multiphasic screening led to no statistically significant difference in health status, bed days, disability days, times hospitalized, or physician visits (28).

The question of a screening program's effectiveness involves a number of separate issues. First, can the program diagnose a disease in a presymptomatic stage? Second, does early diagnosis result in treatments better able to alter long-term survival in a life of sufficient quality? And third, is the cost of the program—in terms of both expenditures and the risk of loss of client control—justified by the benefit? All three of these questions must be answered positively before the usefulness of a screening program can be established.

Breast cancer screening has in recent years become controversial, and there is some evidence that these screening programs have not been demonstrated to be beneficial (1,2,7,11,14,23,37,38). Especially with respect to asymptomatic women under 50 not known to be at elevated risk, the radiation hazards of mammography may be the same order of magnitude as are the benefits (3).

One may wonder what the psychosocial impact of this promotion of increased concern has on the client.

Even with respect to screening for cervical disease with the Pap smear—a procedure whose diagnostic value was considered to be proven—recent data imply that although early detection can be effective, the timing of the need for the test may be much longer than the 1 year which has become common medical practice in the United States. A Canadian task force, the Walton Report, recommends after two consecutive yearly smears, a screening interval of 3 years for asymptomatic women between the ages of 18 and 35 and then smears at 5-year intervals until age 60 (9,10).

One of the ironies of modern medicine is the existence of iatrogenic cancers caused by well-intentioned but not sufficiently researched medical interventions. These include thyroid cancer induced by head and neck radiation popular in the 1930s and 1940s for thymic and tonsillar enlargements and acne, and vaginal cancer in the offspring of women pregnant in the 1940s who were given estrogens to prevent miscarriages (17,22).

With the limited resources which will be devoted to health care in the future, we may find that primary preventive and tertiary services provide a more cost-effective means for promoting health status.

PRIMARY PREVENTION

Primary prevention refers to minimizing hazards in the environment, improving nutrition, and promoting beneficial personal habits.

The first preventive policy—minimizing hazards in the environment—is generally an area which involves enforcement by the government. The decisions as to what should be provided and how it should be provided are based on collective choice; that is, they are group decisions made in the political arena. Because they are political decisions, they are sensitive to powerful, well-financed interest groups who are always more vocal and more well organized than individual consumers. These sensitivities have often resulted in inconsistent treatment of an issue by the legislature. A good example is the tobacco industry. At the same time that HEW is funding an anti-smoking campaign, the Department of Agriculture is promoting the growth of the tobacco industry by supporting prices, developing export programs, and providing systems for grading tobacco.

The case was demonstrated by the fight in California against Proposition 5, the Clean Indoor Air Act, which was defeated in 1978. The tobacco industry in official statements committed $5 million to fight the proposition. (The then current record for spending on a California ballot initiative was $2.6 million.) As of the end of June 1978, 99% of the money raised by the No on 5 campaign had been contributed by the tobacco industry. It is easy to see why they were willing to make this kind of commitment. Tobacco sales in California had amounted to $1 to 2 billion in the preceding year. If the passage of Proposition 5 had resulted in a reduction in cigarette consumption of 10%—an estimate that seems reasonable and even conservative (26,36,40)—the industry would have lost $100 to 200 million in revenues. Parenthetically, the California chapter of the American Cancer Society was supportive of and actively involved in the Committee to Support Proposition 5.

The tobacco industry example is instructive in attempts to understand other areas of environmental pollution control. Primary prevention often costs a powerful interest group something. Individual consumers are unaware or unwilling to become actively involved. With a strong and growing evidence that environmental pollution is a cause of cancer, groups like the American Cancer Society can be important in helping to educate consumers and in joining with environmental groups like the Sierra Club to work for strict enforcement of the Toxic Substance Act.

The other preventive policies—promoting beneficial personal habits and improving nutrition—require individual commitments to modify habits. Educational efforts to convince people of the need for change and to aid them in accomplishing the change are required. Although many have been skeptical of the likelihood of success in changing people's habits, the Stanford Heart Disease Prevention Program concluded that people can be persuaded to alter their life style at reasonable cost (16).

TERTIARY CARE

Once a disease is diagnosed, the current financing and delivery system reacts with treatment. However, with a few notable exceptions, treatment interventions for cancer have been largely ineffective in reducing mortality. Therefore, psychosocial interventions for those diagnosed, to help them to face the realities of their condition and to maintain personal control, may be the major function that the medical system can perform. These caring services have not traditionally been part of a physician's role nor have they had more than minimal coverage by insurance to increase the availability of these types of services. Those professionals specializing in the caring aspects of treatment must be integrated into the delivery model, both professionally and financially. One of the first steps is to find ways to pay those who provide these services.

For the last year we have been involved in an evaluation of an experiment in the Medicare program in Colorado which seems to test, among other things, the impact of clinical psychologists' being directly reimbursed by the program. Our experience with this project has pointed out the rather large political and practical problems involved in providing for nonphysician integration into the current delivery system. It has also pointed up the importance of examining the potential for cost-escalation and designing effective controls. Areas where controls are required are credentialing, reimbursement, defining services to be covered, and peer review.

These areas of interest for defining effective controls may sound familiar because they are the ones which are currently receiving much attention by those designing National Health Insurance. What is important is that these caring services are not added on top of the current system as additional services and additional providers with separate mechanisms, standards, and controls, but that their integration into the delivery system results in a new and different health system which permits joint and equal participation by both those who provide curative services and those who provide caring services.

The resulting health delivery system integration requires the creation of new institutions. Hospice is one possibility currently under discussion. The Hospice concept finds its roots in England, and many are currently under development in the United States. There is a Hospice in the Kaiser Permanente Medical Center in Hayward, California. The first annual meeting of the National Hospice Organization took place in Washington, D.C., in 1978.

Hospice has taken a variety of forms—some are associated with a hospital and some are completely free-standing. The underlying concept is that symptoms are to be managed in a palliative rather than a curative mode in a home-like or home environment by people concerned with the psychological, social, and financial needs as well as the client's physical needs. Clearly the concept has merit.

It is assumed, though no studies have been done, that Hospice costs must of necessity be lower than hospital costs. However, one problem in analyzing these data, even if they were available, is finding comparable hospitalization data on terminal patients.

A small percentage of the population consumes a large percentage of the health expenditures. APT Associates estimates that 1.2% of the United States population consumes 20% of the total national health expenditures (4). Recent work by several authors suggests that a surprisingly large percentage of these high-cost consumers are terminal cases receiving extensive hospital care (12,32). There exist few data on expenditures in the last year of life, but those that do exist suggest that such costs may be staggering. Marian Gornick, examining Medicare data for those persons who died in 1967 and 1969, found—even though the decedent's coverage was not for a full year because they may have died at any time during the year—that reimbursements made in their behalf were much greater than for persons alive at the end of the year. The number who received inpatient hospital benefits in both 1967 and 1969 was about four times as high for decedents as for survivors, and for physicians' services it was nearly twice as high for decedents (21).

Much more work needs to be done in this area. How much are we spending on death rites in American hospitals? How much would we spend with Hospice available? What forms should Hospice take? What should be the proper balance between inpatient Hospice and home care? And how do we insure against the Hospice movement creating but another costly alternative to be developed, along the lines of the end-stage renal disease model?

Hospitals and nursing homes may not be appropriate places to die, but societal changes in the last few decades have made the availability of a family member willing to care for the dying more unlikely. Thus Hospice may provide the answer. Careful evaluation, however, is required.

NATIONAL HEALTH INSURANCE

Private insurance companies insure a client for a specified period of time against an expected risk. They have little or no societal commitment, yet they form the basis of our current health delivery system and to a large extent dictate access to particular kinds of services. Because of this, those diagnosed with cancer find their health and disability insurance policies in jeopardy.

These reasons, along with many others, point to the need for some kind of national health insurance plan. Until we have a national health insurance plan there can really be no comprehensive emphasis on primary prevention. Until we begin to include nonphysician health professionals directly in the delivery system, we will not have tertiary and educational services covered effectively.

Important in the design of National Health Insurance are mechanisms to promote cost control. One proposed mechanism is the HMO or IPA model, and here one can be somewhat optimistic about its potential for promoting prevention. It has incentives to implement cost-effective primary prevention education programs, a tradition of providing secondary preventive care at the same cost as other services, and a history of use of ancillary professionals.

AGENDA FOR RESEARCH

The solutions to many of the problems in the health financing system are political: reforms of the medical care delivery system to make it a health delivery system, support for environmental programs, extension of the role of nonphysician professionals in the delivery of caring services. These all require sound, relevant research data to support policy. We can talk easily about the problems, we can perhaps discuss some tentative solutions, but data are not available to definitively address these issues. What we need is more research to help formulate the answers to these significant policy questions.

Specifically, we need to do studies to identify carcinogens, define their effects, calculate the real costs to eliminate them, the marginal costs to control them, and the benefits ensuing to society from their elimination or control. We need to look realistically at programs to modify environmental and self-imposed risk and evaluate carefully their costs and benefits.

We need to identify effective secondary preventive measures and the most efficient ways of conducting them—by diagnosis, age, and sex class. They need to be measures which provide more benefit than risk, have low rates of false negatives and false positives, lead to appropriate and beneficial treatments that cause improvements in the quality of life, and have savings which exceed the cost. We need to study the kind of client who seeks preventive care and examine the relationship between the use of screening services and other variables including insurance coverage, demographic characteristics, attitudes, and social structure variables.

We need to take a hard look at the integration of tertiary care programs which seem to be beneficial and cost-effective and to investigate methods of integrating them into the financing system. We need more research in the area of estimating medical costs in the last year of life and a detailed analysis of the kinds of expenditures, the kinds of clients, and the benefits of these last-year-of-life expenditures to society.

But most of all we need to think in terms of the allocation of limited resources and using these limited resources in a realistic manner. Promoting the existence of life for its own sake without taking account of its quality is an idea whose time has passed.

One important question for research and discussion on which it is imperative that a dialogue begin is the definition of the societal view of the value of a human life. With hard choices to make, with limited resources to allocate, our society must come to grips in practical terms with just how much we are willing to spend to save a life.

But in our evaluations we should keep in mind Schelling's words (30) from his classic paper:

> Death is indeed different from most consumer events and its avoidance different from most commodities. There is no sense in being insensitive about something that entails grief, anxiety, frustration and mystery as well as economic deprivation. But people have been dying for as long as they have been living; where life and death are concerned, we are all consumers. We nearly all want our lives extended and are probably willing to pay for it. It is worthwhile to remind ourselves that the people whose lives may be saved should have something to say about the value of the enterprise and that we analysts, however detached, are not immortal ourselves.

ACKNOWLEDGMENTS

The author would like to express her appreciation to Steven Snyder, Michelle Swenson, Stan Glantz, Kathy Robinson, and Howard Klechner for aid in securing reference materials, clerical support, and comments on the initial draft of this paper.

REFERENCES

1. Alsofrom, J. (1978): Mammography debate renewed. *Am. Med. News,* Mar. 20.
2. Atkins, Sir H., Hayward, J. L., Klugman, D. J., and Wayte, A. B. (1972): Treatment of early breast cancer: A report after ten years of a clinical trial. *Br. Med. J.,* 2:423–429.
3. Bailar, J. C. (1876): Mammography: A contrary view. *Ann. Intern. Med.,* 84:77–84.
4. Birnbaum, H. (1977): A national profile of catastrophic illness. *Executive Summary,* July. ABT Associates, Cambridge, Mass.
5. Blagg, C. R. (1977): Incidence and prevalence of home dialysis. *J. Dial.,* 1:475–493.
6. Blumberg, M. (1979): Rational provider pricing: An incentive for improved health delivery. In: *Health Handbook 1978,* edited by G. K. Chacko, pp. 1049–1101. North-Holland, Amsterdam.

7. Bunker, J. P., Barnes, B. A., and Mosteller, F., eds. (1977): *Costs, Risks, and Benefits of Surgery.* Oxford University Press, New York.
8. Burney, I., and Gabel, J. (1978): *Reimbursement Patterns Under Medicare and Medicaid.* Paper presented at Conference on Research Results from Physician Reimbursement Studies. Health Care Financing Administration, Washington, D.C. Feb. 21–22.
9. Walton, R. J. (1976): The Task Force on Cervical Cancer Screening Programs. *Can. Med. J.,* 114:981.
10. Walton, R. J., Blanchet, M., Boyes, D. A., et al. (1976): Cervical cancer screening programs. *Can. Med. J.,* 114:1003–1033.
11. Costanza, M. E. (1975): The problem of breast-cancer prophylaxis. *N. Engl. J. Med.,* 293:1095–1098.
12. Cullen, D. J., Ferrara, L. C., Briggs, B. A., et al. (1976): Survival, hospitalization charges, and follow up results in critically ill patients. *N. Engl. J. Med.,* 294:982–987.
13. Cummings, N. B. (1977): *Research in Kidney and Urinary Tract Diseases: Data Book for Fiscal Year 1976.* National Institutes of Health, Bethesda, Md.
14. Evans, K. T. (1969): Are physical methods of diagnosis of value? *Br. J. Surg.,* 56:784–786.
15. Facility Report No. 2 (1976): End-stage renal disease medical information system series 1— The nation reported by network. Medicare Approved ESRD Suppliers. Department of HEW, HFCA, Washington, D.C., Dec. 31.
16. Farquhar, J. W., Wood, P. D., Breitrose, H., et al. (1977): Community education for cardiovascular health. *Lancet,* 1:1192–1195.
17. Favus, M. J., Schneider, A. B., and Stachura, M. E. (1976): Thyroid cancer occurring as a late consequence of head and neck irradiation—Evaluation of 1056 patients. *N. Engl. J. Med.,* 294:1019–1025.
18. Felch, W. C. (1976/1977): Why improve payment for thinking versus doing? *Internist,* 17:16.
19. Freedman, E. A., Delano, B., and Butt, K. (1978): Pragmatic realities in uremia therapy. *N. Engl. J. Med.,* 298:368–371.
20. Gibbon, R. M., and Fisher, C. R. (1978): National health expenditures, fiscal year 1977. *Soc. Security Bull.,* 41:3–20.
21. Gornick M. (1976): Ten years of Medicare: Impact on the covered population. *Soc. Security Bull.,* 39:3–21.
22. Herbst, A. L., Ulfelder, H., and Poskanzer, D. C. (1971): Adenocarcinoma of the vagina. *N. Engl. J. Med.,* 284:878–881.
23. Lewison, E. F. (1963): An appraisal of long-term results in surgical treatment of breast cancer. *J.A.M.A.,* Vol. 186, No. 11, pp. 975–978.
24. McCall, N. (1978): Evaluation of the Colorado clinical psychology/expanded mental health benefits experiment. *First Year Assessment Report Draft,* July.
26. Mead, T. W., and Wald, N. J. (1977): Cigarette smoking patterns during the working day. *Br. J. Prev. Soc. Med.,* 31:25–29.
27. Neuhauser, D. (1977): Cost-effective clinical decision-making. In: *Cost, Risks and Benefits of Surgery,* edited by J. P. Bunker, B. A. Barnes, and F. Mosteller. Oxford University Press, New York.
28. Olsen, D. M., Kane, R., and Proctor, P. H. (1976): A controlled trial of multiphasic screening. *N. Engl. J. Med.,* 294:925–930.
29. Petersdorf, R. (1976): Physicians for our country: A letter to Congress. *Ann. Intern. Med.,* 85:117–119.
30. Schelling, T. C. (1968): The life you save may be your own. In: *Problems in Public Expenditure Analysis,* edited by S. Case. Brookings Institution, Washington, D.C.
31. Schroeder, S., and Showstack, J. (1978): Financial incentives to perform medical procedures and laboratory tests: Illustrative models of office practice. *Med. Care,* 16:289–298.
32. Schroeder, S., Showstack, J., and Roberts, H. E. (1978): *High Cost Hospitalization: A Descriptive Study.* Health Policy Program, San Francisco.
33. Scitovsky, A. A., Benham, L., and McCall, N. (1980): Use of physician services under two prepaid plans. *Med. Care,* 18:30–43.
34. Scitovsky, A. A., and Snyder, N. (1972): Effect of coinsurance on the use of physician services. *Soc. Security Bull.,* 35:3–19.
35. Seldin, D. (1976): Specialization as scientific advancement and over-specialization as social distortion. *Clin. Res.,* 24:245–248.

36. Social Security Administration (1978): SSS Smoking Survey. Baltimore, Md.
37. Their, S. O. (1977): Breast cancer screening: A view from outside the controversy. *N. Engl. J. Med.,* 297:1063–1065.
38. Treatment of early carcinoma of breast (1972): *Br. Med. J.,* 2:417–418.
39. United Kingdom Transplant (1977): *Lancet,* 2:1213–1214.
40. Warner, K. E. (1977): The effects of the anti-smoking campaign on cigarette consumption. *Am. J. Public Health,* 67:645–650.

Psychosocial Aspects of Cancer,
edited by Jerome Cohen et al.
Raven Press, New York © 1982.

Chapter 10

Sociocultural Dimensions Relevant to Preventing Cancer

Thomas A. MacCalla

International Institute for Urban and Human Development, San Diego, California 92110

The purpose of this chapter is to outline a consumer-focused approach to building a social support system for cancer prevention and control. Essential to the task, however, is (a) providing a means of profiling those social and demographic factors that relate to an effective prevention program for a culturally pluralistic society, and (b) identifying the relevant parameters of the consumer–provider–system interfaces. The net result of the undertaking should be a better understanding of some of the psychosocial issues and needs of special populations, especially racial and ethnic minorities who are summarily treated as consumers.

Although race and ethnicity are accidental qualities of human nature, they also tend to be significant determinants of human behavior. To a large extent, what and how people perceive and are perceived determine how they behave and are treated. Their perceptual images reflect the values of family background, subcultural reference group, and societal norms. Consequently, if we are to formulate a culturally sensitive cancer prevention program, we need to clarify some of the attitudes and values associated with special populations and to respond to the sociocultural dimensions of human interaction.

In short, we need to examine the fabric of culture and class and review the points of reference that account for the responses of patients, physicians, and health delivery systems. Since the concept of cultural behavior is relative, it is imperative that we place into perspective attitudes about health and dealing with illness, the importance of knowing, caring, and adapting. Knowing oneself and about others is a prerequisite to responsible action. Caring about others and adapting to new situations, however, complete the process. As Haynes and McGarvey (7) noted in their discussion of physicians, hospitals, and patients in the inner city:

> If people care, it will make no difference if the poor are black or white, Puerto Rican or Indian American, urban or rural. They will be seen as people who need our help and that help will be offered first where it is needed most.

Unfortunately, knowledge, caring, and adapting are not automatic human responses. What we perceive, feel, or act on is a product of our cultural grounding and personality. Our ability to anticipate behaviors and to facilitate desired responses is dependent on our understanding of culture and social behavior of the subcultural groups that make up our pluralistic society. Consequently, to formulate a cancer prevention program that effectively reaches the widest possible audience, we need to examine systematically consumer, provider, and population/social system transactions within the context of pervasive sociocultural influences.

This chapter offers for consideration an applied research tool to identify some of the significant socioeconomic and cultural factors that influence the attitudes and behaviors of special populations. It is a comprehensive, consumer-focused approach to determining the adequacy and appropriateness of the knowledge, skills, attitudes, and behaviors which impact on the planning and management of cancer prevention programs.

The central issues are who the consumers and providers are and what the environmental context is in which they must operate. Because psychosocial research implies dealing with a relatively few knowns and a host of unknown variables determined by culture, education, personality, economic status, and the like, it is important that we have knowledge of these factors and their function in cancer prevention and control. One of the major areas of concern is identifying who (consumer, provider, system) can do what to prevent cancer and to improve the treatment and rehabilitation of cancer patients.

The constant is cancer. The sociocultural variables of behavior become the focus of our research concerns. As such, it is important that we are fully conscious of the target before we attempt to manipulate it. The substantive issues, therefore, should include consumer and provider assumptions on the knowledge of each other's level of understanding, capabilities, and expectations. For example, little is known of race and ethnicity as significant variables, of coping mechanisms of special populations, or of cost and its relationship to cancer prevention compliance. Similarly, information on the relationship of one's social self to one's health status and actions is also lacking. In this regard, attention should be given to the role of sociocultural variance in response to cancer detection, treatment, and rehabilitation programs. We could begin with culture-specific studies on the following:

1. The knowledge base and attitudinal disposition towards health of blacks, Chicanos, and other special populations;

2. The significance, if any, of socioeconomic factors, cultural patterns, or personality traits on the receptivity of cancer prevention information and practices;

3. The levels of understanding health providers have of the psychosocial needs of consumers, especially racial and ethnic minorities; and

4. A profile of internal/external control behaviors related to consumer/pro-

vider value conflicts that impact on planning, communication, and management of effective prevention programs.

TOWARD SOCIOCULTURAL SENSITIVITY

The line between describing group characteristics and stereotyping can become thin; nevertheless, the distinction is real. We seek sociocultural data for proactive planning and prescription and not for programmatic ease and efficiency at the expense of appropriateness and a sensitivity to the realities of a subculture. Stack (11) has commented on the dangers of crossing the line to stereotyping when she discusses the general lack of understanding the reality of black culture:

> Many studies overlook the profound ways that economic and political pressures outside and within the ghetto—the profit motive, the welfare system, the employer, the landlord, the social agency, the school, the physician, the health clinic, the city services—affect cultural patterns, social identity, life chances, and interpersonal relations among the poor.

Billings (2) has also alluded to the pervasiveness of ignorance about black culture, especially the black family as a social system. Discussing the role of family networks and the requirements of survival in a white-oriented society, he cites four concepts as being essential to appreciate the reality of subsocietal life: (a) a social system defined in terms of mutual interaction and interdependence theory; (b) an *ethnic* subsociety as described by Milton Gordon's "shared feeling of peoplehood" and reflecting the many dimensions and variations within the ethnic group; (c) a family structure in which approximately two-thirds of the black families in the United States are nuclear, a quarter are extended families, and a tenth are augmented families; and (d) a family function in which the expectations of society to meet certain responsibilities of the wider society and to provide for the basic needs of family members is the measure of family functioning. Equally important, however, is the notion that the black community as an ethnic subsociety is located variously in the environments created by the intersection of social class and geography.

It should be noted that although blacks are the largest of the many ethnic subsocieties in the United States, they are not the only minority group. A cancer prevention program must consider the universe of special populations (blacks, Chicanos, native Americans, and other non-whites) who make up our culturally pluralistic society. For example, the characteristics of the Latinos in general and the Chicanos in particular need to be examined to determine the different levels of cultural synthesis which depicts the heterogeneity of La Raza. Gomez (6) observes in his treatment of Chicano culture and mental health the breadth of requirements for culturally relevant services to Chicanos.

> Mexican Americans are the well-to-do and the very poor, the well-educated and the illiterate, the migrants from Mexico and the American-born. Then there are the professionals and the agricultural laborers; the successful and those who struggle for survival. Also there are the sober, settled conservatives; the loud, vociferous

activists; and the liberals; the monolinguals in English; and the monolinguals in Spanish; and the bilinguals. There are even those who use strictly Spanish names (Juan, Jose, de la Garza y Menchaca), and those who prefer the American way (Joe William Gonzalez, or Mary Lou Jimenez). It has been pertinent and necessary to have mentioned these differences in order for the reader to understand these divergent characteristics of the Mexican American culture. . . . As we have already mentioned, there is a wide array of differences and contradictions, all of which combine to make the Chicano culture.

With reference to providers and systems in a consumer-focused intervention strategy, Murrell (8) emphasizes the person-environment *fit,* the fit between individual problem management preferences and resources, and the obstacles and opportunities open to the individual by the social system network, as coexisting determiners of an effective social system. We need to keep in mind that sociocultural systems involve people who interact with other people and are influenced by the environment in which they operate. Within this system they exhibit behaviors that are socially learned and socially shared but not always socially performed. As Gillin (5) points out in his discussion of sociocultural integration:

> The situation in which a sociocultural system operates is characterized by features that are given, among them the natural environment, human beings, learned behavior, and foreign influences and features that are produced by the operation of the system, among them social divisions of the population, sociocultural aspects of personality, material features and resultant states.

People also exhibit some behaviors which are inherited and some which are idiosyncratically learned and not shared with others. This phenomenon accounts for the sometimes indistinguishable influences that culture and personality have on human behavior.

In relation to health behavior, we know that there is a positive correlation between socioeconomic conditions, levels of education, and strong motivations toward good health habits. Studies have shown that those individuals who come from a higher socioeconomic bracket and who have a higher level of scholastic achievement are relatively self-motivated toward positive health action and responsive to new health information. Such people are preoccupied with the daily activities of a normal life and are influenced by whatever adds to or detracts from achieving personal goals. However, those individuals who find themselves in a lower socioeconomic level in the society spend more of each day trying to provide self and family with the basic life needs of food, clothing, and shelter. Consequently, there is a tendency on the part of those who feel victimized by the system to react to their plight with a sense of futility, passivism, and resignation to a perceived fate. These observations attest not only to the problem of sociocultural sensitivity, but also to the lack of health education among low income groups:

> Many patients are illiterate and superstitious. They prefer patent medicines, home remedies, or treatment by quacks. They loathe to go to white doctors for fear of

not being treated with dignity or courtesy. They cannot recognize early symptoms of disease because they have never been educated in the detection of illness (9).

The question before us, then, is how do we systematically define the parameters and the relevance of sociocultural dimensions for an effective cancer prevention program.

SOCIOCULTURAL ASSESSMENT

One technique suggested for the required data collection, validation, analysis, and synthesis is based on the functional prerequisites described by Bennett and Tumin (1) as a KEEPRAH system (Table 1). Donoghue's translation of these prerequisites (Kinship, Education, Economics, Politics, Religion, Recreation, and Health) includes two additional categories (Associations and Transportation) (3). The notion of "Associations" is a catchall category which includes peer groups, clubs, and other community organizations; "Transportation" focuses on linkages within and among populations. A third category which is allied to transportation as a prerequisite is Technology, which has become a pervasive force in society.

Taken as a whole, the system can be referred to as KEEPRRHATT (pronounced *kee-prat*), and it can be used as a tool for viewing human (structures, facilities, technology, population, institutions, etc.), natural, and man-made (air, water, life-space, tension, etc.) components of a community or of an individual as a community of one. The bits and sum of information gathered are then categorized and matrixed to determine interrelationships and the implications of these relationships to providers and consumers. It provides baseline information for the planning and management of cancer prevention programs. When the data are collected and analyzed, the prevailing attitudes and patterns of behaviors and environmental forces emerge and demand attention. Procedurally, the principal investigator would enlist and train data collectors as a team of

TABLE 1. *KEEPRAH system*

Functional prerequisites	System
1. Biological reproduction	Kinship
2. Socialization of new members	Education
3. Production and distribution of goods and services	Economics
4. Maintenance of internal and external social order	Politics
5. Maintenance of meaning and motivation	Religion and recreation
6. Maintenance of biological functioning	Health

Adapted from Bennett and Tumin (1).

ethnographers and community contacts. He would prepare them to become cognizant of their own ethnocentrism to ensure accuracy in acquiring data and objectivity in reporting. As indicated above, a tally of coded responses would be matrixed and the data clusters sorted to determine high-frequency patterns and interrelationships. These readings would be checked with reference information from key cultural informants for validation purposes.

The major focus of the KEEPRRHATT technique is profiling a total environment. The rationale for profiling the consumer–provider–system universe is based on a comprehensive approach to community identity. Just as a community can be thought of as a part of a larger system whose life and effectiveness are determined by the flow of goods and services, by linkages and constraints, so can health providers, consumers, and health delivery systems be considered as an interdependent part of a larger whole of human concern (Table 2).

Two other sources that complement the use of the KEEPRRHATT profiling technique are the *Manual of Social and Psychologic Assessment* by Francis and Munjas (4) and the self-instructional text *Psychological Aspects of Cancer Patient Care* by Elizabeth Smith (10). The former is a handbook outlining a five-step process for setting psychosocial norms, collecting data from individuals, making comparisons with the norms, analyzing the data, and validating the conclusions. The latter is a background reference to help the investigator understand the nature of cancer and some of its psychosocial aspects.

The key words associated with the KEEPRRHATT technique are *images, interrelatedness,* and *interdependence.* Images are the perceptions people have of the world in which they live and how they organize experiences. These self-impressions are conditioned by the unique psychological and emotional characteristics of the person and by the socialization process in which one learns to accept and reject certain behavioral qualities based on approval from family, friends, and the meaningful relationships one has with others within his environment. Once these values and habits have been reinforced, they become internalized and are difficult to change. Moreover, they serve as the basis for subsequent modes of behavior. Perceptual images also reflect the values of one's family background, subcultural reference groups, as well as the societal norms.

The interdependence of social status, cultural background, and individual personality sets the stage for realistic appraisals and responses to life situations. These factors also influence one's system of priorities which include attitudes toward health. People are a part of a larger system, a human settlement whose life and effectiveness as a community are determined by the flow of goods and services, the linkages and constraints which enhance or inhibit that flow, and the control points at which materials, energy, people, and information are obtained, prepared, and allocated for their eventual use. Recognizing these dynamics as they relate to the interrelatedness of knowledge and the interdependence of people will enable us to deal with the varying perceptions and points of reference competing for approval as the measure of truth. Understanding the

TABLE 2. *Interdependence of health providers, consumers, and health delivery systems*

	Kinship	Education	Employment	Economics	Politics	Religion	Recreation	Association	Health	Transportation	Technology
Kinship	●										
Education		●									
Employment			●								
Economics				●							
Politics					●						
Religion						●					
Recreation							●				
Associations								●			
Health									●		
Transportation										●	
Technology											●

nature of images and the role of interrelationships in human affairs underscores the meaning of cultural relativity and cultural sensitivity and enhances the usefulness of the technique for cancer prevention programs.

Finally, it should be emphasized that the examination of sociocultural variables associated with the consumer is not the only subject of our concern. We should be equally interested in the survey of the sociocultural dimensions of provider-focused and system-focused research activities that relate to the planning and management of cancer prevention programs. Only then will the summing of the data make for a more significant whole.

REFERENCES

1. Bennett, J. W., and Tumin, M. M. (1948): *Social Life: Structure and Function.* Alfred A. Knopf, New York.
2. Billingsley, A. (1968): *Black Families in White America,* pp. 4–33. Prentice-Hall, Englewood Cliffs, N.J.
3. Donoghue, J. (1972): *An Holistic Approach to Community Development.* International Institute for Urban and Human Development, San Diego.
4. Francis, G. M., and Munjas, B. A. (1976): *Manual of Social Psychologic Assessment,* p. 207. Appleton-Century-Crofts, New York.
5. Gillin, J. P. (1971): Some principles of social integration. *Curr. Anthropol.,* 12:23.
6. Gomez, E. (1978): *Chicano Culture and Mental Health.* Monograph No. 1, pp. 4–5. Centro del Barrio, Worden School of Social Service, OLLUSA, San Antonio, Tex.
7. Haynes, M. A., and McGarvey, M. R. (1969): Physicians, hospitals, and patients in the inner city. *Medicine in the Ghetto,* edited by J. C. Norman, pp. 122. Appleton-Century-Crofts, New York.

8. Murrell, S. (1973): *Community Psychology and Social Systems, A Conceptual Framework and Intervention Guide,* p. 89. Behavior Publications, New York.
9. Seham, M. (1973): *Blacks and American Medical Care,* p. 23. University of Minnesota Press, Minneapolis.
10. Smith, E. A. (1975): *Psychosocial Aspects of Cancer Patient Care: A Self-Instructional Text,* p. 182. McGraw-Hill, New York.
11. Stack, C. B. (1974): *All Our Kin: Strategies for Survival in a Black Community,* p. 25. Harper & Row, New York.

Psychosocial Aspects of Cancer,
edited by Jerome Cohen et al.
Raven Press, New York © 1982.

Chapter 11

Response of the Health Care System to the Psychosocial Aspects of Cancer

Jerome Cohen

*School of Social Welfare, University of California, Los Angeles,
Los Angeles, California 90024*

Efforts to separate mind, body, and the social situations that impinge on both continue to limit our understanding of the human condition in either illness or health. The understanding of human functioning has been divided into parts that suit the conception of scientific method and the interests of scientists in different aspects of a given structure, process, or action. Whereas this may promote accessibility to the study of these phenomena, it may also retard our understanding of the complex interrelationships affecting the human organism. Research as well as clinical experience has identified the multiple impact that cancer may have on the individual and the social environment in which that individual functions. It can disrupt personal functioning, ability to work, marital and family relationships, educational plans, financial stability, and the general life style one aspires to live. Stress reverberates throughout the emotional, physical, social, and economic spheres of life, and patient, family, and society share in the costs. Yet there has been a paucity of research dollars available for the investigation of these aspects of cancer. To what can we attribute this state of affairs? It is unlikely that those associated with the continuum of cancer care have not been aware of the tremendous psychosocial impact of the disease. Perhaps this research is associated with "palliative" rather than curative methods of intervention and seems less urgent to those directing research efforts. Such perspective suggests a conviction that cancer will be cured through interventions aimed at the biological basis of the disease without undue concern about the psychological and social elements that may be involved. At least two major flaws in this perspective stand out clearly. First, the social and physical environments in which humans exist contain a wide variety of potential carcinogenic substances which are not likely to be brought under control in the near future. The only protection against such environments resides in the discovery of a cancer vaccine. It is likely that approaches to early detection and treatment of a more certain nature to retard or stop the disease process as it is discovered will continue to be necessary. Second, the nature of human functioning in regard to health and disease is a holistic one and can be separated into biological, psychological, and social components only for heuristic purposes. In the real world, as opposed to the laboratory experiment, the human acts and is acted on as a single unit in which such elements are interconnecting parts of the whole.

The thrust of the conceptual and empirical work cited in the chapters that follow represents a concern not only for the human values which demand attention concerning the serious psychosocial consequences of cancer, but also to the conviction that we have a scientific responsibility to address these issues as fundamental to the study of cancer in all its forms. Given this perspective, our attention can now turn to the identification of some critical areas of research necessary to understand the psychosocial aspects of cancer through prevention, treatment, and rehabilitation. The chapters that follow are not intended to be exhaustive in respect to all of the psychological and social aspects of cancer. Rather, they represent a reasonable cross section of the efforts currently being addressed.

Chapters 12 through 20 attend to the psychosocial and behavioral issues in cancer treatment, rehabilitation, and continuing care. Marie Cohen examines the meaning of psychosocial morbidity. She views psychosocial morbidity as a changing process analogous to the richly colored, multipatterned and dimensional images within a kaleidoscope. As the handle is turned, all the pieces change their respective and collective positions, each movement bringing a new formation into focus. So it is, she suggests, in a family where someone has been diagnosed as having a malignancy. The habitual transactional patterns of the personal, marital, parental, sibling and social substructures begin to change. These changes do not stop with the catastrophic impact of the discovery of a lump or the confirming diagnosis of another of the warning signs, but continue during the course of the disease, waxing and waning depending on how the individual and available support systems react to the forces of the disease, treatment, and the emotional and physical dysfunction associated with it. She goes on to identify the manner in which the individual and the family's life style and values are disrupted and often irreversibly altered.

Social support systems and the social networks involved in such supports are increasingly being identified as a critical element in the maintenance of health as well as the adjustment to serious illnesses such as cancer. Bloom makes an important contribution to the organization and integration of the diverse and sometimes confusing literature of social support systems. Her attention is focused on the organizing themes in this literature which direct us toward the development of theory and causal explanation. She is concerned with hypotheses about the relationship of social support to decreased vulnerability to disease; the manner in which hazardous health behavior such as smoking can be mediated; and the power to buffer the effect a stresser such as cancer may have on the individual and family. Although there is empirical evidence to support all of these hypotheses to some extent, the process by which social support is translated into better health outcomes is not well understood. Bloom attends to the many forms of social support identified in the literature and the empirical evidence warranting further conceptual clarification and research. A clear and specific research program is suggested.

Joseph and Syme continue the examination of the relationship between social connections and cancer. They review the epidemiological evidence in terms of etiology and attend to the recurrent methodological problems identified in such research. Specifically they are concerned with examination of the rate of cancer among those with and without various forms of social connection to other individuals. Sufficient evidence of a relationship is uncovered so as to suggest the importance of future work. In the conclusion of this chapter they identify the specific reasearch design issues which must be incorporated in order to carry this promising area to a more conclusive set of formulations.

Lazarus' focus is on the manner in which coping styles relate to the course of illness, the individual's continuing morale, and the quality of life during and after the illness has been identified and treated. He identifies coping as any effort, mental or action-centered, designed to manage (master, tolerate, minimize, adapt, perceive) stressful events. Coping is comprised of how the person thinks, feels, and acts in the face of threat to important goals and values. Cancer imposes a particularly heavy threat because of the destructive way it is typically viewed by most people as a "death sentence" or as a harsh way to die. He addresses important questions related to the manner of coping used and the forms of coping that are positive and negative in their consequences. Differential perception of stressive events and the different coping mechanisms used to deal with that stress receive attention as well as the conditions under which a similar coping mechanism may produce a negative or positive outcome. A careful case is made for the relation between coping and health and is supported by systematic empirical research. However, great care is taken to avoid simplistic conclusions about that relationship. He points to the current revival of interest in the manner in which all disease, including cancer, is being considered as potentially psychosomatic although it is recognized that any disease will have multiple causes and the conditions under which psychological and social causation are involved must be carefully proven. Little research has been done on patterns of coping in cancer related to the quality of life experienced. What has been accomplished is provided. These results suggest that coping has much to do with outcome and quality of life but far more needs to be known about the details of this process. Toward this end he suggests the research efforts necessary to describe patterns of coping as employed by different persons in different circumstances of illness and different stages of cancer. The careful development of assessment tools for the measurement of this complex set of mechanisms is a necessary step in carrying out such research. Schmale, in discussing Lazarus' chapter, points to the need for long-term investment in prospective studies. Without such studies, admittedly expensive, we will only repeat the failures of the early interests in the psychosomatic components of disease. Schmale specifies the reasons why cancer is an excellent disease model for the study of stress, coping, and the psychosocial relationships influencing these phenomena. He then goes on to examine some of the elements identified by Lazarus as part of the coping process. Specifically he focuses on the individual components of coping with illness.

In the chapter on work and cancer health histories, Frances Feldman addresses the special and profound meaning that threat to the work role has for the cancer patient and his family. Her report is based on the observations made in a study she recently completed on work and cancer. This involved three studies focusing on (a) white collar workers and professionals, (b) blue collar workers, and (c) the particular work experience and expectations of young people with cancer histories. She discovered occurrences of discrimination as well as work-related psychological, social, and economic problems that have important implications for the prevention, treatment, and control of cancer. Patients, doctors, employers, and union representatives contributed to the study's comprehensive findings. The studies revealed the vulnerability of the cancer patient to the stress produced not only by the negative attitudes of significant people in his life space but also by his own negative attitudes about his ability to work. Fear, shame, and secrecy were characteristic of many of the patient respondents in both their work and personal life circumstances. The centrality of work in our society makes this psychosocial issue critical not only for the patient but for the well-being of the entire family as well.

Focusing specifically on psychological factors and cancer outcome, Panagis addresses the role of premorbid personality attributes as responsible agents in the pathogenesis of cancer as well as the manner in which current mood factors either depress or exacerbate the cancer condition. She examines the state–trait approach concerned with individual differences and the development of cancer. Such studies involve the identification of characteristics of an individual's emotional state related to the onset of the disease or its progression. Although there is a long history of interest in this area of research, poor methodologies deriving conflicting findings have been the rule. Simple relationships between psychological states or traits and cancer outcomes have not been identified. She calls for a conception of outcome research that involves continued interactions between the interplay of biological, social, and psychological forces. Research paradigms are suggested to more effectively attend to this significant issue.

David Kaplan identifies a clinical research issue regarding the timing of intervention strategies necessary to help families cope with the psychosocial consequences of cancer in a member of the family. His research involves families in which there is a leukemic child and those in which there is a woman with breast cancer. Kaplan developed the thesis that prevention of severe psychosocial negative consequences is contingent on having detailed knowledge of the process of adaptation specific to each type of cancer, including the relevant coping tasks and methods of task accomplishment. His concern is with effective intervention based on careful research concerning the psychosocial course of a particular type of cancer. A problem-solving model is developed from the detailed knowledge of the nature of successful coping behavior. Kaplan in his previous work has addressed the specific coping responses necessary to deal with several types of psychosocial crises.

Closing this section, Mantell addresses the issue of sexuality and cancer. This area of psychosocial functioning, although of great significance to cancer patients and their partners, has received little attention in the research literature. As technology allows for prolonged survival, the issue of the maintenance of or improvement in sexual functioning becomes critical to the normalization of daily living patterns. The author organizes what is known about both physiological and psychological factors operating to create sexual problems. Unfortunately, cancer patients must frequently come to grips with an attitude of, "you ought to be glad you're alive," which does not promote confidence in the right to desire a satisfying sexual life. Mantell addresses a wide range of phenomena in respect to issues of sexuality rather than the narrow concern with coitus alone. She examines a variety of cancer sites in terms of their specific consequences for sexual functioning. Implications arising out of the research data are addressed along with preventive educational program suggestions.

Chapters 21 through 23 consider the methodological issues associated with psychosocial research and its evaluation. Three seasoned cancer researchers attend to the issues of design, measurement, and rigorous evaluation of results. Spinetta addresses the importance of matching research design to the research problem. He stresses the necessity for research design to be geared to the specific problem under study rather than to a general notion of a research design most appropriate for all studies. This requires greater precision in the statement of the problem that will allow for empirical testing of the propositions involved. Spinetta is particularly concerned that we do not lose sight of the individual subject while trying to achieve normative conclusions. It is suggested that intraindividual longitudinal designs are as important as normative group research for the investigation of many psychosocial problems. The specific manners in which rigor related to reliability and validity can be addressed in both types of research designs are identified. Bloom and Ross also attend to research design, but focus on measurement issues specifically related to psychosocial aspects of cancer. They are particularly concerned with the biases found in many studies. Careful attention is paid to the underlying assumptions of measurement models with the view to evaluating whether they have been met in the particular model used. Issues of conceptualization and instrumentation are addressed in a similar manner. The special problems of cancer-related psychosocial research are identified. Fox ends this section with an overview and evaluation of psychosocial research in cancer. He identifies the major behavioral issues associated with such cancer research and directs our attention to future requirements.

In Chapter 24 Bloom moves from theory to action. Research utilization is recognized as an important and underdeveloped technology. Much of what we know in the scientific world goes unused even though answers to some critical problems have been identified. The complex problems of research design in the psychosocial research arena are further complicated by our lack of success in communicating our findings to the members of the society whose lives often depend on conviction about those data. Program planning for cancer control is the perfect case in point. The diffusion and adoption of life-saving information have not resulted in the kind of payoff envisioned. Bloom attends to the basis of these limited successes and offers a framework for knowledge utilization in cancer control that may offer a better chance for success.

Psychosocial Aspects of Cancer,
edited by Jerome Cohen et al.
Raven Press, New York © 1982.

Chapter 12

Psychosocial Morbidity in Cancer: A Clinical Perspective

Marie M. Cohen

Wright Institute, Los Angeles, California 90035

An individual diagnosed as having cancer experiences an enormous amount of stress—physical, psychological, and socioeconomic. The term psychosocial morbidity will be used to describe the nature and degree of distress produced by the response to this massive assault on physical and psychological integrity. Only when this kind of distress is understood in both its universal and unique dimensions can health care professionals effectively design and execute interventions to lessen the psychic and social costs of being a cancer patient or a member of such a patient's family.

Psychosocial morbidity is a complex phenomenon composed of societal, interpersonal, and intrapersonal elements. The observations reported are drawn from 5 years of direct service to cancer patients and the families of such patients, representing a variety of diagnoses and situated at different points on the disease trajectory.

The clinician intervenes with a patient and/or family on the basis of responses to the stress imposed by the diagnosis of "cancer." Such interventions are determined by the clinician's assessment of the responses as being "healthy" or "unhealthy." A "healthy" response to the disease can be defined as a response which permits the individual to cope with and master the stresses on him or her in such a way as to increase longevity and at least improve the quality of life (17). The response behaviors are those responses to environmental factors that help the individual master the situation as well as the intrapsychic processes which contribute to the successful adaptation to this stress. Optimally, then, a "healthy" response consists of behaviors which enable the patient to deal effectively with the reality situation and also serve the protective function of keeping anxiety and other emotional distress within tolerable limits (6,15). An "unhealthy" response consists of behaviors which shorten the person's chances for survival and result in their experience of self-defeat, isolation, and profound despair.

These definitions of "healthy" and "unhealthy" responses are influenced by value judgments of how one should confront the fact of one's imminent death. Who can really judge whether it is "healthy" to adopt an attitude based on the *carpe diem* philosophy or that of an ascetic, who renounces all worldly joys in order to search for the "true" meaning of life? In any event, cancer is an organic disease with psychosocial consequences constituting a unique stress to which the person must adapt. Interventions can be related to the nature of the response regardless of the professional's value judgments.

CANCER: ADAPTATION TO STRESS

From a social psychological point of view, it has increasingly become apparent to investigators of stress that adaptation must be considered in terms of the relationship between external physical and social demands on the person and his resources to deal with these demands (8). Successful personal adaptation has at least three components at the individual level. First, the person must have the capabilities and skills to deal with the social and environmental demands to which an individual is exposed, and these can be labeled "coping capabilities." Such capacities involve the ability not only to react to environmental demands, but also to influence and control the demands to which one will be exposed and at what pace. Second, individuals must be motivated to meet the demands that become evident in their environment. Third, individuals must have the capabilities to maintain a state of psychological equilibrium so that they can direct their energies and skills to meeting external as well as internal needs. These capabilities are the mechanisms which facilitate continuing performance and mastery (10). One's abilities to cope with the environment are dependent on the efficacy of solutions provided by culture, and the adequacy of personal preparation.

Cancer may usefully be viewed as an environmental and psychophysical stress. Furthermore, it is not a short-term single stimulus. Rather, it is a complex set of changing conditions—depending on histology of the tumor, clinical and anatomical stage at diagnosis, primary site of lesion, age and sex of patient, co-morbidity with other diseases, and the nature of treatment—that have a history and a future. The person must respond to these conditions through time and must adapt to the changing character of the stimuli. For example, consider the breast cancer patient at the time she first discovers a lump and later, after several months or years, when the doctor tells her that the routine check-up reveals a recurrence. Mastery of this stress is not a static repertoire of skills, but instead an active process over time in relationship to demands that are themselves changing (3,10).

To complicate matters further, many demands are ambiguous and intangible; they are created out of the social fabric and social climate that exist at any time. Challenges are therefore a product of the transactions between the individual and environment, and many of the demands of adaptation are those that involve both aspects. Each person requires other people to respond to his or her responses, resulting in a complex interplay between people. Oncologists have changing expectations of what is a "good" patient. At first it is someone who asks all the questions and takes time as needed, but later in the course of treatment a "good" patient is one who does not take up the physician's time with too many questions.

The final element in viewing adaptation to stress is the notion, popular among clinicians, that successful adaptation requires an accurate perception of reality. But whose perception of reality is the more "accurate": the patient's or the clinician's? We all maintain our sense of self-respect and energy for action through perceptions that enhance our self-importance and self-esteem, and we maintain our sanity by suppressing the tremendous vulnerability we all experience in relation to the risks of the real world (18). Oncologists have been observed "managing" their patients' reality by controlling their access to the "truth" about their medical condition. How then can the patient respond "realistically" in the absence of "reality"? Patients also structure their own reality by their fluctuating level of denial (16). Successful defenses are those which facilitate mastery of the situation at hand. And if those defenses contribute to misperceptions of reality which actually aid the coping and mastery, energize one's involvement and participation in life, and alleviate the pain and discomfort which otherwise would interfere with successful mastery, then they may be useful. Reality is a social construction, and to the extent that perspectives are shared and socially reinforced, they may facilitate adaptation irrespective of their objective truth. If people define situations as real, they are real in their consequences (10). This leads us to examine how cancer is perceived "in reality."

SOCIAL CONSTRUCTION OF CANCER

The "reality" of a cancer patient is quite different from the "reality" of a person with chronic emphysema or coronary disease. One can observe the difference at the moment the person is told the diagnosis. Despite the impressive medical and surgical advances in cancer treatment of recent years, the disease is widely considered a synonym for death. Cancer is often perceived as a mysterious invader, capable of abnormal, incoherent growth, and the person who gets cancer becomes a "cancer victim." Such a person is doomed to die a spectacularly wretched death, robbed of all capacities of self-transcendence, humiliated by fear and agony (14). The prognosis for some kinds of cancer such as prostate or esophageal is better than for some kinds of coronary problems, yet most people are oblivious to that fact. That fear alone can increase the amount of psychosocial morbidity experienced by the person.

Indeed, one can argue that the construction of cancer results in a kind of psychosocial morbidity which is unique to cancer. There are other slow, degenerative diseases such as muscular dystrophy or amyotrophic lateral sclerosis which can produce devastating results physically and psychosocially, but they do not carry the frightening and fatal aura which cancer does. It is not uncommon for a (psychiatrically) depressed patient to insist that she or he has some kind of malignancy (not tuberculosis or another serious kind of illness), or to see throwaway circulars on newstands describing either some new cure for cancer or a new "cause" for it. And it is all too common to learn that what prevented a newly diagnosed cancer patient from going for regular medical check-ups was the fear that the physician would "find something I don't want to know about."

The extent and nature of psychosocial morbidity which is associated with cancer are also influenced by the lack of scientific knowledge about the etiology and biology of cancer. In the absence of factual knowledge, people tend to project their own theories of causation which range from "it's God's will" to "they put something in the water." In this age of psychologizing illness, which is easier to do when the actual etiology is unknown, illness becomes interpreted as more of a psychological event than a physical one. It is something which people can will upon themselves and will themselves out of. In this light, cancer is construed by some as a pathology of energy, a disease of the will (alias "characterological disposition") which occurs because a person has repressed his or her feelings (the work of Simonton, LeShan, and Bahnson, among others, is instructive in this respect). Thus the cancer patient becomes culpable for his or her illness, and also assigned the major responsibility for curing him or herself. The hypothesis that distress can affect immunological responsiveness (by, for example, lowering immunity to disease in some instances) is very different from the view that emotions cause diseases, much less the belief that emotions can produce specific diseases.

Cancer patients are well socialized into this particular construction of reality. One individual said that she is certain that her lung cancer is related to her "cold" personality, which she was told she has had since infancy; another woman with melanoma believes that her use of the Simonton visualization technique was the sole curative agent in her recovery rather than acknowledging at least the partial assistance of the surgery and chemotherapy she received. Also impressive is the social response to (actually the reconstruction of) the cancer patient's identity. Once one has been diagnosed as having cancer, that fact is integrated into one's self-image permanently as with one's families and associates: "I'll never be the same again, I'll always have cancer even when I'm free of signs (symptoms)"; or as the recovered patient with breast cancer who never ceased to identify herself to me or other hospital personnel as being a "mastecto-mommy." Society demands that cancer patients fight "the good fight" against this disease, yet the stigma of being a cancer patient lasts beyond the time of remission. Society makes us culpable for our disease so that we cannot restore any sense of internal equilibrium and thus achieve a sense of mastery. The social environment thus becomes an oppressive entity rather than a supportive one, and pronounces the cancer patient mysteriously and permanently flawed.

CANCER—INTERPERSONAL STRESS

Societal attitudes toward cancer frame the interpersonal experience of the cancer patient and family. The family exercises ambiguous demands on its members, some of which can be met and some of which elude the best attempts. This dilemma is observed in the arena of spousal negotiations about whether and how to alter habitual patterns of nurturance, succor, dependency, initiative, and authority if one spouse is diagnosed with a malignancy. Role expectations and functions are also subject to change because of alterations in the individual's internal self-image and in the altered social context. Parental and spousal system marital goals are altered:

> The adults' life together has been predicated on physical and psychological continuity, with shared spousal, and then parental, tasks. Like the identified patient, the other spouse is also faced with an interruption in his or her expectation of continuity. The marital task divisions are changed, with the experience of weakness, fatigue, confusion, and bodily defect (5).

Cancer clearly challenges all the available coping skills of both members of the marital couple, and poses challenges to both people even after a remission has been achieved. Women who have just had a mastectomy frequently say "I feel mutilated and damaged . . . and my husband looks at me like I am some kind of freak." Of course, this kind of surgery is loaded with all kinds of "extraneous" factors, particularly sexual ones, so that it is difficult to attribute all the problems to the diagnosis of cancer, but women who have had pelvic exenterations for uterine cancer have also spoken about how they feel "contaminated" and are certain that the "invisible killer" is still inside them. People who have undergone amputation of a limb for some other reason do not describe themselves as being similarly contaminated.

The patient wonders about the possibility of recurrence ("having to hear the news all over again, having all this start over again"), and here too demonstrates that altered self-image which is different from that of someone who has a nonmalignant chronic disease. The spouse questions whether or not their mate can resume the customary marital-sexual familial role ("will she always be disabled like this, and will I lose her anyhow and end up alone?"). Again this phrase is usually absent in the conversations of spouses whose mates have been operated on for some other reason. These powerful feelings are often not discussed by the couple and tend to create problems which become exacerbated around the time of every physical re-examination. With ultimate outcome uncertain or ambiguous, one member of the dyad may experience increased dependency while the other strives to stand apart, with resultant marital rift. The following case illustrates such maladaptation and the concept of psychosocial morbidity:

The M. Family

Mrs. M. is a 50-year-old Caucasian mother of two children, ages 21 and 25, who is about to celebrate her 25th wedding anniversary. Sixteen months ago she was diagnosed with a squamous cell carcinoma of the right lung after having received treatment for "bronchitis" for the preceding 5 months. The diagnosis was an incredible shock to both her and her husband and "we cried together morning, noon, and night." Despite their upset, the couple was delighted to hear the surgeons' verdict "we got it all," after Mrs. M.'s lung had been resected. She plunged into a rehabilitation program and made plans to return to work as a bookkeeper. Life resumed its second honeymoon aspect for the couple, "we never had it so good." Mrs. M. even felt able to comfort her husband "although I was the patient."

Right after surgery and her return home, Mrs. M. let her husband assume most of the homemaking responsibilities and allowed him to treat her "like a real queen, which I loved." In 2 months she had returned to work and resumed her duties at home on a full-time basis. Three months later, her husband received an excellent job offer in Eugene, Oregon, and the two of them made plans to move there (the children were away at college) after Mrs. M.'s Los Angeles physician made arrangements for oncological follow-up in Oregon.

At first glance, the move seemed to be an excellent decision for both of them. But Mrs. M. began to experience new symptoms and was frequently ill. She first consulted her new physician in Oregon and then flew down to Los Angeles for confirmation of his findings: she had a recurrence. During this visit to the doctor, husband and wife decided to ask the heretofore unmentionable: how long did Mrs. M. have to live given this new finding? "Less than a year," was the terse reply. The environment had issued a challenge to which Mrs. M. felt unable to adapt. Although she had made some social inroads in Eugene and liked her new life there, she described herself as suddenly unable to further contend with that new life. She began to talk about returning home (to Los Angeles) "to die in my house, with my children and friends." She began to exert subtle and then more direct pressure on her husband to find a new job in Los Angeles. She became more dependent on him for company and sought to keep him home by making innumerable requests of him. At first he willingly compiled and again became the wage-earner and homemaker, but she was unsatisfied and increased her demands without acknowledging his previous efforts.

The symptoms did not abate, and Mrs. M. went to Los Angeles for a brain scan, which revealed cranial metastases. At that point she decided to return to Los Angeles permanently regardless of what her husband wanted. Upon her return she entered the hospital for several weeks in order to receive radiation therapy, and upon discharge she decided to ask her two children to move back home so that they could look after her. Her doctor concurred with the decision because he felt Mrs. M. should not be left alone. Initially the family reunion went swimmingly. Even Mr. M. consented to return home, albeit with great reluctance because his new job in Los Angeles was a step down from his previous position. And he said "I was lonely. It was the first time in 25 years that I had to be alone and I hated it."

Mrs. M. grew increasingly alarmed over her progressive, albeit slow, physical deterioration. She sensed that she could not reverse the disease this time; the intermittent cranial swelling resulted in periods of disorientation which made her feel "crazy." She could not return to her bookkeeper's position, and she was too weak to keep the house as she was accustomed to doing. Those two roles were the sum total of her self-definition and the pillars of her self-esteem. She perceived herself as a valueless burden to her family and began to say to each and all of them "you wish I was dead already, I know. I can't wait to die either!" Her increasing physical dependency alarmed her family as she had never been sick before and had resisted anybody's efforts to take over household tasks. "I took care of everybody always, and I loved it."

Mrs. M. began to increase her demands on family members, testing their willingness to care for her and their wish for her survival. She wanted a greater commitment from her husband who was beginning to back away from this "yawning maw of a woman" who would not leave him alone, and for whom he had no desire. He felt unwilling to recommit and reconnect because "she's going to die anyway; I want this all to be over before we have some ugly blow-up." He felt extremely guilty about feeling this and compensated by doing everything around the house without consulting his wife. She in turn experienced his super-helpfulness as another indictment of her failure as a woman and a wife. She began to wish herself dead as she experienced more and more rejection by her husband and children.

Mrs. M.'s predicament is not an unfamiliar one among cancer patients and their families. Her response to her disease is partly based on her previous style of coping with stress, is partly mediated by her husband's responses to her, and is also affected by the responses of her health care team. In effect, the physician's response to her question about life expectancy and his avoidance of further communication was perceived as a death sentence by Mrs. M., who then proceeded to wait for death to come. Upon reviewing her situation, it is evident that she does not experience her current life style as redeeming in any way. What she lacks is a capacity to see what Daniel Lerner calls "value alternatives" (1). She cannot adapt to her new "freedom" to be other than a superior housekeeper and excellent bookkeeper. She has become too socialized as a cancer patient, who can only sit and anticipate death while renouncing life. Mr. M. appears to cope positively with the tragic circumstances which have befallen him and his wife. Problems ensued when he had completed mourning for her prior to her death and thus had decathected from her. Her fears about abandonment were exacerbated by his withdrawal, which then elicited anger and guilt from him—he then became the overly caring and helpful mate while silently praying for the end to his "sentence" and hers.

Children and their parents also experience cancer as an interpersonal stress, which can produce psychosocial morbidity. Society decrees that parents shall protect their offspring from all conceivable harm, and furthermore, children represent one's future caretakers. When a child becomes ill with leukemia or one of the "solid" tumors, parents often interpret the illness as their failure to be good parents and assume that "God is punishing me for a reason." Overwhelmed with guilt and pity, parents may single out this child to receive Christmas (presents) in July; or they refuse to discipline this child as they would their other children.

Believing that children cannot understand the implications of the diagnosis, parents often seek to shield them from any awareness of the prognosis by tailoring conversations with them or trying to modify the environment so that they are "protected." Health care team members are often forbidden to discuss the illness with these children; the parents isolate them from others in the outpatient clinic waiting room. Some parents are so overwhelmed by the shameful associations they have with cancer that they keep their child home from school even when attendance is not a health hazard. Or a mother may insist that her 5-year-old son wear a wig all the time, when the boy appears perfectly content to go around bald (the hair loss being a consequence of chemotherapy and radiation).

The results of such drastic changes in the parent–child relationship are children who are extremely depressed and withdrawn and often say, "My parents don't like me anymore [and] they act funny," or "Mommy doesn't yell at me when I do things that are wrong." The children are all too aware of what is wrong with them and often have rather sophisticated ideas about the disease and what can and cannot be done for them. They quickly perceive that some people can listen to their concerns and some cannot, and they correspondingly edit their conversations with the latter group, which often includes their parents. "Mommy gets sad when we go to the clinic, so I don't ask her questions that make her more sad." That girl's mother was certain that her child had no idea about what was really wrong: "Oh, I just told her she had some weak blood cells and the doctors are giving her new blood and medicines to make her stronger." Another child was acutely aware of how much her parents had fought since her illness began, and so stopped taking her chemotherapy, reasoning that if she died quickly her parents would soon feel better.

INTRAPSYCHIC SPHERE

Having observed the interactions in the marital and parent–child dyads to identify types of adaptation to the stress of cancer, we focus now psychosocial morbidity as it is reflected within the intrapsychic sphere. This area has commanded the most attention from researchers and clinicians who have generated a wealth of literature—among others, Bahnson, LeShan, Shneidman, Ninton, Weisman, Eisler, and Pattison—about the intrapersonal reactions to cancer and the consequences in terms of psychosocial morbidity.

Hinton [7], Schmale [12], Schneidman [13], and Weisman [17] state, as do so many others, that the individual who receives a diagnosis of cancer hears it as a death sentence, which produces an "ego-chill." What could possibly produce any more disabling distress than the knowledge that one has a (potentially) fatal disease? One is forced to grapple with the "universal negative"— that event which repudiates the objectives so sought in life. What may ease the distress and permit positive adaptation is the realization that one cannot prevent death, but one can influence one's way of life until that time. Following the initial treatment, the anxiety and dread concerning dying disappear and are replaced by a strong sense of relief and the belief that everything is going to be all right [10a,16]. Such beliefs can persist even in the face of the most discouraging medical reports. The patient or the family has often been heard to comment to the effect that, "I feel so good now I know they were wrong,

I don't have cancer." Denial can function effectively until evidence appears of metastases, and even then one can continue although one denies the implications of such evidence. Finally, if the disease is terminal, the person will come to acknowledge that event, but still only intermittently (16). This kind of intermittent awareness is typical of both children and adults with cancer.

A "positive" response to having such a diagnosis appears to consist of alternating between the acceptance and denial of the disease and its implications, and being able to experience satisfaction in the area of marital/family relationships, in the area of relations with friends, and in the area of work or school. The definition of what is positive rests on what the patient perceives as a worthwhile quality of life and kind of life style. Again, the social and interpersonal context will influence the person's response and consequently affect the occurrence of psychosocial morbidity. Consider the woman with breast cancer. She is faced with the problems of re-establishing satisfying emotional and sexual connections with her partner, accepting the loss of her breast, and reintegrating her self-image as one who is worthy of love and the rewards of life. Our society tends to devalue women when they lose one or more physical tokens of sexuality and in this manner challenges a woman's self-worth and adaptation.

If she cannot redefine herself as a sexual person, if she continues to focus only on the loss of her breast, if the depression which accompanies the discovery of a lump and, later, the biopsy/surgery does not substantially lessen within 2 months of the procedure (2,8), then this woman is "at risk" for psychosocial morbidity.

The clinician's values can influence the diagnosis of psychosocial morbidity in a patient. If the patient adopts a self-percept which conflicts with the projected image of the clinician, she or he may label that self-percept as a morbid adjustment. For example, a woman who has made an excellent physical recovery from mastectomy 3 years previously has a new career as a public speaker to cancer support groups, women's groups, and the like. She has created a new self-definition of "actively dying" and she tells people that she is dying. She is happy in her new career and would contend that she has a good quality of life. As a clinician I feel uncomfortable with her new self-concept, because it conflicts with my value judgment about people who make a career out of being a "dying person."

My value system and clinical perspectives are more in synchrony with another woman who had a mastectomy almost 4 years ago. She wants her family to acknowledge that she has had cancer, but not to treat her as a "cancer victim." She has re-evaluated her life goals and values with a subliminal awareness that she has less time available than prior to her diagnosis. She views her coping with cancer as a modeling experience for her 19-year-old daughter and is determined to do it well, since her daughter comes from a family with cancer in all the females on both sides. Although this woman has become something of an existentialist, she is not insistent that her family adopt her stance—only that they acknowledge her need to do so.

Pediatric cancer patients must also cope with this immense disruption in their lives affecting school and play activities, as well as relationships with friends and family. In the section on interpersonal stress, the interpersonal precipitants of psychosocial morbidity in children were discussed. At this time it would be useful to focus on the intrapersonal precipitants in children.

The child's emotional and cognitive capacities are still plastic and immature; hence sickness, separation, and death mean different things to a child than they do to an adult. The child who manifests a positive response to having cancer is the child who can choose one or more persons to confide in and/or play out his fears, anger, and depression about being confined, separated from family and friends, and subjected to the numerous painful procedures and physical changes which accompany cancer. Children describe the (correct) rationale for bone marrow biopsy. They know the difference between "red death" (adriomycin) and "the stuff that makes you pee red" (cyclophosphamide), and they can tell just how sick they are and where they are on the stages-of-illness continuum.

The children to be concerned about are those who will not go back to school, refuse to see even their best friends, will not talk to anyone about what is happening to them, and/or totally withdraw. "I'm bad, so I got sick," is a statement often heard from pediatric patients. Children are "at risk" if they cannot relinquish such thoughts throughout the course of the illness.

CONCLUSIONS AND IMPLICATIONS FOR RESEARCH

Psychosocial morbidity in cancer patients results when the person cannot cope with and master the immense distress of being diagnosed with a malignancy. The individual's response is governed by a variety of factors including societal attitudes toward cancer (its etiology and so on), and the person's ability to master stress on the intrapersonal and interpersonal levels before and after diagnosis. The positive response to having cancer is that collection of attitudes and behaviors which appear to prolong the person's survival and improve the quality of life, while the negative response foreshortens one's life. Those individuals who had always experienced life as a series of alienating, depriving, depressing, and destructive episodes appear to fare worse than their peers who hold a different world view and self-concept.

It is my belief that the psychosocial morbidity associated with cancer patients is unique and is different from that found in other degenerative, chronic diseases. However, research efforts need to be directed toward understanding the unique nature of the psychosocial morbidity associated with cancer. In line with that is the need for meticulous, longitudinal work on the subtle and more evident changes in the cancer patient's self-image: the areas of doing, feeling, and becoming. Medical treatment has extended the potential life expectancy for cancer patients, but their personal response to the disease still appears to control actual longevity. Much of the past and current research stops at the 1- or 2-year mark. What are cancer patients doing later in life, and do they still consider themselves "patients" who engage in "illness behavior"?

Such research could promote a clearer understanding of the individual factors among cancer patients which promote positive or negative responses to the disease. It could also refine the psychotherapeutic interventions used with patients and their families because cancer does have unique meanings in our society and results in repercussions which are different from those found in other diseases.

The cancer patient's emotional state is not linear, as Kübler-Ross initially suggested; rather, it involves the constant interplay of disbelief and hope, and against these as background, a waxing and waning of anguish, terror, acquiescence and surrender, rage and envy, disinterest and ennui, pretense, daring and taunting and even yearning for death—all these in the context of bewilderment and pain. "Traditional" psychotherapy might label such affects as "negative" and seek to mollify or modify them. The clinical examples related in this chapter are intended to demonstrate that such emotions can be "positive" given their origin. The clinician working with cancer patients needs to develop an empathic frame of reference toward these individuals which validates their difficult predicament at each stage of the illness.

The need for such research and psychotherapeutic interventions is imperative and immediate as these concerns have direct bearing on the quality of life and prospects for survival for each of us.

REFERENCES

1. Antonovsky, A. (1972): Breakdown: A needed fourth step in the conceptual armamentarium of modern medicine. *Soc. Sci. Med.,* 6:537.
2. Asken, M. J. (1975): Psychoemotional aspects of mastectomy: A review of recent literature. *Am. J. Psychiatry,* 132:1.
3. Dubos, R. (1965): *Man Adapting.* Yale University Press, New Haven.
4. Friedman, S., Chodoff, P., Mason, J. W., and Hamburg, D. A. (1963): Behavioral observations on parents anticipating the death of a child. *Pediatrics,* 32:4.
5. Gottlieb, F. (1976): Family force fields in health care. In: *Family Health Care: Health Promotion and Illness Care,* edited by R. C. Jacobson and J. Morton. University of California Press, Berkeley.
6. Hamburg, D. A., Hamburg, B., and de Goza, S. (1953): Adaptive problems and mechanisms in severely burned patients. *Psychiatry,* 16:1.
7. Hinton, J. (1975): The influence of previous personality on reactions to having terminal cancer. *Omega,* 6:2.
8. Jamison, K. R., Wellisch, D. K., and Pasnau, R. O. (1978): Psychosocial aspects of mastectomy. I. The woman's perspective. *Am. J. Psychiatry,* 135:4.
9. McGrath, J. (ed.) (1970): *Social and Psychological Factors in Stress.* Holt, Rinehart & Winston, New York.
10. Mechanic, D. (1974): Social structure and personal adaptation: Some neglected dimensions. In: *Coping and Adaptation,* edited by G. Coelhoe, D. Hamburg, and J. Adams. Basic Books, New York.
10a. Pattison, E. M. (1974): Help in the dying process. In: *American Handbook of Psychiatry, Vol. 1, revised Ed.,* edited by S. Arieti. Basic Books, New York.
11. Schmale, A. H. (1972): Giving up as a final pathway to changes in health. *Adv. Psychosom. Med.,* 8:86.

12. Schmale, A. H. (1976): Psychological reactions to recurrances, metastases, or disseminated cancer. *Int. J. Radiat. Oncol. Biol. Phys.,* 1:4.
13. Schneidman, E. S. (ed.) (1976): *Death: Current Perspectives.* Jason Aaronson, New York.
14. Sontag, S. (1977): *Illness as Metaphor.* Farrar, Straus & Giroux, New York.
15. Visotsky, H. M., et al. (1961): Coping behavior under extreme stress: Observations of patients with poliomyelitis. *Arch. Gen. Psychiatry,* 5:423.
16. Weisman, A. D. (1972): *On Dying and Denying.* Behavioral Publications, New York.
17. Weisman, A. D., and Worden, J. W. (1975): Psychosocial analysis of cancer death. *Omega,* 6:11.
18. Wolfenstein, M. (1957): *Disaster: A Psychological Essay.* Free Press, New York.

Psychosocial Aspects of Cancer,
edited by Jerome Cohen et al.
Raven Press, New York © 1982.

Chapter 13

Social Support Systems and Cancer: A Conceptual View

Joan R. Bloom

Department of Social and Administrative Health Sciences, School of Public Health, University of California, Berkeley, Berkeley, California 94720

Increasing evidence points to the central role that social support plays not only in preventing disease and maintaining health, but also in alleviating the impact of illness on both the stricken individual and those close to him. We seem to be riding the crest of a wave of research and development efforts into the nature and use of social support systems. Unhappily, it may be more accurate to say that we are on the verge of drowning in this rapidly accumulating literature. More important, are we any closer to knowing what social support is and what is "supportive" about support?

What is both intriguing and confusing about the literature on social support systems is its immensity and diffuseness. Integration of this literature discloses both conceptual weakness and research richness. Foregoing the "good scientific method" of beginning with the issue of definition, the issue of what evidence exists on the effect of social support can be explored to see how such support fits into treatment and rehabilitation concerns for the cancer patient. Definitional and theoretical issues can then be confronted. Finally, attention can ¹ ᴜ directed to research gaps and priority areas of inquiry. By moving away from isolated studies and toward organizing themes, we move toward causal explanations. By pointing to conceptual and theoretical gaps, we build toward precision and provide directives for future work. And by developing a theoretical basis of explanation, we can assist clinicians and practitioners in the development and construction of social support systems that may modify poor health outcomes.

SOCIAL SUPPORT AND HEALTH

The process by which social support (undefined) is translated into better health outcomes is not well understood. Knowledge claims have been put forth suggesting that social support (a) decreases vulnerability to disease, (b) buffers between the individual and poor health habits such as overeating, smoking, and drinking, and/or (c) facilitates the adjustment by the individual and those close to him or her to a stressor such as the diagnosis of cancer. The evidence presented below suggests that all three of these knowledge claims have some empirical basis.

Social Support and Host Resistance

An incidental finding of many statistical surveys of mortality and morbidity is the importance of marital status. Contrary to general impressions, marital status is a stronger predictor of age-adjusted mortality ratios than are those for ethnicity (white/nonwhite) or gender (male/female) (56). Mortality ratios for chronic health conditions such as vascular lesions and arteriosclerotic heart disease, cancer at some sites (leukemia, lung cancer, cancer of the digestive organs), tuberculosis, and cirrhosis of the liver are higher for the divorced and widowed men than for married men. Other social indicators such as death from suicide, homicide, and traffic accidents are also higher for the single, the widowed, and the divorced than for the married. Many of these findings, however, do not extend to married women; the often-stated conclusion is that marriage may be protective of men but not of women.

The same pattern of findings is also found in data collected by mental health planners (40). In one study, using 1960 data from 13 states, age-adjusted first admissions to state and county mental hospitals ranged from 16.0 to 29.0 per 100,000 for the married, while for the separated and the divorced they ranged from 109.0 to 124.1; age-adjusted admission rates were intermediate for the single and widowed. Even when admitted, the married are the soonest to be discharged, and once discharged their recidivism rates are the lowest (2,40,64,76). These data suggest that the institution of marriage increases one's resistance to chronic physical and emotional disease and to death due to other social indicators. Exactly how the institution of marriage might increase host resistance is not clear, but data from two recent studies begin to build toward a causal explanation. First, in a study of psychiatric disturbance of women, Brown and his colleagues (11) found that having a confidant (either a spouse or a boyfriend) mitigated the effects of a traumatic event or a major difficulty and the onset of a psychiatric disorder. In this sample, 38% of those who suffered a stressful event with no husband or boyfriend as confidant had onset of disturbance; fewer than 4% of those with a confidant reported such a disorder. This relationship did not hold for those reporting a mother, sister, or friend seen weekly. Thus the quality or intensity of the relationship seemed to be a key factor in protecting the woman from objective life circumstances (11).

In a second study, Berkman (6) studied the effect of social ties on the risk of mortality. Data came from a random sample in Alameda County who completed a questionnaire concerning their health and life style for the California Health Department in the early 1960s. Ten years later a considerable number of the sample had died. Using death certificates and the information from the questionnaire, Berkman was able to determine the effect of social participation on risk of mortality. Like other investigators she found that being married decreased risk of mortality from all causes of death, including cancer. However, in the absence of marriage, other modes of social participation—belonging to a church group, having other family and friends, belonging to formal clubs or groups—also provided protection from premature death to the individual.

The data described above suggest that social support, operationally defined as social ties, does have an effect on outcome. In these data social support decreased the vulnerability of the host. In the latter two studies some hints as to what social support means are also found. For Brown, it is not only having social ties in times of crisis that is important, but the quality of those relationships—having a confidant. Berkman suggests that over the long run social ties of all kinds are important. For those without marital partners, other ties are functional equivalents.

Another type of evidence documenting the importance of social support in the host's resistance to illness comes from studies in which the loss of social support is related to morbidity and increased mortality. In one study Gore (32) followed a group of men after a factory in which they had been employed closed. Those who did not perceive their spouses to be supportive suffered more illness symptoms, higher cholesterol levels, and greater self-blame for their unemployment than did men who were also unemployed but perceived their wives to be supportive. Gore's findings validate those of Brown suggesting that the nature of the support provided by the marital institution is important. In another study, Parkes (59) also ascertained that loss of support can increase emotional morbidity. While investigating psychiatric admissions in two hospitals in England, he discovered that 30 adult patients during a 2-year period had been widowed within 6 months prior to admission. This is six times the rate of newly bereaved individuals one would expect to be admitted. In another study Parkes and his colleagues (60) have shown that mortality for a group of widowers aged 55 and older was 40% greater than expected within the first 6 months following bereavement. With time this rate decreased so that within a year after the death of a wife the survivors' rates were no different from those of a comparable group of married men. The principal excesses in deaths by cause were found to be for coronary thrombosis and "other arteriosclerotic and degenerative heart diseases."

These studies provide some confirmatory evidence of the role that social support plays in decreasing host resistance. During a crisis, such as a loss of job, Gore (32) finds lack of social support is related to physiological changes. These changes are consistent with a picture provided by Parkes and his colleagues (60) of excess of mortality due to degenerative cardiovascular disease.

Social Support as a Buffering Mechanism

Good health habits have been related to increased longevity and poor ones to increased risk of morbidity and mortality (4,5). Thus Belloc and Breslow found that individuals following four of seven rules for good health—some examples of this index are eating breakfast, not eating between meals, sleeping 8 hours and having adequate physical activity, having no more than four drinks at a time—lived longer than those who did not follow these rules of health. In other words, good health habits lead to good health. The obverse also appears to be true. The relationship of smoking to increased risk of lung cancer and other health problems, such as bladder cancer, coronary heart disease, and emphysema, has also been demonstrated (70). The controversial links between nutrition and cardiovascular disease (38) have recently been augmented with hints that nutrition might also be related to cancer (27). The relationship between nutrition and morbidity has received increasing attention. These concerns have been brought to the attention of the media as a result of senatorial review of a National Cancer Institute budget (14,17). Previously, nutrition and its relationship to cardiovascular disease was as newsworthy.

Germane to our discussion of the role of social support as a buffer between poor health habits, such as drinking, smoking, and overeating, and health outcomes are the findings of two community studies—Alameda County, California, and Roseto, Pennsylvania. Interest in the latter community was triggered by findings of a surprising low death rate from coronary heart disease among the population of Roseto, Pennsylvania, when compared to that of several surrounding communities. Roseto is a small community settled by Italians emigrating to this country at the turn of the century. Of interest was not only the low death rate (especially among males) during a 7-year period, but also the life style of the population, which seemed contradictory—their diet was high in calories, animal fats, and alcohol, and resulted in a population with a high proportion of obesity (69). In an effort to understand the conditions under which these contradictory social facts coexisted, a study of the life style of this community was undertaken (12). Although his conclusions relating dietary fat to coronary heart disease may be controversial (38), Bruhn's description of life style differences between the Rosetans and their neighbors is intriguing. He found that the Rosetans participated more in community social organizations than did citizens of neighboring communities. Less residential and social mobility among citizens of this town maintained cultural and ethnic continuity. Rosetans also scored lower on a religiosity scale, suggesting more conservative religious values. And when crises occurred, they were met by the joint efforts of family members, with additional support from relatives and friends. Bruhn's description of this community seems close to what Tonnies (77) has characterized as *Gemeinschaft*. A *Gemeinschaft* community maintains close bonds between individuals, a set of common values, and mutual dependence between the individual and the community (58). The *Gemeinschaft* community buffers the potential impact on the individual of known cardiovascular risk factors such as obesity and a diet high in calories, animal fats, and alcohol.

Data coming from a community study of Alameda County, California, validate and extend Bruhn's findings. Participants were surveyed on their health habits and ways of living in 1965; 10 years later, Berkman used death certificates to study the effect of health habits on mortality. She found that individuals with many social ties (her index was composed of marital status, family, religious, and community factors) and poor health habits (4,5) had lower mortality than individuals with relatively better health habits and few social ties. Thus individuals with many social ties who were overweight, had limited physical activity, were heavy drinkers, or were smokers had lower mortality than a comparable group who were of normal weight, had moderate physical activity, or were nonsmokers and nondrinkers but had few social ties (6). In some yet unspecified way, social support seems to protect the individual from poor health habits. These two examples suggest the importance of exploring the process by which social integration buffers and protects one's health.

Social Support and Adaptation to Illness

&Of particular relevance is the effect of social support systems on treatment and rehabilitation outcomes. Adaptation is defined to include both a psychosocial component, involving the person's re-evaluation of self, and a behavioral component, indicating an acceptance of change or loss such as compliance with the medical regimen or efforts at physical rehabilitation (47,79). Adaptation is often used interchangeably with adjustment and may also mean the absence of psychosocial morbidity (9).

In a study of the physical rehabilitation of 208 persons, adjustment was measured by the speed of achieving an independent level of function in activities of daily living (68). The authors found that, when an individual contributed sufficiently to the family so as not to make the work of others all-consuming and psychologically disturbing, there was a greater willingness to keep the member within the family and to work toward a favorable rehabilitation outcome. Individuals who played important roles within their families and had a high motivation to return to role responsibilities were not admitted for hospitalization as early as those who played peripheral roles. The authors concluded that for long-term recovery the family context was more important than was either the patient's personality characteristics or physical condition.

The posthospital adjustment of men recovering from myocardial infarction was also related to the degree of support the men received at home (20). For Finlayson (25) a favorable postmyocardial infarction outcome consisted of the husband's return to work and the wife's definition of the cessation of the illness. Initial examination of the data suggested social class differences, but upon a closer evaluation these reflected differences between the types and amount of support the families received immediately after the crisis and 1 year later. Families with favorable outcomes had received more assistance initially and over the long term than had families for which outcomes were less favorable. Assistance included both socioemotional and material sources of support and was provided by children, relatives, and friends. Families with favorable outcomes received the greatest amount of support from their children.

Families' reactions to having a disabled child were the focus of a study by Dow (22). He found that extensive networks of interaction and obligation such as found in large families enabled balanced reactions to the child's illness; whereas small families with contracted social networks were characterized by extreme reactions. The author speculates that the extensive network is functional in inhibiting excessive preoccupation with, hence extreme reaction to, any one unit within the network.

When talking about the cancer patient, one must by necessity talk about the health care system and how providers interrelate with patients. Social support by the health care system also affects adaptation as demonstrated in the following examples. In an intervention trial, Pless and Satterwhite (63) experimented with the use of lay counselors in providing social support to families with chronically ill children. Although this sample size was small, the findings are of interest. They recruited women to work with these families who had had personal experience with chronically ill children. One year later, the psychological status of children whose families received supportive counseling was more improved than that of children whose parents did not receive supportive counseling. This example reinforced Finlayson's findings of the importance of providing support to family members that indirectly affects the patient.

Social support by the health care system may determine adaptation to illness by affecting the amount of health care information and skills of adherence that the person learns. Caplan and his associates (15) pilot-tested a social support intervention for hypertensive patients to determine its effectiveness in encouraging adherence to medical regimens. Compared to a control group, members of the social support group were more motivated to adhere and were more likely to take medication. Given the complexity and complications associated with the treatment regimens of cancer patients, further work on the relationship of social support to absorption of information and adherence appears worthwhile.

In another example of how social support increases adaptation to illness, Bloom et al. (9) reported the use of an oncology counselor working with a group of women with breast cancer from the time of diagnosis until 2 months after mastectomy. The counselor provided information about cancer and its treatment as well as social support. Compared to a group of women not receiving these services, the supported group was more emotionally labile during the immediate postsurgical period, but by the end of 2 months felt more efficacious than the untreated group.

Currently, a vast literature exists describing social support programs designed for cancer patients. Volunteers (such as the American Cancer Society's Reach to Recovery group), social workers, nurses, psychologists, and physicians advocate their roles in the provision of support. Who should provide support, when it should occur, and what is the most effective intervention have been frequent topics in the literature (43). However, because of limited systematic research in this area, answers to these questions have usually been determined by the tastes and professional biases of the provider rather than by science. Improvement both in the design and in the delivery of services to the cancer patient will occur through the linking of research on social support with clinical intervention. Until clinical intervention is based on a foundation of research, improvements may be due more to chance than to the systematic application of knowledge.

"Social Support" as Nonsupport

Not all well-intended social interchange is supportive; that is, some "social support" may actually hinder the individual in reaching his goal. This may occur when the "supportive" source encourages the individual to move toward another and opposing goal—eating, for example, when one is on a diet and should reduce eating. The behavior of a peer group in hindering an individual from reaching his goal, whether to lose weight, stop smoking, or stop drinking, is well known.

A second problem can occur when social support is perceived as pressure by the individual. In a study of doctoral students taking preliminary exams, Mechanic (49) notes that anxieties and tension experienced by the students could be reduced by their spouses. A statement such as "Do the best you can" was perceived as more supportive than one such as "I'm sure you are going to do well." In this latter example, the statement increased rather than decreased the individual's anxiety and discomfort as the loss of respect in the spouse's eyes as well as personal disappointment must be considered.

A third consideration, optimum timing, also affects attempts at supportive interchange. At least two issues are related to the timing of the social support attempt. First, the provider or relative must be able to conceptualize the illness process from the victim's perspective. According to Payne and Kraut (61), many providers are unable to do this. Second, the patient/provider communication may not be synchronized—the provider may be ready to listen when the patient is not ready to tell (1). Maguire's large-scale study (45) of women coming to a surgery clinic with a breast complaint indicates the high frequency with which patients display emotional response that is undetected by both nurses and physicians.

A fourth problem arises from a situation in which individuals desire social supportive exchanges but perceive few sources of support for their deepest thoughts, feelings, or fears. This problem is well illustrated by Friedman and his associates (29) who examined parents' responses to their children's fatal illnesses (leukemia). The authors noted that parents rarely turned to their own parents for social support. They explained this as due to the grandparents' denial of their beloved grandchild's life-threatening illness. The parents were then forced to "defend" the medical diagnosis and prognosis rather than be able to relate their own fears and sense of helplessness. A potential source of support had thus been eliminated.

These examples indicate that social support as a construct consists of ways to alter behaviors toward the target individual as well as his perception of these behaviors. Without *mutuality* between the behavior and its perception, a well-intentioned act may not be received as such. Thus good intention is not a sufficient condition for the provision of social support. In fact, training of well-intentioned volunteers, including recovered cancer patients, and providers is essential if efforts to provide social support are to be effective.

SOCIAL SUPPORT AND RESEARCH

Problem of Precise Definition

One of the difficulties in integrating this literature is that the authors have been reluctant to use each other's definition of the concept. In addition to new and novel ways of defining social support, many authors let the reader intuit the intended meaning of the construct. This lack of precision inhibits development of cumulativeness in our knowledge of social support and in making predictions as to the effects of social support. Recently, several authors have alluded to the multidimensionality of the construct (15,53,62,78). The most common definitions include (a) maintenance of social identity, (b) emotional support, (c) material aid and services, (d) information, and (e) social affiliation. Although these categories are somewhat overlapping, they seem to move us toward the "essence" or connotative meaning of the construct.

Maintenance of Social Identity

This dimension can be viewed as a system or network of social ties to which the individual is connected—a macro-perspective, or as the interaction between individuals that compose the system—a micro-perspective. Since both perspectives are important, each will be considered in turn.

From the macro-perspective, this dimension is defined as the degree to which an individual is integrated into the larger society. Classic scholars such as Durkheim (23) and Simmel (66) hypothesized that the loosening of ties between an individual and the social structure resulted in "anomie." Anomie, or the breakdown in social integration, results in an unhealthy state of isolation and loneliness such as is often expressed by the cancer patient. Social ties, then, help maintain one's identity and seem to be particularly important in the face of a crisis. In addition to describing the degree to which an individual is integrated into the larger society, classification can be made along a dimension of local to cosmopolitan. Locally oriented are those whose interests and personal associations are restricted to the communities in which they work and live. Their ties are many and long-lasting. An illustration of a group which is local in orientation is the Rosetans described earlier (12). The entire community was described as local in orientation, with multiple and enduring ties to family, friends, and the community. On the other hand, a cosmopolitan-oriented individual tends to maintain interests and friendships outside the local community. In either case, the social ties of the individual reinforce his sense of "who am I."

From the micro-perspective, interaction between the target individual and the support system reveals the process by which an individual's social ties provide social identity feedback. Feedback is of at least two types. First in importance to an individual, especially when facing a new situation, is the knowledge that the experienced feelings are not unique but are experienced by others facing a similar situation. The commonality of the experiences helps reduce any initial sense of isolation. Often the temporary disorganization of the individual accompanies a crisis situation. We must remember that in a brief period of time an individual may move from a state of apparent health through a series of transitions. Outcomes of diagnostic examinations are awaited; then, if cancer is diagnosed, uncertainty continues as treatment recommendations are made and carried out. Once more the individual is placed in a state of uncertainty as the effectiveness of the treatment modality is evaluated. Often, the uncertainty itself is problematic for the individual. The importance of maintaining some social identity during periods such as these appears critical.

The second aspect of social identity support is the provision of feedback by others on the inappropriateness of current behavior patterns. As Cassel (16) explains, changes in the environment may make previously adaptive behavior patterns lead to unanticipated and potentially detrimental consequences. Both types of feedback reinforce the individual's sense of identity and resulting competence expected in the new role one must assume owing to changes in self or environment.

Emotional Support

Emotional support refers to behavior which assures the individual that he is loved and valued as a person regardless of achievement. It is especially significant for the individual who is experiencing emotional distress, such as the cancer victim. These expressive needs of the individual are usually met by the primary group. In addition to meeting the expressive needs of its members, the primary group is characterized by the permanency of social ties among its members and by the opportunities it provides for face-to-face interaction (18). While the family is the prototype, primary groups composed of neighbors, friends, or other helping persons can assume this role for the individual.

Emotional support has been linked to adjustment to cancer as well as other types of chronic illness. Support from one's family has been related to the arthritic patient's adherence to use of a hand splint (55), to return to work after congestive heart failure regardless of actual disability (42), and to adherence to a hypertension treatment program (13,15). Yalom (82), among others, has experimented with the use of peer support groups for women with metastatic breast cancer. Preliminary analysis of longitudinal data collected indicates that, compared to a control group of randomly selected women, the participants in the peer support group were less anxious and depressed. These findings are, perhaps, more surprising in light of information suggesting that members of the peer support group were initially in poorer physical condition than the controls.

Tangible or Environmental Support

Tangible or environmental support refers to resources at one's disposal such as someone from whom one can borrow money, get a needed ride to a medical appointment, or obtain assistance with housework or babysitting. This type of support has also been linked to adaptation to chronic illness. Thus, as Finlayson reported, patients with the most favorable postmyocardial infarction outcomes were those whose spouses received tangible support provided by children, relatives, and friends continuously from immediately after the illness to 1 year later. Although others have found the ability to get emergency resources is critical in a crisis situation, this study suggests that for the chronically ill, long-term support may be even more important.

Information

Information as a type of support includes directions to a proper street address or assistance in finding a job, as well as information about the diagnostic and treatment options for a cancer patient. Although tangible and environmental support is often provided by family, kin, and close friends, informational support is often better provided by more casual acquaintances. Both meet instrumental needs of individuals. The strength of these "weak" ties has been described by Granovetter (33). If you are looking for a job, the information provided by close ties is less helpful than information provided by casual acquaintances because your close friends usually have the same information that you do. McKinlay (44) and Friedson (30) have studied social networks as "lay referral systems" that influence individuals' use of services. McKinlay's observations reinforce those of Granovetter—underutilizers of medical services had a higher frequency of interaction within a limited group of acquaintances than did utilizers. To summarize, casual acquaintances may have different and better information than close acquaintances in seeking assistance in finding a job or in finding a source of medical care.

Health providers are another source of information. The purpose of a study by Bloom and colleagues (9) was to evaluate the extent to which an intervention program of informational support improved patients' adjustment to mastectomy relative to a comparison group that received standard medical care. The intervention program was predicted to increase the woman's sense of efficacy as a consequence of providing her with information about breast cancer, treatment options, and her role in making treatment decisions. Immediately after surgery, both groups had comparable scores on a health locus of control scale that measured their perceptions of control over health matters. Two months later, the intervention group members perceived themselves to have greater efficacy than did the group not receiving the intervention.

Several other studies suggest that when health providers offer patients information about illness and its treatment, the quality of patient care is enhanced. Some of the ways this can happen are by increasing acceptance of the diagnosis (72); promoting patients' trust in physicians and their prescriptions (39); increasing patients' compliance with therapeutic regimens (21,41,71); heightening patients' satisfaction with their medical treatment (39); and reducing physiological, psychological, and behavioral indices of stress (24,36).

Social Affiliation

Social affiliation refers to the mutual dependence between people and institutions, or, colloquially speaking, people's need for other people. In the *Gemeinschaft* communities such as Roseto, Pennsylvania, the individual's affiliative needs are more easily met than in communities characterized as *Gesellschaft*, where links between individuals and institutions are looser.

The importance of social affiliation has been examined in studies of the Japanese culture and what happened to the Japanese-American during assimiliation (46,48). These studies suggest that social affiliation is a socialized value—one is the product of one's cultural environment. In Japan the mutual dependency of individuals and institutions, primarily the place of employment, is highly valued; in this country the "rugged individualist" reminiscent of frontier days remains the norm. These studies also suggest that the support derived from group affiliation is health protective. Once the Japanese have emigrated to this country and have assimilated, with consequent changes in life style, including diet and relationships to institutions, this protective force ceases. Assimilated Japanese-American health profiles on cardiovascular disease incidence as well as breast and bowel cancer rates begin to resemble those of the rest of the population (17).

Social affiliation affects the individual through the processes of social exchange and social conformity. Using Homan's notion (35) of social exchange, there is an interchange of ideas and support. Yalom (82) calls this the giving-and-receiving cycle and feels that this interchange is the key to the success of peer support groups for metastatic cancer patients. Social conformity is defined as the psychological force exerted by members of a group on an individual to elicit expected behavior. If cooperation is a group norm, then the member will be expected to become cooperative and to meet other behavioral and role expectations as well. We may see the empirical effect of social conformity processes as a decrease in the variance of the responses of group members as membership in an identifiable group is observed over time.

Like information, new opportunities for social affiliation are more likely to be made through one's casual acquaintances and through acquaintances of acquaintances than through closer ties. New social contacts meet affiliative rather than instrumental needs and are particularly important when an individual's previous sources of social support are reduced as in the case of the death of a spouse, or unused as in the case of a cancer patient who does not perceive the availability of support from family, kin, and close friends (29,78). Such support can be provided through the peer support group. When people face a stressful situation, they are motivated to affiliate with others confronting the same threat. Because peer group members are in the same predicament, they can exchange information, obtain reassurance, and reduce feelings of isolation and loneliness. Significant decreases in helplessness and powerlessness were found after 3 months in one group therapy program for the terminally ill; decreases in the variance of the group members responses were also found (7).

Developing More Precise Explanations

In the foregoing section, we considered the multidimensionality of social support and at least five components of the concept. These include, first, social support as feedback to the individual on "who am I" and "what is expected of me." A second, more traditional, definition of social support concerns the expression of affection and acceptance of the individual. A third conceptualization deals with tangible and material support. A fourth definition is social support as information. Finally, the fifth dimension concerns the interventional or affiliative aspect of social support. Even though social support includes at least these five components that seem conceptually distinct, it is not clear whether they are operationally distinct. The studies cited suggest that if some of the conceptual fussiness is removed, different predictions can be tested. For example, Bloom (7) predicts that providing information about treatment options and increasing involvement in one's own treatment should decrease feelings of powerlessness. Her data confirm this prediction. In a similar vein, several studies have considered the effects of emotional support on behavioral adaptation to illness, such as compliance with the medical regimen. One of the difficulties in separating out the components of social support is the lack of conceptual clarity of the term "adjustment" or "adaptation." In the work reported, this term has been used in at least three different ways. Thus more precision is needed in conceptualizing social support for use in future research and in selecting appropriate outcome measures. Precision is also mandatory in the development of successful intervention strategies which can be generalized to other populations.

Constructing Powerful Explanations

Evidence has been presented here that provides an empirical basis to three knowledge claims asserting that social support affects health outcomes by (a) decreasing vulnerability to disease, (b) mitigating the effects of poor health habits, and (c) facilitating adjustment of the individual and his family to a stressor such as cancer. Missing are explanations about the process by which social support is translated into these outcomes. The first two of the knowledge claims posit that support is related primarily to mortality, although some evidence has been presented suggesting its relationship to morbidity as well. One claims the importance of a change in the level of perception of social support; the other that a biological or psychological stressor is the intervening factor. Both differ from the third knowledge claim which assumes illness and predicts increased health.

Three theoretical approaches, at different levels of analysis, provide at least partial explanations of the translation process. At an individual level of analysis, a biophysiological theory has been asserted. At an interpersonal level, social networks provide a partial explanation of the phenomena to be explained. Finally, an ecological approach asserts that the person in relation to his environment explains outcomes.

Biophysiological Theory of Social Support: An Individualistic Explanation

Following Selye (65) and Wolff et al. (81), Cassel (16) explains the process by which changes in interpersonal relationships have neuroendocrine correlates that control the individual's vulnerability to disease agents. These agents may be either physiological or microbiologic (and may already be present, albeit dormant, in the host) or may be ones to which he is subsequently exposed. Thus highway and other accidents, alcoholism, psychoses, suicide, cancer, and cardiovascular disease all describe symptom syndromes for which the disease agent is already present by virtue of genetic potential and/or prior experience and exposure, and susceptibility appears more a matter of the state of the host; however, the presence of social support increases the resistance of the host to the stressor. Either the introduction or the removal of social support affects the homeostatic mechanism. Presumably, the former enhances host resistance and the latter suppresses it. Once the disease process is introduced, the theory does not specify if the course of the disease process can be altered or how this might occur. Literary critic Norman Cousins' (19) description of his own battle with disease suggests that there are ways to alter the course of the disease— in his case, by laughter. And the Simontons' (67) purported success in the use of visualization for cancer also suggests that the direction and progress of the course of the disease are by no means inevitable.

Others, notably Syme (73) and later Antonofsky (3), suggest that an individual's disease should not be the focal point of the investigation. The wide range of disease entities related to features of the social environment leads them instead to hypothesize that people break under situations of stress. How they break and to what extent vary greatly from one individual to another. According to Syme, the understanding of this brokenness is critical rather than the display of the brokenness as psychosis, suicide, cardiovascular disease, or whatever.

This theory predicts illness for an individual. Missing is the link between the general mechanism and the specific disease outcomes. Why does one individual develop cancer and another ulcers? Gore (31) suggests that, under conditions of high stress and high wife hostility, individuals will have more flare-ups of their ulcers than if wife hostility is low. In a similar vein, she suggests that wife support is critical in the relationship between work stress (job termination) and cardiovascular symptomatology. Although she does not go quite as far as saying that social support is the determination between whether one's "stomach aches" or one's "heart aches," this is certainly implied.

To accept this biophysiological theory, one must also assume that all stressors are of equal magnitude and equally problematic for the individual; that is, one must equate biophysiological, genetic, environmental, and social stressors. Further, one must assume that they are equally likely to trigger a response in the neuroendocrine system. A recent study examining the relationship between social support, social stress, and pregnancy complications provides further insight into this issue (54). Data were collected on 170 primiparas between 18 and 29, of similar social class, and delivered by the same obstetrical service. Neither stressors nor social supports alone were related to complications of pregnancy. However, when these factors were considered jointly, 91% of the women with high levels of social stress and low levels of social support had one or more obstetrical complications. Only a third of the women who had high life-stress scores as well as high social support scores had pregnancy complications. At least two important issues are suggested by this study. First, stressors are of different magnitudes—one cannot equate pregnancy as a social stressor with, for example, loss of a loved one. And social stress may be a triggering mechanism only under certain conditions. One of these may be the presence of more than one source of stress; thus, for a pregnancy to be a sufficient condition to be a triggering mechanism, other sources of stress must also be present, whereas death of a spouse may be sufficient by itself. Data being analyzed in conjunction with research on women's adjustment to diagnosis and treatment of breast cancer provide some support for this contention (8). The unsupported woman who is already under stress experiences psychosocial problems following mastectomy—the last straw.

In our efforts to understand the theory of social support, we need to consider the conditions under which the relationship between social support and adaptation might be found. Specification of such conditions is important not only in the development of a theory of social support but also in its application. If a condition were found to hold up after more definitive study, the application to the clinical setting would be straightforward. We could, for example, separate those individuals at risk for psychosocial morbidity from those who are not. Intervention could then be targeted for this vulnerable group.

Social Network Theory

A social network is simply a description of the links between people in social situations. Social exchange theorists such as Homans (35) and Thibaut and

Kelley (75) view society as structured by its transactions rather than by its institutions, and the network describes the form and content of these transactions.

All links that lead to and from an individual or an entire community can be plotted (10,50,51). The network is usually described in terms of its configuration or structure, such as the number and directness of associations as well as the interrelations between associations. The configuration of a network suggests the *accessibility* of social support and is a necessary condition for the provision of support (37). For example, if one is seeking informational support, a network which is diffuse, with lots of indirect or bridging connections, is preferable to a dense network in which the links are interrelated (33,78). A second descriptive property of a social network is the interaction between links that suggests the content of social support. This includes frequency and duration of interactions, the reciprocity of exchanges, and the closeness or intensity between links. Using these two properties, Kaplan and his associates (37) hypothesized that the structural availability of social supports is a necessary condition for health protectiveness, and that the stronger the support functions of the *content* between the links, the more health protective the network.

Social network theory is appealing as both an analytic and a methodological tool. As an analytic tool it has been developed from the perspective of sociometric methods (51) and graph theory (26,50). As a methodological tool it has been used to describe the configuration and interaction of the various linkages. Perhaps its greatest attractiveness has been in its application to professional activities. Individual practitioners have used social network theory to focus attention on the social links between clients and their significant others in an effort to expand intervention beyond the isolated client.

Much of the difficulty in the use of social network theory is due to imprecision in its features and definitions. Its adaptability for study of both micro- and macro-systems becomes a source of weakness because the necessary imposition of boundaries to the network becomes a restriction. As Wolfe (80) has pointed out, the network can be described for a person, a category of people, a set of actions, an organized role system, or a content of exchange (for example, economic or political networks).

Theories Relating People to Their Environments

French and his associates (28) studied the relationships of individuals in organizational settings and developed a theory based on this work, which they termed the Person-Environment Fit. They report that objective stressors are translated into psychological strains that affect the individual. In the work setting, these might include overwork, role conflict, or role ambiguity. These strains have physiological correlates for the individual and, if they long endure, health consequences. Like the biophysiological theories described by Wolff (81), Selye (65), and Cassel (16), the Person–Environment Fit model is based on a psychopathological model of stress and strain.

Living on opposite sides of the world and with differing terminology and predictions, Antonofsky (3,3a) and Syme (73) have come to amazingly similar conclusions as to the consequences of stress in the relationship between the individual and his environment. Antonofsky is intrigued by data from a population of women who survived concentration camps, suggesting that fewer than might be expected have become ill. He argues that instead of asking what makes a person ill, one should ask how a person remains healthy in situations of great adversity. Critical to his formulation is the conception of a health/illness continuum. In the medical world, we usually conceive of a dichotomous state—one is either healthy or ill. If one is ill, medical treatment takes place. Antonofsky, however, argues that the individual exists in a state of only relative health or illness.

Key to his thinking are three "generalized resistance resources" that derive from one's social relations and prevent breakdown of the individual. The first is adaptability, which can be defined as a psychological, sociological, or anthropological construct. Psychologists have usually defined adaptability by its opposite—rigidity, dogmatism, authoritarianism. Anthropologists talk about empathy, or the ability to see value alternatives. And socially, we can discuss the individual's freedom to define and modify roles as necessary. The second resistance resource is profound ties to others. The availability of this resource increases one's strength whether or not the resource is actually activated. Finally, ties between an individual and his total community constitute a significant resistance resource. Not only are such ties important, but the extent to which they are institutionalized, that is, the extent to which the institution is responsible to the individual, is critical.

In a more recent formulation, now called salutogenesis, he argues that an individual develops a "sense of being under control," and this feeling prevents breakdown. A sense of being under control is defined as a "global orientation expressing a pervasive, enduring though dynamic feeling of confidence that one's internal and external environments are dependable, and that there is a high probability that things will work out as well as can reasonably be expected" (4).

Sifting through study after study of mortality and morbidity, Syme and Berkman (74) conclude that "persons in lower-class groups have higher morbidity and mortality rates of almost every disease and illness." They conclude that an overall explanation of illness vulnerability is necessary, and that research should be focused on the "more generalized ways in which people deal with problems in their everyday lives." Individuals develop a sense of themselves as winners or losers, and this is manifested in how they solve the problems that they face. Winners are confident in the ability to master the environment, whereas losers accept their lot. This mastery can be based on profound religious beliefs as well as on one's prior experience of success. Those who possess this sense of confidence in facing and solving daily problems of living are less susceptible to illness than those who do not (Syme, *personal communication*). How this sense of confidence develops and how it is translated into decreased rates of disease are as yet unanswered in his theoretical concept.

Neither Antonofsky nor Syme considers adaptation to illness. However, one can easily imagine that the individual with either Antonofsky's "sense of being under control" or Syme's sense of confidence that things will work out will do better than individuals without the self-beliefs. Observations by clinicians seeing patients prior to diagnosis and during their treatment suggest that previous patterns of adaptability are good predictors of adjustment. Validation of these observations comes from a 2-year longitudinal study recently completed in England. Morris and her associates (52) followed 160 consecutive admissions for breast biopsy, 43% of which proved malignant. A third of the women having mastectomies sought psychiatric assistance postsurgically. Elevated emotional lability and depression scores presurgically predicted poorer postsurgical adjustment 2 years later. In another study, interview data obtained from 60 married, terminally ill cancer patients and their spouses revealed that the capacity to face problems, a sense of life-fulfillment, and a positive marital relationship were associated with an easier adjustment to dying (34).

FUTURE DIRECTIONS

After reviewing an extensive literature that reports the importance of social support in illness and health, it is incumbent on the author to summarize the gaps perceived in this research and to make some suggestions as to areas where further work may improve the treatment and rehabilitation of the victim of cancer.

- The "theoretical approaches" to social support need further development. The basic concepts are not well defined, and major propositions in many instances are not specific. For the most part, where propositions have been specified, the conditions under which they are likely to hold have not been addressed. Although this area of basic social science research may not have immediate payoff, it is clearly an important area where funding should be focused. In the long run, this line of research can potentially assist in the design of intervention programs as well as in the definition of persons at risk (those having inadequate or nonexistent support systems).
- Precision in the development of a concept or its dimensions is necessary for the development of appropriate measurement and for theoretical development and application. Therefore, it appears that research on specific and global measures is a priority area. When current measures of social support were analyzed using the five dimensions delineated earlier, their limitations were striking. Most measures contain several of the dimensions, but none can be called either global or specific. For example, Berkman's (6) measure is primarily social affiliation (quantity and frequency). Gore (31) measured emotional support (from wife, friends, and relatives), affiliation (frequency and sociability), and expressiveness. A measure currently under development by Panagis (57) consists primarily of indicators of emotional support.
- Most of the current support intervention programs have been accepted

under the premise that doing something is better than doing nothing, and they have rarely undergone the scrutiny of evaluation. Evaluation may be seen as either a threat, a way of eliminating a program—or an opportunity, a way of improving a program. We need to take a good look at what we are doing currently and to make adjustments in practice based on rigorous evaluation. However, this should not be accomplished atheoretically, for when a program is considered to be successful, its atheoretical nature may cause difficulties in its transferability. It is usually necessary to make some adjustments in a program when it is adapted to a new location. During this process, the critical features of the program may be modified or eliminated, resulting in an ineffective program. We need to evaluate what we are doing currently to determine whether it makes any difference at all and, in the process, to determine what features are critical to success, thereby improving the transferability of the intervention.

• In a time of limited dollars for medical care, the cost of intervention must be carefully considered. The level of credentialing of key personnel, and the length of time and when in the course of the disease process an intervention should be offered are all important factors that will affect cost estimates. Therefore, another suggested priority area of research is determination of cost-effectiveness of various intervention models. This may not be "innovative" research; it is, however, imperative.

In summary, understanding what social support is and the process by which it operates will facilitate the development of (a) methods for defining individuals at risk, (b) ways to mobilize resources for individuals and groups defined to be at risk, (c) alternative sources of social support, and (d) cost-effective ways to provide such support to the cancer victim and the family.

REFERENCES

1. Abrams, R. D. (1966): The patient with cancer: His changing pattern of communication. N. Engl. J. Med., 274:217–322.
2. Adler, L. M. (1955): Patients in a state mental hospital: The outcome of their hospitalization. In: Mental Health and Mental Disorder, edited by A. Rose, pp. 501–523. W. W. Norton, New York.
3. Antonofsky, A. (1972): Breakdown: A needed fourth step in the conceptual armamentarium of modern medicine. Soc. Sci. Med., 6:537–544.
3a. Antonofsky, A. (1979): Health, Stress and Coping, Jossey-Bass, San Francisco.
4. Belloc, N. (1973): Relationship of health practices and mortality. Prev. Med., 2:67–81.
5. Belloc, N., and Breslow, L. (1972): The relationship of physical health status and health practices. Prev. Med., 1:409–421.
6. Berkman, L. (1977): Social Networks, Host Resistance and Mortality: A Follow-Up Study of Alameda County Residents. Unpublished dissertation. University of California, Berkeley.
7. Bloom, J. R. (1978): Psychological Aspects of Breast Cancer. Annual Report, Project NO1-CN-55313 (DHEW), National Cancer Institute (August). SRI International, Menlo Park, Cal.
8. Bloom, J. R. (1979): Social and Behavioral Predictors of Adjustment to Breast Cancer. Paper presented at annual meeting of the American Sociological Association, Boston (August).
9. Bloom, J. R., Ross, R. D., and Burnell, G. M. (1978): Effect of social support on patient adjustment following breast surgery. Patient Counsel. Health Educ., 1:50–59.

10. Boissevain, J. (1974): *Friends of Friends.* Basil Blackwell, London.
11. Brown, G. W., Bhrolchaim, M. N., and Harris, T. (1975): Social class and psychiatric disturbance among women in an urban population. *Sociology,* 9:223–254.
12. Bruhn, J. G. (1965): An epidemiological study of myocardial infarctions in an Italian-American community. *J. Chronic Dis.,* 18:353–365.
13. Caldwell, J. R., Cobb, S., Dowling, M. D., and de Jongh, D. (1970): The dropout problem in antihypertensive treatment: A pilot study of social and emotional factors influencing a patient's ability to follow antihypertensive treatment. *J. Chronic Dis.,* 22:579–592.
14. *Cancer Letter* (1978): Cancer Letter, Inc., Reston, Va. (June 23).
15. Caplan, R. D., Robinson, E., French, J. R., Jr., Caldwell, J. R., and Shinn, M. (1976): *Adhering to Medical Regimens: Pilot Experiments in Patient Education and Social Support.* Report, Institute for Social Research, Ann Arbor, Mich.
16. Cassel, J. (1976): The contribution of the social environment to host resistance. *Am. J. Epidemiol.,* 104:107–123.
17. Clark, M., Hager, M., and Gastel, B. (1978): Cancer and our diet. *Newsweek* (July 24): 85–86.
18. Cooley, C. H. (1955): Primary groups. In: *Small Groups: Studies in Social Interaction,* edited by A. P. Hare, E. F. Borgatta, and R. F. Bales, pp. 15–19. Alfred A. Knopf, New York.
19. Cousins, N. (1976): Anatomy of an illness (as perceived by the patient). *N. Engl. J. Med.,* 295:1458–1463.
20. Croog, S., Levine, S., and Lurie, Z. (1968): The heart patient and the recovery process: A review of the directions of research on social and psychological factors. *Soc. Sci. Med.,* 2:111.
21. Davis, M. S. (1968): Variation in patients' compliance with doctors' advice: An empirical analysis of patterns of communication. *Am. J. Public Health,* 58:274–288.
22. Dow, T. E. (1965): Family reaction to crisis. *J. Marriage Fam.,* 27:363–366.
23. Durkheim, E. (1951): *Suicide: A Study in Sociology.* Free Press, Glencoe, Ill.
24. Egbert, L. D., and Bartlett, M. K. (1964): Reduction of postoperative pain by encouragement and instruction of patients. *N. Engl. J. Med.,* 270:825–827.
25. Finlayson, A. (1976): Social networks as coping resources. *Soc. Sci. Med.,* 10:97–103.
26. Fischer, C. S. (1977): *Networks and Places.* Free Press, New York.
27. Fox, B. H. (1976): *Premorbid Psychological Factors as Related to Incidence of Cancer: Background for Prospective Grant Applicants.* Mimeograph. National Cancer Institute (Oct. 16).
28. French, J. R. P., Rodgers, W., and Cobb, S. (1974): Adjustment as a person environment fit. In: *Coping and Adaptation,* edited by G. V. Coelho, D. A. Hamburg, and J. E. Adams, pp. 316–333. Basic Books, New York.
29. Friedman, S. B., Chodoff, P., Mason, J. W., and Hamburg, D. A. (1963): Behavioral observations of parents anticipating the death of a child. *Pediatrics,* 32:610–625.
30. Friedson, E. (1960): Client control and medical practice. *Am. J. Sociol.* 65:374–382.
31. Gore, S. (1973): *The Influence of Social Support in Ameliorating the Consequences of Job Loss.* Unpublished dissertation. University of Michigan, Ann Arbor.
32. Gore, S. (1978): The effect of social support in moderating the health consequences of unemployment. *J. Health Soc. Behav.,* 19:157–165.
33. Granovetter, M. S. (1976): The strength of weak ties. *Am. J. Sociol.,* 78:1360–1380.
34. Hinton, J. (1975): The influence of previous personality on reactions to having terminal cancer. *Omega,* 6:95–111.
35. Homans, G. C. (1961): *Social Behavior: Its Elementary Forms.* Harcourt, Brace, & World, New York.
36. Johnson, J. E. (1975): *Altering Patients' Responses to Threatening Events: Surgical Study I.* Paper presented at N.L.N. Convention, New Orleans (May).
37. Kaplan, B. H., Cassel, J. C., and Gore, S. (1977): Social support and health. *Med. Care,* 15 (5), supplement (May).
38. Keys, A. (1965): Arteriosclerotic heart disease in a favored community. *J. Chronic Dis.,* 19:245–254.
39. Korsch, B. M., Gozzi, E. K., and Francis, V. (1968): Gaps in doctor/patient communication: Doctor/patient interaction and patient satisfaction. *Pediatrics,* 42:855–871.
40. Kramer, M. (1967): Epidemiology, biostatistics and mental health planning. *Psychiatric Research Report #22,* pp. 25–44. American Psychiatric Association (April).
41. Leventhal, H. (1975): The consequences of depersonalization during illness and treatment: An

information-processing model. In: *Humanizing Health Care,* edited by J. Howard and A. Strauss. John Wiley & Sons, New York.

42. Lewis, C. E. (1966): Factors influencing return to work of men with congestive heart failure. *J. Chronic Dis.,* 19:1193–1209.

43. Lewis, F. M., and Bloom, J. R. (1979): Psychosocial adjustment to breast cancer: A selected review of literature. *Int. J. Psychiatr. Med.,* 9:1–10.

44. McKinlay, J. B. (1973): Social networks, law consultation and help-seeking behavior. *Soc. Forces,* 51:275–295.

45. Maguire, P. (1975): The psychological and social consequences of breast cancer. *Nurs. Mirror,* 140:54–58.

46. Marmot, M. G., and Syme, S. L. (1976): Acculturation and coronary heart disease. *Am. J. Epidemiol.,* 104:225–247.

47. Matson, R. R., and Brooks, N. A. (1977): Adjusting to multiple sclerosis: An exploratory study. *Soc. Sci. Med.,* 11:245–250.

48. Matsumoto, Y. S. (1970): Social stress and coronary heart disease in Japan: A hypothesis. *Milbank Mem. Fund Q.,* 48:9–36.

49. Mechanic, D. (1962): *Students under Stress: A Study in the Social Psychology of Adaptation.* Free Press, New York.

50. Mitchell, J. (1969): The concept and use of social networks. In: *Social Networks in Urban Situations,* edited by J. C. Mitchell, pp. 1–50. Manchester University Press, Manchester, England.

51. Moreno, J. L. (1955): Contribution of sociometry to research methodology in society. In: *Small Groups: Studies in Social Interaction,* edited by A. P. Hare, E. F. Borgatta, and R. F. Bales, pp. 99–106. Alfred A. Knopf, New York.

52. Morris, T., Greer, H. S., and White, P. (1977): Psychological and social adjustment to mastectomy. *Cancer,* 40:2381–2387.

53. Murawski, B. J., Penman, D., and Schmitt, M. (1978): Social support in health and illness: The concept and its measurement. *Cancer Nurs.,* 1:365–371.

54. Nuckolls, K. B., Cassel, J. C., and Kaplan, B. H. (1972): Psychosocial assets, life crisis and the prognosis of pregnancy. *Am. J. Epidemiol.,* 95:431.

55. Oakes, T. W., Ward, J. R., Gray, R. M., Klarber, M. R., and Moody, P.M. (1970): Family expectation and arthritis patient compliance to a headresting split regimen. *J. Chronic Dis.,* 22:757–764.

56. Ortmeyer, C. E. (1974): Variations in mortality, morbidity and health care by marital status. In: *Mortality and Morbidity in the United States,* edited by C. E. Erhardt and J. E. Berlin, pp. 159–188. Harvard University Press, Cambridge, Mass.

57. Panagis, D. (1977): *Perceived Social Support Scale.* Mimeograph. West Coast Cancer Foundation, San Francisco.

58. Panzetta, A. F. (1971): The concept of community: The short circuit of the mental health movement. *Arch. Gen. Psychiatry,* 25:291–297.

59. Parkes, C. M. (1964): Recent bereavement as a cause of mental illness. *Br. J. Psychiatry,* 1:198–204.

60. Parkes, C. M., Benjamin, B., and Fitzgerald, B. G. (1969): Broken heart: A statistical study of increased mortality among widowers. *Br. Med. J.,* 4:740–743.

61. Payne, E., Jr., and Kraut, M. (1969): The psychosocial aspects of advanced cancer: Teaching people interviewing techniques and record-keeping. *J.A.M.A.,* 210:1238–1242.

62. Pinneau, S. R. (1975): *The Effects of Social Support on Psychological and Physiological Strain.* University of Michigan Press, Ann Arbor.

63. Pless, I. B., and Satterwhite, B. (1972): Chronic illness in childhood: Selection, activities and evaluation of nonprofessional family counselors. *Clin. Pediatr.,* 11:403–410.

64. Rosen, B. M., Anderson, T. W., and Bahn, A. K. (1968): Psychiatric services for the aged: A nationwide survey of patterns of utilization. *J. Chronic Dis.,* 21:167–177.

65. Selye, H. (1946): The general adaptation syndrome and diseases of adaptation. *J. Clin. Endocrinol. Metab.,* 6:117–230.

66. Simmel, G. (1950): *The Sociology of George Simmel,* edited by K. H. Wolff. Free Press, New York.

67. Simonton, O. C., and Simonton, S. S. (1975): Belief systems and management of the emotional aspects of malignancy. *J. Transpers. Psychol.,* 7:29–45.

68. Slater, S. B., Sussman, M. B., and Stroud, M. W. (1970): Participation in household activities as a prognostic factor for rehabilitation. *Arch. Phys. Med. Rehabil.,* 51:605–611.

69. Stout, C., Marrow, J., Brundt, E. N., and Wolf, S. (1964): Unusually low incidence of death from myocardial infarction. *J.A.M.A.,* 188:845–849.
70. Surgeon General of the United States Public Health Service (1964): Report of the Advisory Committee on Smoking and Health (DHEW). U.S. Government Printing Office, Washington, D.C.
71. Svarstad, B. (1976): Physician/patient communication and patient conformity with medical advice. In: *The Growth of Bureaucratic Medicine,* edited by D. Mechanic, pp. 220–238. John Wiley & Sons, New York.
72. Svarstad, B., and Lipton, H. L. (1978): Informing parents about mental retardation: A study of professional communication and parent acceptance. *Soc. Sci. Med.,* 11:645–651.
73. Syme, S. L. (1966): *The Clinical Bias in Epidemiology.* Paper presented at meeting of the American Public Health Association.
74. Syme, S. L., and Berkman, L. S. (1976): Social class, susceptibility and sickness. *Am. J. Epidemiol.* 140:1–8.
75. Thibaut, J. W., and Kelley, H. H. (1959): *The Social Psychology of Groups.* John Wiley & Sons, New York.
76. Thomas, D. S., and Locke, B. Z. (1963): Marital status, education, and occupational differentials in mental disease. *Milbank Mem. Fund Q.,* 41:145–160.
77. Tonnies, F. (1957): *Community and Society: Gemeinschaft and Gesellschaft,* translated and edited by C. P. Loomis. Michigan State University Press, East Lansing.
78. Walker, K. N., MacBride, A., and Vachon, M. L. S. (1977): Social support networks and the crisis of bereavement. *Soc. Sci. Med.,* 11:35–41.
79. Wright, B. (1960): *Physical Disability: A Psychological Approach.* Harper, New York.
80. Wolfe, A. W. (1970): On structural comparisons of networks. *Can. Rev. Soc. Anthropol.,* 7:226–244.
81. Wolff, C. T., Friedman, S. B., Hofer, M. A., and Mason, J. W. (1964): Relationship between psychological defenses and mean urinary 18-hydroxycorticosteroid excretion rates. I. A predictive study of parents of fatally ill children. *Psychosom. Med.,* 26:576–591.
82. Yalom, I. (1977): Group therapy with the terminally ill. *Am. J. Psychiatry,* 134:396–400.

Psychosocial Aspects of Cancer,
edited by Jerome Cohen et al.
Raven Press, New York © 1982.

Chapter 14

Social Connection and the Etiology of Cancer: An Epidemiological Review and Discussion

Jill Gregory Joseph and S. Leonard Syme

Program in Epidemiology, School of Public Health, University of California, Berkeley, Berkeley, California 94720

It is the purpose of this chapter to examine the relationship between social connection and cancer etiology. There are numerous published reports of an association between a particular type of social connection or disconnection and cancer; to be most useful, these studies need to be drawn together, compared, and assessed. This task is made more urgent by the current popularity of research on social support and social networks (1,2,20,29). Fortunately, sufficient work is now available to permit a review of the epidemiological evidence in terms of the etiological question. In addition to a discussion of the results that have emerged, recurrent methodological problems can be highlighted by such a presentation. In this way, future research goals can be more readily identified and addressed.

SOCIAL CONNECTION AND CANCER: THE RESEARCH EXPERIENCE

Bloom (Chapter 13) has documented the extensive possible links between social support and disease etiology, treatment, and prognosis. This chapter will be limited to a discussion of the epidemiology of cancer and social ties; it is our intent to introduce as little theoretical structure as possible and, instead, to examine the rates of cancer among those with and without various forms of social connection to other individuals. Excellent work elsewhere attempts to explore models of causality or examine the detailed sociology of social networks (5,27,37). We are only asking the question: Is there adequate reason to call for further research on the relationship between social connection and cancer? In order to answer this question, evidence concerning marital status, divorce and widowhood, object loss, and group affiliation will be examined.

One of the most obvious forms of social connection is marriage. Table 1 summarizes the results of 10 studies of marital status and cancer. With the

TABLE 1. *Marital status and cancer: published results*

Authors	Data base	Results of interest
Registrar-General's Office (36) Peller (33)	Vital statistics, England and Wales Vital statistics, Great Britain	For women ≥ 25 years old ("age-equated" rates): widowed and divorced RR 1.14 for cancer mortality For women at all ages:
Herring (11)	Vital statistics, U.S.A.	widows experience "significantly higher" cancer mortality For women: reproductive site and other cancer mortality divorced and widowed > single and married
Lombard and Potter (21)	Retrospective, case-control study of cervical cancer Cases N = 523 Controls N = 670	For women: divorce or separation ~ 3 times more common in cases
Shurtleff (40)	Vital statistics, U.S.A.	For men and women: *in general* divorced > widowed > single for site-specific cancer mortality
LeShan and Worthington (17)	Vital statistics, U.S.A., England, Australia	For women: widowed > divorced > single > married for cancer mortality
Kraus and Lilienfeld (15)	Vital statistics, U.S.A.	For men and women, ages 20–44: widowed experience increase in total cancer mortality
Snell and Graham (41)	Retrospective, case-control study of breast cancer Cases N = 352 Controls N = 670	No difference between cases and controls by marital status or number of separations, divorces
Lilienfeld et al. (19)	Vital statistics, U.S.A.	For men and women: in all geographic areas, for both whites and non-whites, the single, widowed, and divorced experience an excess cancer mortality
Moss (28)	Prospective cohort study, N = 2,170	For men and women: marital separation or recent divorce associated with excess risk of cancer mortality (RR ~ 3); widowhood resulted in no significant cancer mortality increase

exception of two case-control studies and one cohort study, results are based on available national mortality statistics. All were conducted within the United States, Great Britain, or Australia. It is necessary, therefore, to be cautious about generalizations concerning cancer incidence or extremely dissimilar societies.

As the data in Table 1 show, as early as 1931 it was observed that widowed and divorced women in England and Wales died 14% more frequently of cancer than "spinsters" and married women (36). These figures were reported to be "age equated." Work by Peller (33), using data from all of Great Britain available during 1932, indicated widows experienced "significantly higher" cancer mortality than single women. Work in the United States by Herring (11) during this same period confirmed high cancer mortality for the divorced and widowed; this was true of cancer of reproductive sites as well as all other cancers. A case-control study subsequently compared women diagnosed as having cancer of the cervix with matched controls (21); approximately three times as many cancer patients had "at some time" been divorced or separated. Other findings were reported by Shurtleff (40), using 1949 to 1951 United States census data for both men and women. He concluded that, in general, the divorced have cancer mortality rates higher than the widowed and that the single fare better than either group. This pattern was true of all cancers except four: leukemia and aleukemia for men, and cancer of the buccal cavity and pharynx for women.

In contrast, LeShan and Worthington (17) reported female cancer risk in the United States, England, and Australia to be highest in the widowed, lowest in the married, and intermediate for the single or divorced. Kraus and Lilienfeld (15) confirmed higher cancer mortality for a group of widowed men and women aged 20 to 44. Several forms of death, such as those due to arteriosclerosis, demonstrated a much more dramatic increase; nonetheless, cancer mortality still was approximately doubled in this group. The authors were particularly careful to discuss possible bias in their findings. They conclude that their findings are probably not explainable by economic or age differences between the widowed and married, nor by the unhealthy marrying one another.

Negative findings were reported by Snell and Graham (41) in a case-control study of breast cancer; they reported no differences between cases and controls in either marital status or the number of separations and divorces. These results may be partially explained by the fact that more than half the controls had cancer of another site. Marital status may represent a risk factor for multiple forms of cancer; the use of other cancer patients as controls would, therefore, obscure the impact of this shared risk factor.

More expected results were reported by Lilienfeld et al. (19) in their report of 1949 to 1961 cancer mortality in the United States: for both men and women, both whites and non-whites, in all geographic areas, excess mortality was demonstrated for the single, widowed, and divorced. They further concluded that differences in smoking habits could not fully account for the observed differences. Important additional evidence comes to us from one of the few studies to view cancer prospectively. Moss (28) has recently reported coronary heart disease and cancer mortality in Alameda County residents followed for 9 years by the Human Population Laboratory. Extensive baseline information on demographic characteristics, health status, and certain behaviors or attitudes was available to him. He found that individuals experiencing marital separation or recent divorce had a three fold increased risk of dying from cancer; this excess was not attributable to smoking or physical health (including pre-existing cancer). This difference was statistically significant for both men who smoke and women who do not. Insufficient numbers of male nonsmokers and female smokers were available to draw conclusions concerning these groups.

We have reviewed 10 studies that dealt with marital status as a categorical description; yet the very words "widowed" and "divorced" imply a change of status across time. It is noteworthy that people who experience a loss of social connection are so often reported to experience an increased risk of cancer. The effects of such loss are examined more directly in work dealing with bereavement; let us now turn to available evidence linking bereavement and cancer. Unfortunately, this evidence is sparse, as most of the work in this area has reported only total mortality. For a general discussion of health and bereavement, the reader is referred to an excellent review article by Jacob and Ostfeld (13).

In 1940 Ciocco (3) reported work dealing with "homogamy," the tendency of like to marry like; his data were based on examination of the 1898 to 1930 Washington County (Maryland) death records to determine husband-and-wife cause of death. Although not interested in excess mortality following bereavement, he did report that husbands and wives died of the same cause more often than expected. This was true for cancer as well as infectious disease and heart disease. More relevant for our purposes is work by McNeill (25) using data concerning 9,247 men and women widowed in Connecticut during 1955. He demonstrated an excess cancer mortality for women, although only during the second 6 months following bereavement. He did not detect any cancer excess for widowers. Parkes et al. (32) have reported a slight excess cancer mortality in 4,486 widowers at least 55 years old followed for 9 years. This excess was observed only in the first 6 months following bereavement, was minimal (relative risk = 1.15), and did not achieve statistical significance. Previously discussed research by Moss (28) reported similar findings: a slight excess in cancer mortality after the death of a spouse was found in the Alameda County cohort; this excess also failed to achieve statistical significance.

The case-control study by Snell and Graham (41) also failed to detect any differences in "deaths among household and other family members" in the 5 years preceding diagnosis of cancer. The caution about their choice of controls needs to be kept in mind, however.

It is apparent that studies concerning marital status and bereavement yield contradictory results. What can we then conclude about the general topic of social connection and cancer? Before answering, let us turn to further work on this question.

There is a tradition of psychological and psychoanalytic research on the antecedents of cancer; special emphasis is often placed on actual, threatened, or symbolic object loss (16,17,39). Green (9) reports, for example, a pattern of such loss 4 years preceding the diagnosis of cancer; however, this impression is largely clinical and derived entirely from retrospective data. Two prospective studies examine more systematically the loss of personal relationships and cancer. Kissen (14) reported data obtained from patients admitted to the chest services of three English hospitals. All patients were interviewed prior to diagnosis; cases and controls were thus determined after data collection. Analysis of interview data revealed that the death of a parent during childhood was more frequently observed (at statistically significant levels) in cancer patients.

Thomas and Duszynski (43) prospectively studied 1,337 Johns Hopkins medical students who graduated between 1948 and 1964. Twenty individuals who reported the subsequent diagnosis of cancer were matched with appropriate controls. No differences were observed in the frequency of parental death or divorce during the subjects' childhoods. However, the authors did find a "marked lack of closeness" to parents as assessed by baseline questionnaire data. This pattern is different not only from controls, but also from those who commit suicide or develop mental illness, hypertension, or coronary heart disease. Such emotional distance may, of course, represent another aspect of social disconnection.

One can also examine the effects of social connection to the broader organization or group. In this regard, one study of sociocultural mobility and two of certain religious denominations are of interest. Sociocultural and geographic mobility has long intrigued the cardiovascular epidemiologist (23,42). Less work has been done on such mobility and cancer. Haenzel et al. (10) reported, however, on lung cancer and mobility. They concluded that there was an association between lung cancer and mobility which was not explained by smoking alone. Those who were born outside the United States or in rural areas but moved to urban centers were especially likely to develop cancer of the lung. This association could be explained many ways; nonetheless, the disruption of broadly based social ties is certainly a common feature of mobility and may contribute to this finding.

Although religious participation certainly influences key health habits, it also provides a form for social contact and connection. Aspects of Mormon and Seventh-Day Adventist religious observances which probably influence health outcomes are compared in Table 2. Enstrom (4) reported that Mormon men experienced extremely low rates of those cancers associated with tobacco use, such as cancer of the lung. Of greater interest is that cancer of sites not affected by smoking was also less common—about two-thirds of the U.S. average. The rates used for calculation apply to white men and are appropriately age-adjusted. Phillips and Kuzma (34) reported similar results in a study of Seventh-Day Adventists. Because of their doctrines on food and drug use, cancers of both diet and smoke-related sites must be analyzed separately; such site-specific rates

TABLE 2. *Religious habits that may affect health*

Religious group	Avoidances	Diet
Mormons	Tobacco, alcohol	No special diet
Seventh-Day Adventists	Coffee, tea, alcohol, tobacco	Ovo-lacto-vegetarian

are extremely low, as expected. Just as in the Mormons, other cancers are also less frequent—approximately 70% of that expected. Thus not only advantageous health behaviors but group participation itself may influence cancer incidence in Seventh-Day Adventists and Mormons. Further support for this notion is derived from the observation that the more active members of both groups have lower rates than the less active members.

To this point we have reviewed cohort studies, case-control studies, and studies using vital statistics; authors have ranged from statistical to psychoanalytic in their orientation; the data bases vary between small interviewed samples and nation-wide mortality figures. The results are not uniform; they are, however, remarkable. From 40 years of diverse work conducted in such divergent manners on a controversial topic, we begin to see a pattern. Social connection as defined by marital status seems related to the likelihood of cancer. Social connection to parents in childhood, the religious group, and the broader social milieu may be related to cancer. Bereavement does not seem to increase cancer mortality.

Although the findings available are important, the conclusions that can be reached from this study must be tentative. There are numerous and often competing explanations for such findings. At a minimum, there seems ample justification to explore the association between cancer incidence and socioeconomic status, acculturation to Westernized urban society, "life events," and psychological and behavioral characteristics. This last category is itself a potpourri of specific psychological states (such as depression), particular behaviors (as in the type A-B literature), styles of cognitive appraisal or affective reponse, and coping.

In any case, the need for further work on social connection seems real; the results to date justify this answer. The next question is how best to proceed. An approach to this question is considered in the remaining sections of this chapter.

PSYCHOSOCIAL EPIDEMIOLOGY AND DESIGN ALTERNATIVES: THE RESEARCH DILEMMA

One research dilemma is that concerning the prospective study of a cohort versus the retrospective study of cases and controls. Each design alternative is fraught with well-documented difficulties (18,24). Prospective studies are expensive, take years of investment in surveillance, and yield few cases of disease. The Human Population Laboratory cohort used by Moss (28) consisted of 2,170 persons and yielded 67 cases of cancer after 9 years of follow-up. There were, therefore, 2,103 "controls" for these 67 cases. To be sure, some of these persons developed coronary heart disease or stroke, but most people remained well. It should be noted that Moss reported on a cohort 45 to 64 years old; participants were, therefore, experiencing more disease than younger and thus even healthier individuals. Balanced against these problems is the useful contribution of prospective results to causal influences. Information obtained prior to the development of disease is not subject to erroneous or biased recall. This is a compelling advantage.

The alternative is a retrospective case-control design; by selecting individuals already ill and their appropriate controls, a less expensive and more rapid assessment of possible risk factors can be made. To avoid the problems of biased recall, some authors have attempted to interview patients after hospitalization but before diagnosis. Fox (6) presents an excellent discussion of the likely failure of this approach to achieve its aims with the cancer patient. He concludes that such patients are not diagnostically naive, and, indeed, are probably preoccupied with the possibility of cancer. In addition, retrospective studies cannot recreate physiological variables of interest, nor assure accurate recall of remote events. The reference here is not to biased recall but to the normal inadequacies of memory.

Another problem compounds these difficulties. Because of both professional experience and budgetary constraints, investigators tend to choose a variable or two of interest. One becomes intrigued with life events, another with socioeconomic status or social support. Study design is, therefore, further limited by these choices. At most, we may examine the interactions of two psychosocial variables, such as stressful life events and social support (8,20).

A consequence of this style of work is that few "critical" (in the classic sense of that word) social epidemiological studies are ever designed. Each of us pursues a particular slender thread of evidence, tending to believe in our own schema for understanding psychosocial risk. Yet socioeconomic status and coping style and acculturation and social support and life events do not everywhere produce the same prediction concerning risk. Such areas of conflict have elsewhere in the history of science led to crucial experiments, and thus to a more advanced or unified theory. For example, debate between a general and specific model of stress produced extensive research to the eventual benefit of all.

Finally, social epidemiology is often limited to one-time assessment of the independent variables. This is by definition true of the retrospective study and usually true of the prospective. In cardiovascular epidemiology, for example, we determine acculturation status or available social support based on an interview or questionnaire administered once. We seldom obtain longitudinal data concerning the variables we have chosen to study. Data from a typical cohort of 3,000 to 4,000 individuals are difficult enough to accumulate, reduce, and analyze from one assessment.

In summary, what we are most often left with is the single-time assessment of one or two variables in a cohort from which little disease will develop. Alternatively, there exists the case-control design with its attendant problems. In contrast to this intentionally bleak picture of current efforts, there exist widely discussed standards for future work. Within this volume itself there is remarkable consensus about the design of psychosocial research. There is general agreement that truly excellent epidemiological work entails the following characteristics:

1. Research on psychosocial factors must be conducted prospectively (see Chapter 16). This does not exclude a role for well-conducted retrospective studies to explore potential risk factors.

2. Research on psychosocial factors must include longitudinal assessment with repeated measurement of salient participant behaviors, characteristics, or attitudes (see Chapters 7 and 15).

3. Research on psychosocial factors must examine multiple variables that no doubt interact in critical and as yet poorly understood ways (7).

The contrast between these standards and currently available research strategies makes the research dilemma clear.

Additional difficulties are associated with the choice of dependent or outcome variables. Epidemiological investigations usually are concerned with binary outcome categories. Participants are dead or alive; they have disease or they are well. There may be intermediary categories ("probable ischemic heart disease") or multiple outcomes (cancer, suicide, heart disease), but customary outcomes are generally binary. This is, of course, largely a consequence of available technology. Unable to easily determine the extent of arteriosclerosis, one must await a frank myocardial infarction. Unable to conveniently document premalignant changes in the lung, one needs a tissue diagnosis of bronchogenic carcinoma. It is important to remind ourselves, however, that physiological reality is continuous instead of binary. It seems most likely that progression toward disease is not uniform; throughout periods of seeming health, there is probably movement in and out of physiological states that are precursors to illness. Continuous predisease outcomes might better reflect underlying physiological reality. Yet, as mentioned, current psychosocial epidemiology is concerned with binary distinctions in trying to identify risk factors for disease or death. This is an unfortunate focus since few of those we study become ill or die. Yet once ill with cancer or coronary heart disease, return to premorbid health is rare (C. Schaefer, *personal communication*).

It would seem more productive to identify risk factors for predisease states that are particularly injurious or suspect. Such research might push the time frame of our concern further away from disease and toward health maintenance. Recent interest in cancer and immunosurveillance represents such thinking (7,35). Although this specific technique may not prove useful, we need to remain alert to similar possibilities.

Psychosocial epidemiology repeatedly confronts research dilemmas. This chapter has discussed two such problems: design issues related to the investigation of independent variables, and limitations on our assessment of outcome. No real response can be made to the second point. At best, investigators can only remain alert for developing techniques that would permit a continuous predisease outcome measure. Fortunately, the problem of design can be addressed more successfully. In the next section, we will examine a specific proposal for future directions in psychosocial epidemiology.

CASE-CONTROL SUBSAMPLING FROM A PROSPECTIVE STUDY: A RESEARCH PROPOSAL

A large prospective cohort was developed by Paffenbarger and co-workers (30,31) in their study of 40,000 former college students. Those who remained well in the cohort vastly outnumbered those who were ill. From this large undiseased group Paffenbarger and his colleages selected a much smaller number of controls. Published analyses compared such subsamples of controls with these few cases. Hexter (12), working to compare infant deaths with successful deliveries, used a similar method. Mantel (22) subsequently formalized the statistical methods appropriate for this strategy, while arguing that such an approach permits more comprehensive and imaginative analysis. Work in Norway by Miller et al. (26) applied this technique to the study of coronary heart disease and lipoproteins. In this study, sera from all participants were frozen after basic analyses. Subsequently, only serum samples from cases and selected controls were ever submitted for complex and expensive lipoprotein studies. For this reason Miller et al. described their work as a "prospective case-control study."

There is, then, a tradition of what Brand *(personal communication)* calls "case-control subsampling from a prospective study." This design has usually been developed to lessen the burden of analyzing data from massive numbers of controls or to reduce costly laboratory procedures. It is an alternative design which could hold special promise for psychosocial epidemiology. Baseline assessments of a large prospective cohort could be "frozen," unanalyzed, much as Miller did with plasma samples. The data would simply be stored in their original form without further reduction. Only information from those who develop disease and their appropriate controls would be subject to review, coding, and entry into computer-based data files. The immediate benefits of such a design are primarily financial. For the social epidemiologist it represents, however, a remarkable opportunity for more thorough and exciting research. As discussed earlier, both effort and expense traditionally are devoted to the one-time study of a few variables in a huge cohort. With case-control subsampling, resources could be redirected to the analysis of multiple longitudinally sampled variables in a much smaller subsample. This would permit the development of a more useful and appropriate data base for the investigation of psychosocial hypotheses.

There are, of course, human limits to any process. Participants cannot be endlessly queried. Investigators cannot comfortably familiarize themselves with every psychosocial variable. Nonetheless, this broader and longitudinal approach would permit us to understand the interaction of risk factors, to design "critical experiments," and to observe change across time. There is nothing new about the criteria for excellent psychosocial research discussed earlier. Case-control subsampling from a prospective study may, however, bring us closer to realizing these objectives.

CONCLUSIONS

In conclusion, available research has been reviewed and discussed. This review points to the potential of further work on the relationship between social connection and cancer etiology. Many different studies, with a variety of designs and addressing particular forms of social connections, suggest in provocative fashion that an association exists between these two factors. It is now time to improve research methods so that sharpened and more informed inferences can be drawn. From the findings available to date, it seems clear that the problem is worth our best efforts.

ACKNOWLEDGMENTS

We acknowledge with special appreciation the work of Catherine Schaefer, Richard Brand, and William Satariano, whose comments and suggestions were instrumental in the development of this chapter.

REFERENCES

1. Berkman, L. F., and Syme, S. L. (1979): Social networks, host resistance, and mortality: A nine-year follow-up study of Alameda County residents. *Am. J. Epidemiol.,* 109:186–204.
2. Cassel, J. (1976): The contribution of the social environment to host resistance. *Am. J. Epidemiol.,* 104:107–123.
3. Ciocco, A. (1940): On the mortality in husbands and wives. *Hum. Biol.,* 12:508–531.
4. Enstrom, J. E. (1978): Cancer and total mortality among active Mormons. *Cancer,* 42:1943–1951.
5. Fischer, C. S., Jackson, R. M., Sueve, C. A., Gerson, K., and Jones, L. M. (1977): *Networks and Places: Social Relations in the Urban Setting.* Free Press, New York.
6. Fox, B. N. (1978): Premorbid psychological factors as related to cancer incidence. *J. Behav. Med.,* 1:45–133.
7. Fraumeri, J. F., and Hoover, R. (1977): Immunosurveillance and cancer: Epidemiologic observations. *Natl. Cancer Inst. Monogr.,* 47:121–126.
8. Gore, S. (1978): The effect of social support in moderating the health consequences of unemployment. *J. Health Soc. Behav.,* 19:157–165.
9. Green, W. A. (1966): The psychosocial setting of the development of leukemia and lymphoma. *Ann. N.Y. Acad. Sci.,* 125:794–801.
10. Haenzel, W., Loveland, D. B. and Sirken, N. (1962): Lung cancer as related to residence and smoking histories. I. White males. *J. Natl. Cancer Inst.,* 28:947–1001.
11. Herring, R. A. (1936): The relationship of marital status in females to mortality from cancer of the breast, female genital organs and other sites: A statistical study. *Am. Soc. Control Cancer Bull.,* 18:4–9.
12. Hexter, A. (1977): *Parameter Estimation in the Synthetic Retrospective Study.* Unpublished Ph.d. dissertation, University of California, Berkeley.

13. Jacob, S., and Ostfeld, A. (1977): An epidemiological review of the mortality of bereavement. *Psychosom. Med.,* 39:344–357.
14. Kissen, D. M. (1966): The significance of personality in lung cancer in men. *Ann. N.Y. Acad. Sci.,* 125:820–826.
15. Kraus, A. S., and Lilienfeld, A. M. (1959): Some epidemiological aspects of the high mortality rate of the young widowed group. *J. Chronic Dis.,* 10:207–127.
16. LeShan, L. (1966): An emotional life-history pattern associated with neoplastic disease. *Ann. N.Y. Acad. Sci.,* 125:780–793.
17. LeShan, L., and Worthington, R. E. (1956): Personality as a factor in the pathogenesis of cancer. A review of the literature. *Br. J. Med. Psychol.,* 29:49–56.
18. Lilienfeld, A. M. (1976): *Foundations of Epidemiology.* Oxford University Press, New York.
19. Lilienfeld, A. M., Levine, M. L., and Kessler, I. I. (1972): *Cancer in the United States.* Harvard University Press, Cambridge, Mass.
20. Lin, N., Simeone, R. S., Ensel, W. N., and Kuo, W. (1979): Social support, stressful life events, and illness: A model and empirical test. *J. Health Soc. Behav.,* 20:108–119.
21. Lombard, H. L., and Potter, E. (1950): Epidemiological aspects of cancer of the cervix. *Cancer,* 3:960–969.
22. Mantel, N. (1973): Synthetic retrospective studies and related topics. *Biometrics,* 29:479–486.
23. Marmot, M. G., and Syme, S. L. (1976): Acculturation and coronary heart disease in Japanese-Americans. *Am. J. Epidemiol.,* 104:225–247.
24. Mausner, J. B., and Bahn, A. K. (1974): *Epidemiology.* W. B. Saunders, Philadelphia.
25. McNeill, D. N. (1973): *Mortality Among the Widowed in Connecticut.* Unpublished M.P.H. essay. Yale University, New Haven.
26. Miller, N. E., Førde, O. H., Thelle, D. S., and Mjøs, O. D. (1977): The Fromsø heart-study: High-density lipoprotein and coronary heart-disease: A prospective case-control study. *Lancet,* 1:965–968.
27. Mitchell, J. C. (1969): *Social Networks in Urban Situations.* University of Manchester Press, Manchester, England.
28. Moss, A. (1979): *Specific Risk Versus General Susceptibility: Social and Psychological Risk Factors for Heart Disease and Cancer Mortality in a Nine-year Prospective Study.* Unpublished Ph.D. dissertation. University of California, Berkeley.
29. Nuckolls, K., Cassel, J., and Kaplan, B. (1972): Psychosocial assets, life crises and the prognosis of pregnancy. *Am. J. Epidemiol.,* 95:431–441.
30. Paffenbarger, R. S., and Asnes, D. P. (1966): Chronic disease in former college students. III. Precursors of suicide in early and middle life. *Am. J. Public Health,* 56:1026–1036.
31. Paffenbarger, R. S., King, S. H., and Wing, A. L. (1969): Chronic disease in former college students. IV. Characteristics in youth that predispose to suicide and accidental death in later life. *Am. J. Public Health,* 59:900–908.
32. Parkes, C. M., Benjamin, B., and Fitzgerald, R. G. (1965): Broken heart: A statistical study of increased mortality among widowers. *Br. Med. J.,* 2:740–743.
33. Peller, S. (1940): Cancer and its relation to pregnancy, to delivery and marital and social status. *Surg. Gynecol. Obstet.,* 71:1–8, 181–186.
34. Phillips, R. L., and Kuzma, J. W. (1977): Rationale and methods for an epidemiological study among Seventh-Day Adventists. In: *Epidemiology and Cancer Registries in the Pacific Basin.* NCI Monograph 47, U.S. Department of Health, Education and Welfare, Washington, D.C.
35. Prehn, R. T. (1974): Immunological surveillance: Pro and con. *Clin. Immunobiol.,* 2:191–203.
36. *Registrar-General's Decennial Supplement. England and Wales, Part II* (1931): Her Majesty's Stationery Office, London.
37. Satariano, W., and Syme, S. L. (1979): Life change and illness in the elderly: Coping with change. Paper presented at the National Academy of Science Conference on Biology and Behavior, Woods Hole, Mass., June 22–24.
38. Schmale, A. (1958): Relationship of separation and depression to disease. *Psychosom. Med.,* 20:259 ff.
39. Schmale, A., and Iker, H. (1966): The psychological setting of uterine cervical cancer. *Ann. N.Y. Acad. Sci.,* 125:807–813.
40. Shurtleff, D. (1955): Mortality and marital status. *Public Health Rep.,* 70:248–252.
41. Snell, L., and Graham, S. (1971): Social trauma as related to cancer of the breast. *Br. J. Cancer,* 25:721–736.

42. Syme, S. L., Borhani, N. O., and Beuchley, R. W. (1966): Cultural mobility and the occurrence of coronary heart disease. *J. Health Hum. Behav.,* 6:178–189.
43. Thomas, C. B., and Duszynski, K. R. (1974): Closeness to parents and the family constellation in a prospective study of five disease states: Suicide, mental illness, malignant tumor, hypertension and coronary heart disease. *Johns Hopkins Med. J.,* 134:251–270.

Psychosocial Aspects of Cancer,
edited by Jerome Cohen et al.
Raven Press, New York © 1982.

Chapter 15

Stress and Coping as Factors in Health and Illness

Richard S. Lazarus

*Department of Psychology, University of California, Berkeley,
Berkeley, California 94720*

Psychosomatic medicine, which made an enthusiastic beginning in the 1920s, had lost much ground as a scientific discipline by the mid-1950s. As Lipowski puts it, "The field suffered a sharp drop in popularity and credibility and seemed to be heading for the annals of medical history" (43, p. 235). Fortunately, in recent years there has been a remarkable revival of interest and activity in the links between stress phenomena and disease. We now seem again at the threshold of making important advances in our understanding of the complex relationships on the one hand between stress processes and, on the other, adaptational outcomes such as somatic illness, social functioning, and morale (see also 12,13,58). In the current revival of interest, however, all disease, including cancer, is being considered as potentially psychosomatic in the cause-and-effect sense, the main restriction being that any single disease is also considered to have multiple causes and that the case for psychological and social causation in cancer must be proved.

This chapter is designed to examine some important issues underlying the relationship of stress and these adaptational outcomes from the perspective of psychological stress theory. We include social functioning and morale among relevant outcomes which must be considered along with somatic ones because a positive outcome in one area frequently occurs at the expense of a positive outcome in another, as when denial or avoidance through heavy drinking helps to maintain morale, but at the expense of physical health and social functioning. Furthermore, this chapter considers illness generally, rather than cancer specifically, on the reasonable assumption that whatever applies to the former is also relevant to the latter, although the specifics will vary.

Author's note: Portions of this chapter were originally prepared for publication elsewhere.

Certain broad independent issues stand out as particularly interesting, important, and underdeveloped with respect to an examination of stress and coping as factors in health and illness—namely, how mediating cognitions, emotions, and coping processes, respectively, affect such adaptational outcomes, and how research should be designed to evaluate such effects. These topics will be taken up in order, but the subject of coping, because of its extraordinary importance in life-threatening illnesses such as cancer, will receive the greatest attention.

MEDIATING COGNITIONS

The key feature that distinguishes psychological stress from stress at the social and physiological levels is the assumption that cognitive activity—evaluative perceptions, thoughts, and inferences—is used by the person to interpret and guide every adaptational interchange with the environment. The person appraises each ongoing and changing transaction (or bit of commerce) with the environment with respect to its significance for his or her well-being. This appraisal includes judgments (conscious or unconscious) about environmental demands and constraints as well as about the person's resources and options for managing them. At the human level, cognitive appraisal processes are complex and symbolic, permitting us to distinguish among actual harm-loss, (future) threat, and challenge, and to make many other subtle cognitive distinctions that give our lives their highly rich and complex emotional qualities.

There is elaborate empirical support for the mediating role of cognitive processes in psychological stress (32,33,35,36). The general principle seems not to be greatly challenged or held in doubt by most recent writers (10,11,45). However, the nature of the link among cognitive processes, adaptational behavior, and physiological outcomes remains obscure. It is here that some of the most interesting and significant research issues concerning the role of stress in somatic illness, social functioning, and morale appear to lie. We shall concentrate on whether different dimensions of appraisal have different adaptational consequences.

First it is necessary to distinguish carefully between the actual nature of a potentially stressful circumstance and the matter of appraising that event. Many of the research reports now available do not make this distinction. Thus Holmes and Masuda (26) see illness as the result of the general mobilization required in order to adapt to the change, and do not address separately the psychological valence of the change itself. The assumption is that individual appraisal of the nature of these events is not relevant or does not vary enough to contribute to differences in adaptive consequences.

Selye (59) has made a distinction between "good" stressors, such as commitment to accomplishment, and "bad" ones, such as frustration and resentment. In our terms, these are not stressors, but reactions whose nature depends on the appraisal of transactions with the environment. Further, the same event or set of circumstances (e.g., an examination) could clearly be seen as a "good" stressor by one person and a "bad" stressor by another. Some persons appear to appraise environmental demands as largely threatening while others, seeing mainly a positive potential in engaging them, appraise such demands as challenging. Although the environmental conditions themselves may provide a basis for this difference in cognitive appraisal, personality factors seem also to be important; that is, some persons feel more frequently challenged while others most often feel threatened.

The possibility that threat and challenge have different adaptational outcomes makes the distinction in this example important. The "common sense" expectation would be that those who are disposed to see environmental demands in positive rather than threatening terms have two major advantages. First, they are apt to have higher morale than those who feel threatened, since they can see things in a positive light even when others would be dysphoric; second, they are likely to perform better under pressure because they are more confident, less emotionally overwhelmed, and more capable of drawing on their resources than those who are inhibited or blocked.

There are, however, some arguments against this common sense view of differences in cognitive appraisal. Clinical observers often assume that the person who seems to think positively is actually involved in self-deception, using denial or reaction formation as a defense. Such defenses could conceal conflicted inner states and actually increase the individual's psychological vulnerability. Moreover, self-deception may require considerable adaptational energy, as expressed in Otto Fenichel's lovely phrase, "silent internal tasks" (15). These tasks supposedly leave the individual with reduced energy resources, a clinical syndrome once referred to as neurasthenia.

These negative outcomes of defensively positive thinking may indeed occur in some persons, but the empirical case is not strong. Even less empirical support can be generated for the alternative proposition that challenge appraisals result in more benign or protective somatic processes than do threat appraisals. Thus at present it is still an open question whether health, morale, and social functioning are harmed by or benefit from an accent on the positive in the face of demanding or unfavorable life conditions.

EMOTION

Emotions are intricately intertwined with the processes of cognitive appraisal and coping. For example, the way a person construes (appraises) his or her plight influences the quality and intensity of the emotional reaction. How effectively a person copes with troubled social relationships, and with associated affective distress and somatic disturbance, also influences that reaction. Moreover, the relationship between cognitive activity and emotion also operates in the other direction, as when strong emotions interfere with adaptive thought and skilled performance, alter the appraised significance of what is happening, or serve as rewards and punishments that have current emotional as well as developmental significance.

There have been two major approaches to the study of the link between emotion and somatic illness: the generality model and the specificity model. The generality model assumes that the nature of the stress itself and the particular forms of coping used are less important than the general mobilization accompanying any emotion; it is this mobilization which precipitates tissue damage or increased vulnerability to illness through the direct and indirect effects of associated neuroendocrine activity.

Psychosomatic medicine, however, actually began with a version of the specificity model. It held that each illness—hypertension, gastric ulcers, colitis, or whatever—has its own distinctive stress dynamics (2,43). Faulty management or discharge of anger, for example, was said to be implicated in hypertension, whereas concealment of dependency urges predisposed the person to duodenal ulcers. The logic of this position is not unreasonable if one assumes, for example, that psychodynamic variations can lead to different chronic or recurrent emotional patterns and, further, that different emotions have distinguishable physiological response patterns.

The argument over generality and specificity has continued through the last several decades. In the 1950s and 1960s the generality position was still being seriously entertained, although it was losing ground as new research began to suggest that there were different emotional correlates of epinephrine and norepinephrine, and divergent patterns of autonomic nervous system end-organ response. The dominant outlook today, moreover, seems to favor a strong generality position. One reason for this is the seminal influence of Selye. Another is the weakness of the early research on specificity, for example, data linking fear to epinephrine secretion and anger to norepinephrine (17). A third is that autonomic nervous system patterns in these emotions have been shown to be highly overlapping. Still another is a view which is probably incorrect, that is, emotion considered as a generalized form of arousal, distinguished qualitatively only by the cognitive label a person puts on the situation; in effect, if one is aroused in an anger-centered situation, one thinks and feels anger, whereas the same arousal in a euphoric situation is labeled and felt as euphoria (57). Such a stance, however, equates emotion with the external social context and fails to deal with the internal mediating psychological processes that shape emotion. Besides, this research did not test whether or not these emotion–context patterns had similar physiological response profiles.

Evidence that general arousal theory is wrong or at least overstated comes from a number of important directions. First, studies involving more than one autonomic end-organ reaction have demonstrated negligible or very low correlations between them. For example, when skin conductance goes up, heart rate or blood pressure may or may not be dropping. Lacey's impressive work on the specificity of autonomic end-organ reactions to different types of stressful situations (31) should have brought about the demise of general activation theory. Lacey showed, among other things, that although skin conductance always rose under stimulating or stressful conditions, heart rate rose simultaneously when a person was seeking to avoid stimulus input or trying to engage in mental work despite interference from the outside, but fell sharply just before the occurrence of an anticipated, time-locked stimulus. In effect, somatic responses may reflect the psychological impact of the person–environment relationship. At best, the relationships among diverse physiological measures are also quite modest (41). Such findings fail to support activation or arousal theory.

One reason that the case for specificity has not impressed researchers and theoreticians on the psychophysiology of emotion is methodological. Because of technological complications and high costs, the laboratory has tended to study either autonomic end-organ reactions using electrophysiological instruments, or catecholamines by means of blood or urine measures, or corticosteroids also assessed in the blood or urine. Rarely if ever does a single laboratory simultaneously examine somatic patterning across multiple hormonal or organ systems, that is, catecholamines and corticosteroids and autonomic nervous system reactions.

Thus, although it is not a distortion to state that the present evidence is weak for somatic response specificity in qualitatively different emotions such as fear, anger, depression, guilt, anxiety, joy, love, or exhilaration, it would indeed be cavalier to assert that the whole body responds in essentially the same way regardless of the emotion involved. Such a claim would require that research include multiple somatic response systems and multiple research settings, and entail better methods for assessing the quality of an emotional response and of the changing patterns of emotion and coping activity occurring in the ordinary course of adaptation. Nothing approaching this has been done until recently by Mason (48) and Mason and colleagues (49), whose work we shall discuss below.

These endocrine researchers have provided a useful model for how the relationships among emotion, coping processes, and somatic response patterns might be profitably addressed. They obtained measures of many different endocrines and assessed their profile of response to a variety of physical stressors in both monkeys and humans. Physical stressors such as heat, cold, exercise, and fasting were compared, and particular efforts were made to control for any psychological threats that might have been confounded with these physical stressors. For example, any sudden change of temperature was avoided in the heat and cold situation; and in fasting, the experimental monkeys were given placebos in order to prevent the psychological distress they would have experienced on seeing the other animals being fed. In the human exercise situation, threats connected with doing poorly or with perceived physiological reactions were eliminated or at least reduced by keeping the exercise demand modest.

Two findings are of interest: first, corticosteroid output in the absence of psychologically based threat did not necessarily rise with physical stressors;

second, a different profile of hormonal response was found for each type of physical stressor. In short, there was a high degree of stimulus specificity, but little evidence of an overall, general response as predicted by Selye's General Adaptation Syndrome theory.

Mason has not yet tested systematically the relationships between hormonal patterns and specific emotional response qualities, although he is convinced that his data suggest such relationships will be found (Mason, *personal communication*). He has studied the hormonal response of monkeys in situations that should have quite distinctive psychological implications, for example, those characterized by unpredictability and which generate coping efforts. The inferred psychological factors seem to produce distinctive hormonal secretion patterns. Summarizing this work (48), he writes cautiously:

> Research on psychological stimuli has so far, then, yielded only preliminary and limited indications that different, relatively specific emotional states may be correlated with different, specific patterns of multiple hormonal responses, although several promising leads along these lines appear worthy of further study.

Clearly, what is needed is research designs in a variety of environmental contexts using a sufficient diversity of somatic response measures to construct patterns or profiles while simultaneously varying the key mediating psychological processes in stress, emotion, and illness, including appraisal, coping, and the emotion quality (32,34). We think future research will show that quite divergent, although perhaps overlapping, somatic response patterns are associated with different emotional states. Such findings would again bring to the fore the earlier notion that psychodynamic factors do have causal significance in individual differences in psychosomatic disease etiology.

There is another fascinating aspect to the generality-specificity issue that has received little serious attention, and yet is potentially of great importance. It is a variant of the distinction made earlier in this chapter between positively toned and negatively toned emotions. There has been some interest in positive emotions but mainly from the standpoint of psychological well-being or marital happiness. However, the unresolved practical issue implied in this discussion is whether or not adaptation is affected by the positive emotions which enter or predominate in a person's life. It is widely assumed (although not conclusively demonstrated) that negatively toned emotions may result not only in low morale and social disability, but also in diseases of adaptation through the hormones they produce. Our question is whether positive emotions might have the opposite—that is, a positive or constructive—effect at the physiological as well as the social and psychological levels, possibly helping to prevent, ameliorate, or cure stress-linked disorders.

Norman Cousins, former editor of the *Saturday Review,* has raised this provocative question in an article in the *New England Journal of Medicine* (9) in which he describes his bout with a collagen disease the normal course of which is severe and rapid deterioration. He suggests that his self-generated program of laughter and positive affect significantly helped him to overcome his illness. Although recognizing that such a single case could have little scientific validity, he writes engagingly of this as follows:

> The inevitable question arose in my mind: What about the positive emotions? If negative emotions produce negative chemical changes in the body, wouldn't the positive emotions produce positive chemical changes? Is it possible that love, hope, faith, laughter, confidence and the will to live have therapeutic value? Do chemical changes occur only on the downside?

The idea suggested by Cousins is, of course, not new. It forms part of the belief system of the field commonly referrred to as "holistic medicine," the essence of which is to emphasize the whole person rather than the diseased tissues per se. It is found in most or all of the current crop of inspirational guides to living through relaxation, meditation, and the search for a greater sense of unity and connection with the environment. Unfortunately, the potential value of this belief system is limited by the failure to test and discover the rules by which ongoing psychological processes such as emotional states affect health and illness. It is time, however, for serious researchers to take up the challenge posed by layman Cousins' well-stated question. We think that there are substantial theoretical and empirical grounds for believing that such research could yield important insights into psychosomatic theory and practice.

In the above discussion of the links between emotions and physiological responses, we have been talking about short-range outcomes—momentary or acute changes in physiological functioning due to psychological stress or emotional states. However, mammals are constructed to be capable of "emergency reactions." Although such reactions in themselves are not disease, one important issue is whether they are, as Levi and Kagan (42) have intimated, "precursors" of disease. For example, blood pressure can rise sharply under stress, but hypertension represents a long-term change in tissue activity. Similarly, duodenal ulcer and colitis are diseased tissue states, and many diseases involve irreversible changes. The crucial question here concerns the process by which an acute, short-range emergency reaction or pattern of physiological mobilization becomes transformed into chronic or recurrent disease. The answer to this question is really not known, since research has not been designed to attack concurrently both the psychosocial and physiological processes contributing to illness and the emergence, exacerbation, or cessation of illness.

Epidemiological studies using such longer-range outcomes have shown the importance of psychosocial factors in rates of disease and overall mortality. For example, Marmot and Syme (47) demonstrated the importance of acculturation among Japanese-Americans in explaining differential rates of myocardial infarction and angina pectoris. Low socioeconomic status has repeatedly been found to be a risk factor for many diseases, as has the status of being unmarried (65). Bereavement, too, has been cited as an antecedent of many diseases. In fact, the evidence supporting these psychosocial variables as risk factors in widely varying disease outcomes has led at least one investigator, Syme (64), to propose that such an observation supports a generality model. It is Syme's contention that these psychosocial factors as well as others create a raised susceptibility to all disease.

The problem with this idea, in our view, is that it leaves unexamined the mechanisms underlying such phenomena as increased or decreased probability of illness that may accompany low socioeconomic status, acculturation, or being unmarried. After all, all three of these imply a large number of associated psychological and social factors that might be at work in producing the relationship to illness. What is needed is research which would establish the link between the correlations observed among momentary or acute phenomena and longer range, population relationships. This "missing link" has been remarked on by a number of researchers, including Luborsky et al. (44), Stahl et al. (62), Herd (24), and Lazarus (35). The case is most easily made for the example of hypertensive cardiovascular disease, where, to quote Herd:

> We have some knowledge concerning the mechanisms whereby psychological processes may influence cardiovascular function during short periods of time. However, we do not know the mechanisms whereby a susceptibility to transient elevations in blood pressure may convert to sustained arterial hypertension. Finally, we do not know what psychological and physiological characteristics might predispose an individual to develop hypertensive cardiovascular disease when exposed to certain environmental situations over long periods of time.

Omitted here is the possibility that recurrent or stable psychological characteristics, regardless of the environmental situation, entail certain physiological consequences which might eventually result in disease. If, for example, one observed repeated patterns of appraisal, emotion, or coping among the same individuals over time and across diverse environmental situations, one might find that, depending on the content of the repetitious behavior, this group of individuals also had distinctive adaptational outcomes. This is one way to conceptualize the possible connection between momentary or acute phenomena and longer range or chronic disease-related ones. Discovery of such mechanisms requires certain measurement and design innovations which we will discuss later under methodological issues.

COPING PROCESSES

It is beginning to be widely recognized that coping processes, set in motion when a person is having a stressful transaction, greatly affect adaptational outcomes at the social and physiological levels, including the prospect of somatic illness. Some coping processes can increase the risk of maladaptation or illness whereas others decrease it, although the psychophysiological mechanisms underlying these effects are far from clear.

COPING AND INCREASED RISK OF ILLNESS

There are at least three ways in which coping can add to the risk of social, psychological, or physical malfunctioning. The first is by direct damage to tissues. Obvious examples of this include smoking, drinking, overeating, and undereating. Such behavior, often generated as ways of dealing with stressful conditions of life, can result in damage to morale or social relationships or in physiological damage, e.g., to the liver, lungs, or the cardiovascular system—which in turn may increase general vulnerability to disease or directly result in disease itself, as in esophageal or lung cancer or cirrhosis of the liver.

A second way is more indirect and involves the bodily effects on the internal milieu of the mobilization often required for coping. Epidemiological research implicates such mobilization under conditions of life stress in disorders such as hypertension (52,63). The well-known findings concerning the relationship between type A behavior and coronary heart disease belong in this category (54). Type A behavior is a coping response arising from the socialization process in a society emphasizing the Protestant ethic. Note that type A behavior is an extremely stable, self-induced response in individuals exemplifying it. We can speculate that it is the repeated physiological mobilization associated with this behavior pattern which leads to the bodily changes that eventually result in increased risk of coronary disease and infarction. Research is just beginning on the situations that do or do not elicit type A behavior, the physiological mechanisms linking it to the long-term atherosclerotic process, and the immediate, short-term events surrounding a heart attack (20).

In any case, the hormonal secretions that accompany mobilization can cause direct damage, as in one element of Selye's General Adaptation Syndrome (GAS) triad of the alarm stage, namely, ulceration of the gastrointestinal tract (60); or they can cause indirect damage, as illustrated by another GAS element, shrinkage of the thymus gland and reduction in the number of lymphocytes in the blood. This mechanism, which weakens the capability of the immune system to resist infection, thereby increasing the likelihood of illness, is favored by some (6) in explaining the damaging effects of unfavorable social relationships on morbidity and mortality.

Less obvious is a third mode of effect in which coping processes interfere with adaptive behaviors that could help preserve life or normal adaptive functioning. Katz et al. (30) have observed many women who, on finding a suspicious breast lump, denied its serious health implications and delayed seeking medical attention. Similar observations have been made by Von Kugelgen (66) with respect to men experiencing the symptoms of a heart attack. And Hackett and Cassem (21) have described cases of men who, during a heart attack, did vigorous pushups or ran up a flight of stairs, reasoning that they could not be experiencing a heart attack since the exertion did not cause their death. These palliative uses of coping, that is, those whose function is to decrease feelings of threat and distress, increase the vulnerability of these persons to truly life-threatening illness by interfering with or delaying actions that might save or prolong their lives. Similar examples could be cited of palliative coping which interferes with psychological health or social relationships.

COPING AND DECREASED RISK OF ILLNESS

The major reason why coping has been gaining center stage in the study of stress and illness is the growing evidence that some forms of coping decrease morbidity and mortality. In effect, they appear to reduce vulnerability or are highly beneficial to the person's well-being. It will be instructive to examine briefly some of the major examples of research that demonstrate this.

Nuckolls et al. (51) obtained information on life stress and psychosocial coping assets from women early in their first pregnancies. The prognosis for pregnancy complications was predicted most accurately for women who had high life crisis scores along with low assets to cope with crisis. On the other hand, women with equally high life stress levels who were characterized by high psychosocial assets had only one-third the complication rate of their peers with low psychosocial assets.

Other studies, while also not addressing the mechanisms by which somatic illness might have been influenced, nevertheless demonstrate quite clearly the potent role of coping. One of the most interesting is a study by Aldrich and Mendkoff (1) of coping and mortality in aged persons who were moved from one institution to another. In this type of dislocation it is customary to find great increases in mortality rates (53), and indeed this was observed by Aldrich and Mendkoff. However, when the ways in which these aged people coped with the dislocation were taken into account, large differences in mortality rates were noted. Those who did most poorly were the manifestly psychotic, and those responding with depression were not far behind. The lowest mortality rates were found for persons who reacted to the move philosophically, and nearly as favorable rates were observed for those who responded with anger; so it is not just a matter of controlled arousal. It is quite possible that the major mechanism underlying these relationships involved life maintenance behavior, such as eating and caring for themselves in other ways, rather than the hormonal secretions associated with mobilization for coping with stress. Although the mechanisms remain obscure, again we see the profound consequences that coping has for somatic health/illness, in this case operating on the most severe criterion of adaptation, survival itself.

In another study of coping, Cohen and Lazarus (8) assessed how patients were coping with the threat of surgery the night before their operation. The interviewer determined how much the patient knew about the illness, the nature of the surgery, and the extent to which information was sought or avoided. Patients were found to vary greatly, from one extreme of avoidance to the other extreme of vigilant search for information. The score on this "dimension" of coping was then related to a variety of measures of outcome, including the number of days spent in the hospital, the extent of negative psychological reactions, pain medication, and minor medical complications. The vigilant group showed a poorer picture of postoperative recovery than the avoiders, especially in regard to the outcome criteria of number of days in the hospital and the extent of minor complications.

If we ask why the avoiders should have the best postsurgical outcome, one possible speculation is that continual vigilance to signals of trouble and search for active ways of coping are likely to lead nowhere in the hospital setting, where passivity and conformity are highly valued and where literally nothing constructive can be done through efforts at active mastery. In a postsurgical hospital stay, as perhaps distinguished from other stressful contexts, avoidant modes of coping seem to be a more adaptive solution than are vigilant modes. Here, too, the psychophysiological mechanisms involved are unknown. It is possible that the difference in recovery indices for the two groups reflects more on features of the institutional setting and on social behavior than on hormonal or other tissue processes. For example, physicians may be quicker to release patients who are anxious to leave and who seem comfortable than those who are vigilant worriers. And since in this hospital pain medication was given more or less on demand, we would expect that avoiders demanded less medication than did the vigilant patients. In sum, assuming the replicability of this finding, a variety of biological, social, and psychological mechanisms could easily be operating.

Another illustration of the role of coping comes from recent research by Weisman and Worden (69) with patients suffering from advanced cancer. These researchers were interested in differences in coping between two groups of patients: those who survived longer than expected on the basis of the severity of the disease, and those whose outcomes were unexpectedly poor. Weisman and Worden found that longevity depended heavily on coping. For example, survival was longer among patients "who could maintain active and mutually responsive relationships, provided that the intensity of demands was not so extreme as to alienate people responsible for the patient's care." On the other hand, survival was poorer for patients who showed long-standing alienation, deprivation, and depression and maintained destructive relationships with others extending into the terminal stages of the illness. The latter group displayed these social and interpersonal difficulties in despondency, desire to die, contemplation of suicide, and inordinate complaints, all of which increased their isolation and feelings of self-defeat.

Here, too, as in the Aldrich and Mendkoff study (1), the psychophysiological mechanisms underlying earlier or delayed death were not assessed. Moreover, behavioral and social processes may offer good prospects for understanding health outcome. That is, they may have to do with coping behavior that is damaging to health, such as failing to do what is necessary for survival as opposed to increasing or ameliorating the destructive effect of the hormonal secretions associated with stress emotions. Present evidence does not permit us to determine the mechanisms operating in these relationships between coping and adaptational outcomes or even to be sure of the cause-and-effect link between them. Nevertheless, a considerable body of observation suggests strongly that coping processes are central factors in adaptational outcome.

Several studies seem to indicate that successful coping can affect levels of stress hormone production which, if elevated chronically or repeatedly over a long time, might produce "diseases of adaptation." One example is a study by Wolff et al. (70) of coping in parents facing the tragedy and stress of having a child dying of leukemia. Through psychological assessment, the parents were rated on the extent to which they were well defended (usually through various forms of avoidance or denial), and a high correlation was found between this rating and corticosteroid production. The most well-defended parents showed the lowest levels of adrenal cortical hormone production during the period preceding the death of the child. Although unfortunately this study confounded the measure of coping with evidence of distress, it does support the idea that successful coping can be inversely related to the somatic stress response. Later studies (25) of the same group of parents have suggested that those who showed low corticosteroid levels before the child died were more disturbed 6 months later, which raises the question about the costs of coping and highlights the problem of time in evaluating coping outcomes.

Weiner et al. (67) exposed hypertensives and normotensives to an emotional interview and found, paradoxically, that the hypertensives had lower blood pressure than the normotensives during the interview. Clinical assessment suggested that this was the result of a process the authors refer to as "insulation." The hypertensives defended themselves against threatening interactions with the interviewer to which they were especially vulnerable by remaining "consistently impersonal, distant, and wary" (56,61).

We have defined three broad areas that we believe are both interesting and important for an understanding of the relationship between stress and adaptation: mediating cognitions, emotion, and coping. We have also made a number of distinctions and raised issues within each of these areas, namely, the importance of differing appraisals, coping that increases the risk of illness versus coping that decreases it, and the generality-versus-specificity issue, where particular attention was given to the distinction between positive and negative emotions. These distinctions and issues must be explored if we are to understand how psychological stress affects health, illness, morale, and social functioning.

It would be both simplistic and misleading, however, to consider each of these areas separately when in reality they are interdependent. For example, emotion is a response to cognitive appraisal; feelings of fear, guilt, excitement, or exhilaration each follow different cognitive appraisals. Appraisal and emotion, in turn, affect coping by influencing the choice of coping strategy and the effectiveness with which it is utilized. Finally, the feedback about the success of coping influences further appraisals, stimulating the entire process again. When we consider appraisals, emotions, and coping and their relationship to outcomes, we are in fact speaking of a complex, interrelated set of ongoing processes; these processes must be examined if we are to understand how psychological factors mediate the relationship between person and environment, and between stress and adaptational outcomes. Such psychodynamic research requires certain approaches in measurement and design which are addressed in the next section.

FUNCTIONS OF COPING

One major difference I have with the cognitive behavior therapists and with the traditional psychiatric approach is with respect to their assumption that the best coping strategies are necessarily "realistic." If one assumes that the pathology of emotional life rests on false or irrational beliefs about life, then therapy must try to make such beliefs realistic, and coping must ultimately be predicated on the accurate testing of reality. One can agree, of course, that action undertaken in order to change a troubled relationship with the environment (or deliberate *in*action, sometimes mislabeled "passivity") is often of crucial importance to the outcome, especially under conditions in which there is some possibility of preventing the harmful confrontation. However, in encounters in which little or nothing can be done even when we have obtained all the available information about a problem, living optimally or even adequately requires a high tolerance for ambiguity, or even that we engage in some self-deception (23). Therefore, to the problem-solving or instrumental function of coping we must add another important function, in a sense the antithesis of instrumentality, namely, the self-regulation of emotional distress.

Two major functions of coping must therefore be considered: first, to change the situation for the better if we can, either by changing one's own offending action (focus on self) or by changing the damaging or threatening environment; and second, to manage the somatic and subjective components of stress-related emotions themselves, so that they do not get out of hand and do not damage or destroy morale and social functioning. These functions are sometimes, but not always, contradictory, and when they are there is danger of maladaptation. For example, we make ourselves feel better in the face of harm or threat by palliative modes of coping, such as by denying, intellectualizing (achieving detachment), avoiding negative thoughts, or taking drugs (e.g., alcohol, pain killers, and tranquilizers). These make us feel better although they do not change the actual person-environment relationship. Under certain conditions, when such palliative modes of coping do not countermand needed adaptive actions, they may help greatly.

Although the two functions of coping—problem solving and regulation of emotional distress—are sometimes in opposition, especially when the palliative function preempts adaptationally necessary actions, often one supports the other. For example, if one is not too distressed during an examination or a performance before an audience (through the use of a tranquilizer or some intrapsychic process that lowers anxiety), performance can be much improved or at least less impaired. Since we know little about normal optimal functioning, we may make the unfounded assumption that palliation is necessarily pathological because it produces poor adaptational outcomes, when it is quite possible that such a generalization does not apply to people who are getting along well. It is therefore a worthwhile hypothesis that, despite the high value our society places on reality testing and direct action, effective copers typically engage in forms of coping that achieve both of these functions, and that effective copers use both direct actions and palliative coping modes.

The Alcoholics Anonymous "Serenity Prayer" captures this theme well. It states: "God grant me the serenity to accept the things I cannot change, courage to change the things I can, and the wisdom to know the difference." A cynic might substitute for the last phrase, "and the good luck not to foul up too often."

Emotions are not always negative or pathological, as is widely assumed in psychology and psychiatry in general; there is no room in such an analysis for positively toned emotions, nor is their value in general adaptation given widespread credence. If we obtain our understanding exclusively from the clinical context of maladaptation, we are in danger of maintaining a one-sided and incorrect conception of effective adaptation as manifested in the lives of people who have never been in treatment. A fuller understanding and appreciation of normal, ordinary adaptation, and even optimal adaptation, requires that we learn much more about the ways people and peoples in our society manage their lives, and about the place of both positive and negative emotional experiences in their lives. This is a theme that my colleagues and I have strongly expressed elsewhere (39).

COPING MODES

In a recent treatment of coping (40) four main coping modes were identified, each serving both problem-solving and emotion-regulatory functions, each capable of being oriented to the self or the environment, and each concerned with either past or present (harm/loss) or future (threat or challenge). The four modes are information seeking, direct action, inhibition of action, and intrapsychic processes.

Information seeking involves scanning the characteristics of a stressful encounter for knowledge needed to make a sound coping decision or to reappraise the damage or threat. In addition to providing a basis for action (problem-solving function), information seeking can also have the function of making the person feel better by rationalizing or bolstering a past decision (27,28). Ironically, this palliative function is contrary to the assumptions usually made about decision making by information-processing researchers (16). Palliation often calls for ignoring the negative implications of what one knows or of information one receives or seeks. Moreover, the regulation of emotional distress often requires accepting ambiguity (the obverse of information) as a natural feature of living. At times such ambiguity or uncertainty can be a balm rather than a source of anxiety.

For example, it is no accident, nor is it necessarily a self-protective conspiracy, for a physician not to provide all the gruesome details of the patient's condition, including the recovery process after surgery and what could go wrong, a negative prognosis, a statement of the probable duration of life in a terminal illness, and so on. When little can be done to change the situation, the preservation of uncertainty can facilitate hope, morale, and involvement with living and help the person tolerate or relieve pain and emotional distress. On the other hand, failure to be totally honest can also do great damage in ultimately destroying credibility or preventing the patient from coming to terms with death or some other distressing fate. Therefore, the recognition that uncertainty can be used positively should not be read as a prescription for professional deception.

The most sensitive physicians look to the patient for cues about what is needed, cues that are presented when the patient turns away from further information that is tentatively proffered or seeks to pin down what is happening more precisely. Such physicians also know that what might be avoided or sought at one point in the personal crisis might change at a later point. Still, we must not forget that there are other ways of coping with threat than wanting to know all, and that the uncertainty afforded a patient by a lack of detailed information can have utility in his or her overall coping strategy. We know too little about the probably wide variation in successful patterns of coping to make the unequivocal assumption that accurate reality testing is always best for all persons and under all conditions.

Anything one does (except cognitively) to handle stressful transactions falls within the rubric of direct action. Such actions are as diverse as the environmental demands and personal goals people have to manage, including expressing anger, seeking revenge, fleeing, committing suicide, building storm shelters, taking medication, jogging to preserve health, and the like. The list is virtually endless. Direct coping actions can be aimed at the self or the environment, since either is potentially capable of being changed, thereby altering the stressful person-environment relationship for the better. The action can be aimed at overcoming a past injury, as when a grieving person becomes buried in work or seeks a new love relationship, or at a future danger. In the light of their great importance in human adaptation, too little attention has been devoted to anticipatory coping actions.

It may seem strange to cite inhibition of action as a coping mode since it implies inaction, but effective coping often calls for holding back action impulses that will do harm rather than taking action that poorly fits the requirements of a transaction. In a complicated social and intrapsychic world, every type of action is capable of coming into conflict with moral, social, or physical constraints and dangers, and choice is possible only if strong natural impulses to act (as in anger and fear) can be held back in the interest of other values.

All the cognitive processes designed to regulate emotion—the things people say to themselves, as it were—are included in intrapsychic modes, making this, too, a highly varied category. Not only does it encompass self-deceptive mechanisms or defenses, such as denial, reaction formation, and projection, but it also includes avoidance and efforts to obtain detachment or insulation from a threat in order to achieve a feeling of control over it. These modes are mostly palliative in that they make the person feel better by reducing or minimizing emotional distress. As in the case of the other coping modes, they can be oriented to the past (as in the reinterpretation of a traumatic event) or to the future (as in the denial that one is in danger). They can also be focused on the self ("I am not adequate or evil") or on the environment ("The symptom is not a danger").

DIFFICULTIES IN ASSESSING COPING

The assessment of coping processes requires strategies of measurement and research that are quite different from those employed by personality assessors to measure coping styles or traits. One must develop means of describing what the person is doing and thinking in specific encounters. Most measures of coping currently available are trait oriented, that is, they inquire about what a person usually does rather than what he or she did in a specific encounter (50). They are also usually focused on a limited class of coping modes, for example, specific intrapsychic dimensions such as repression-sensitization or, in some cases, a cluster of intrapsychic or defensive modes. Almost never do they cover the full ground of the four modes cited above, namely, information search, direct action, inhibition of action, and intrapsychic processes.

There are a number of difficult problems to face if one is to assess coping as it takes place (as a process) in naturalistic settings. A few of the major ones will be treated here, albeit briefly: specifically, coping as a constellation of many acts, obtaining information about how people cope, ambiguities in the definition of coping processes, and evaluating coping effectiveness.

Coping as a Constellation of Many Acts

As noted earlier, coping is not a single act but a constellation of many acts and thoughts engendered by a complex set of demands that may stretch over time. There are undoubtedly styles or patterns of coping that are more or less characteristic of an individual, but such styles, too, involve a combination of many acts and thoughts. Thus what is needed is a way of describing the many things a person, or particular kinds of persons, did or thought over the period of an encounter or a series of encounters. Such pattern description could then be used to compare one person or group with themselves and with others. It is one thing, for example, to note that a person used avoidance, denial, or intellectualization, and quite another to be able to describe the pattern of thoughts and acts employed in the different stages of an encounter, contexts, and instances.

A stressful encounter can be relatively simple or quite complex, short-lived, or extended. But even in relatively simple instances, thoughts and actions may be directed toward more than one person, and there is apt to be more than one interchange in which coping thoughts and actions are brought to bear. Before we can summarize what happened through simplifying generalizations, we must be in a position to say which of many possibilities have actually occurred. For example, in a quarrel with a loved one, the person under investigation may have used humor, denial, threats, assaults, anger, martyrdom, attempted detachment, information-seeking, avoidance of implications, self-depreciation, tears, passive dependency, escape from the situation, expressions of love with or without irony or criticism, and so on.

If we, as systematizers of coping, cannot describe these various interpersonal and intrapsychic maneuvers, we will not be able to take the next step of describing the constellation of coping processes used by an individual in any given encounter, whether this takes place over minutes, hours, days, or months. The assessment task requires recording both details and combinations of details as the process unfolds; only then can we abstract about an overall constellation and style. The clinical setting has a tradition of doing this sort of thing. For example, in Berne's transactional analysis (3) types of interchanges are described and given names that reflect the motivation or function of the interpersonal game being played. The problem is not that such description has not been attempted, but that what has been done is not systematic or measurement-oriented so that it can ultimately be used in research on the determinants and adaptational outcomes of coping, or on the measurement of stability and flux of coping patterns across diverse stressful encounters. There is presently no existing method for handling this assessment problem systematically, although my associates and I are currently trying to develop such methods, both for specific encounters and across encounters, intraindividually and interindividually, and to find ways of effectively analyzing ipsative-normative data.

Obtaining Information about How People Cope

We cannot expect most people to tell us how they coped, that is, whether they used denial, intellectualization, or whatever in a given encounter. However, we can ask them to tell us whether they did or thought this or that. For example, they can tell us if they felt the need to act even though such action could not change the situation; if they joked, tried to put a good face on things, saw the situation as hopeless, tried not to think about the problem, and so on. For our research on coping we created checklists describing dozens of such tactics based on our own rational classificatory scheme and on research and clinical reports, and we focus on some specific stressful encounters that our research subject chooses from the immediate past. At the same time, through in-depth interviews we use trained clinicians in order to observe independently and evaluate what, through their observer eyes and ears, they believe the person was doing.

Assessment of the coping process will always have to face the issue of self-report versus observational and inferential sources of knowledge. This issue can be faced only when we are in a position to correlate self-report coping patterns with inferential, observer-based sources. In addition, such patterns can be related to outside criteria, for example, adaptational outcomes such as health/illness, morale, social functioning, general personality descriptions by observers and by the person being studied, and by other criteria such as reported patterns of emotion and appraisals.

Ambiguities in the Definition of Coping Processes

When we speak of denial, avoidance, and other specific intrapsychic coping processes, it is as though we know clearly what these processes are and how they are to be assessed. Such clarity, however, does not exist, and in practice their assessment is filled with ambiguity and confusion. This is easily illustrated in the case of denial and avoidance. The problem has at least two facets, both stemming from faulty conceptualization.

First, denial and avoidance are quite different psychological processes, yet they are easily confused and often hyphenated to suggest similarity. Denial is the attempt to negate a problem; the person states that he or she is not angry, not dying, not in danger, or whatever. Avoidance, on the other hand, accepts the reality of the threat but involves a deliberate effort not to think about it. A person may deny that he or she has a serious illness, or, when such denial becomes impossible, that he or she is not dying, and ultimately, if Weisman (68) is correct, that this does not mean extinction (believing that in some sense he or she will live on). In avoidance, the person does not deny the facts or implications of the illness, but under certain conditions refuses to talk or think about it. The problem is that often in research on the subject, especially when the assessment process is superficial or mechanical, the fact of avoidance may lead the researcher to classify the process as denial although there is really no negation.

Second, and more important, our typical trait-centered, static research paradigm leads us to treat denial as a permanent, established mode of coping, in which case we tend to speak of deniers rather than denying. This is misleading because rarely does a process such as denial become so fully consolidated as a mode of coping that it is no longer subject to uncertainty, challenge, or even dissolution in the face of the evidence. Consider, for example, this familiar scenario that takes place on the cancer ward of a hospital. The patient spends an entire interview giving direct evidence to the clinical worker (physician, psychologist, social worker, nurse) that he is denying his imminent death. The clinician, having listened to the denial-based affirmations, feels sure that the patient is denying. If he or she were a research worker, perhaps studying coping, she might then classify the patient as a denier. Yet almost immediately upon leaving her office and turning a corner of the corridor, the same patient sees another member of the staff whom he knows, and bursts into tears, sobbing and crying out that he is dying. What happened to the denier?

We can offer two kinds of speculation. On the one hand, perhaps, the first clinician tended by his manner and personal vulnerabilities to encourage denial in a manner described insightfully by Hackett and Weisman (22). Physicians, friends, family, and visitors to the dying patient encourage denial by being unable to acknowledge what is happening without evident distress. Instead, they mouth platitudes, protecting themselves but believing they are protecting the patient. They are already distancing themselves somewhat from the person who soon will no longer be around. The patient, already frightened by imminent death, is further threatened with the loss of important human relationships. The sight of a more accepting and less vulnerable person in the corridor releases what is really in his mind. The earlier denial was only skin deep. Weisman (68) has elaborated richly on the concept of "middle knowledge" in which a patient seems to believe one thing on the surface but somehow "knows" at some dim and perhaps even unverbalized level that he or she has cancer, that death is imminent. A second possibility is that in the first interview the patient is really trying to see the situation in favorable terms, that is, he is making an effort at denial, but an unsuccessful one. Having heard his own statements, he is no longer able to believe the self-deception.

Herein lies the conceptual confusion. We treat a process of coping as a static state of mind rather than as a constant search for a way of comprehending what is happening, a way that simultaneously seeks to test reality and retain hope. Depending on the moment, the circumstances, the evidence, the social pressures, the personality, such a construction remains always in flux. Only severely disturbed persons display well-consolidated defenses that consistently resist uprooting. If we look at the problem as a continuous effort at meaning (18,19) we come closer to the way Erikson (14) views the struggle in aging to achieve integrity rather than despair. One does not usually arrive fixedly at one or the other pole of thought, but is constantly in tension between the two. As Erikson (1956) states it:

> . . . identity *formation* neither begins nor ends with adolescence; it is a lifelong development largely unconscious to the individual and to his society . . . an *evolving configuration*—a configuration which is gradually established by successive ego syntheses and resyntheses . . . integrating *constitutional givens, idiosyncratic libidinal needs, favored capacities, significant identifications, effective defenses, successful sublimations, and consistent roles.*

Not only does this idea of constant tension between the polarities—of constant struggle to construe what is happening in one's existence—represent a dramatically different view of coping than the more traditional emphasis on trait, style, or achieved structure, it also calls for a different research strategy. One must observe the coping pattern employed by an individual again and again, at diverse moments, across different types of encounters, and over time in order to make an accurate description. Our mistake has been prematurely to freeze people into postures and styles; not that styles cannot be identified, but that for such a style to be a valid representation, one must study the individual in greater depth and breadth of encounter than is possible in a single sampling, and then be ready to recognize the frequently transient nature of the coping process and pattern.

Evaluating Coping Effectiveness

The final difficulty meriting comment is perhaps the most complex and tenuous of all, and it is also the aspect of adaptation theory that has been given the least attention. The problem is made more simple if we limit ourselves to the reduction of existing pathology, since in the clinical setting we know the person is hurting and relatively ineffectual, and we can perhaps justify any efforts to ameliorate the unwanted symptoms. Even here, however, we may be treading on dangerous ground. For example, those involved in efforts to eliminate type A behavior because it predisposes to greater risk of cardiovascular disease than does the behavior of persons less pressured, aggressive, and achievement-dedicated, often forget that for the type A person the alternative may be to give up a social value to which he or she has made a lifelong commitment in favor of another value which, for that person, is anathema. On the other hand, as the findings of Clark (7) seem to suggest, aging persons who cannot relinquish the forms of coping suitable to youth carry far greater risk of being institutionalized for emotional problems than those who take on coping patterns more suitable for older people.

There is no longer any doubt that values are inextricably tied to the evaluation of coping effectiveness. We have to ask: Coping effectiveness for what? And at what cost? The stakes include somatic health/illness, morale, and social functioning, and sometimes one is achieved at the expense of the other. Thus the virtues of being type A include living up to a deeply entrenched social and personal value, but at the expense of an increased risk of somatic illness. On the other hand, being insulated in human relations might facilitate somatic health but decrease emotional satisfactions and positive involvements that help make life worthwhile.

The dilemma is that, just as we have little descriptive knowledge of the patterns of coping employed by most people, including diverse subgroups within the society, we also do not know the patterns of coping that work for given types of persons, the ways these patterns work, and the specific sets of circumstances under which they work. In treatment settings, the issue tends to be almost entirely begged (55), but the therapist can at least hope for improvement in the dysfunctional areas which brought the patient into treatment. In prevention— whether primary, secondary, or tertiary—the absence of rational guidelines poses an even more serious handicap. As Bower (4) has put it:

. . . lack of knowledge alone does not seem to deter action [to ameliorate psychopathology]; all kinds of halfway or inadequately documented therapies are visited upon the mentally ill—perhaps because the need is critical and the person is hurting. It is humane to try to help the ill despite our doubts about what we are doing. One cannot make such a case for primary prevention.

We must make efforts in coping theory and research to evaluate the adaptational effectiveness of the diverse patterns of coping, but obviously this can be done only after we have done the basic work of identifying such patterns as they appear in all sorts of individuals, populations, and conditions.

RESEARCH DESIGN AND MEASUREMENT

Several important implications for research design and measurement emerge clearly from the theoretical issues raised above concerning the roles of mediating cognitions, different kinds of emotion, and coping processes in adaptation (35,38). These implications stem especially from two features of the way we look at stress. First, we treat stress as a relational concept referring to transactions between person and environment that are characterized by harm–loss, threat, or challenge. Second, to understand stress relationships and their adaptational consequences in people requires that we consider the role of two related mediational psychological processes, namely, cognitive appraisal and coping. These shape the flow of each transaction and the adaptational outcome. We shall now discuss briefly some of the main methodological implications of our theoretical perspective and of the substantive issues we have raised.

LABORATORY VERSUS NATURALISTIC FIELD STUDY

Although laboratory studies are useful in evaluating the relationship between stressors and short-range physiological responses such as elevated blood pressure, they fail to tell us enough of what we need to know about the psychological, social, and physiological mechanisms underlying longer-range disease processes and other adaptational outcomes. There are at least three serious limitations of laboratory research. First, adaptational outcome measures such as changes in physical health, social functioning, and morale usually take time to evolve; experiments with humans cannot put us in touch with this long developmental process or with the concurrent social and psychological processes affecting it. Second, it is not possible, ethically or practically, to produce in the laboratory levels of stress and disease comparable to those brought about by serious life crises and chronic, everyday stress-inducing hassles (38). Nor is the laboratory well suited to create the rich variety of positive and distressing emotions we spoke about earlier that are so much a part of normal living, or to permit the person to utilize the full range and pattern of coping normally available in real-life stress. Third, we cannot discover in the laboratory the ordinary sources of stress, and the coping patterns used by different kinds of persons and groups in their natural settings. If we depended only on the laboratory, we would remain ignorant of stress and coping processes throughout human life. For these reasons, laboratory research on the substantive issues we have raised must be supplemented by field research centered on stress-related events and processes occurring naturally.

LEVELS OF ANALYSIS

In the past, stress research has been characterized by restriction to a single level of analysis, say, physiological stress, social stress, or psychological stress, and confusion has occurred when processes at one level are taken automatically to stand for those at another in some form of reductionism. The three levels of stress analysis are to a degree independent, and they refer to different conditions, concepts, and mechanisms. If one level led automatically to another, we would not need coordinated interdisciplinary research but could reduce stress to the lowest usable common denominator of explanation, the cellular or biochemical level, or perhaps ultimately the molecular or atomic level. However, the links between these levels are largely unexplored, tenuous, and complex, primarily because they have not been studied within the same research design.

Consider the form of social stress in which a social unit, for example, the family, is undergoing disruption in its functioning, as in divorce between the parents. Because of the divergent characteristics of the individual family members, this social stress may be psychologically and physiologically stressful for one member but benign or stress-reducing for another. Therefore, one cannot take stress at the social level to stand automatically for stress at the individual psychological or tissue level. Or, to take another example, Mason and his colleagues (49), whose work we cited earlier, note that psychological stress is often confounded with physiological stress, and that the effects are attributed to the latter when in reality they are determined, at least in part, by the former. Only by measuring stress inputs and reactions at both levels within the same research framework can this source of confusion be eliminated.

The methodological implication of this, and of the fact that each level plays a crucial part in understanding the relationship of stress to adaptational outcome, is that the most thorough research must be designed to assess all three concurrently (44). Only then will the interrelationships be properly evaluated and understood.

We believe that most of the important sources of stress in human life arise from the social context of living, from social arrangements based on shared meanings, in effect, from troubled interpersonal relationships. Social demands have their effects on any individual via cognitive appraisal and coping processes determining how that individual views, reacts to, and handles them. In turn, outcomes are first noted through changes in psychological or social functioning, or through the operation of diverse physiological mechanisms in short-range physiological changes, and only later in long-range disease processes. These physiological effects can wax and wane as the social context changes, as psychological coping processes alter the troubled person–environment relationship, and as physiological mechanisms exacerbate or ameliorate the development of more permanent disease processes.

PROCESS AND FLUX

The essence of adaptation is change. That is, when confronted with a dangerous or demanding situation, the person copes, thus altering the stressful person–environment relationship and, in turn, the physiological disturbance or disease process. Person–environment relationships are always in flux, emotions rising and falling and changing in quality, with attendant changes in tissue reactions. The way a person appraises what is happening is also constantly changing with changing circumstances and with his or her own cognitive and behavioral activity. Effective coping also requires that the person be attuned to the specific demands of the situation. The successfully adapted person does not do the same thing, or react in the same way, from one stressful encounter to another, although there are undoubtedly some things about that person's tendency to react that are comparatively stable. Research into the relationships between stress and adaptational outcomes must be designed to allow us to determine flux and change as well as stability. What is called for is a new type of assessment technology, namely, the measurement of process in contrast to most current practices of sampling traits or environmental conditions on a single occasion and assuming this will be stable over time or across occasions.

Process measurement, which implies flux or change, can be illustrated briefly both for person traits and for environmental characteristics. A number of personality assessment scales are available to measure certain coping traits or styles. These scales emphasize how a person might usually respond psychologically, say, by vigilantly seeking information so as to permit order and control over events, or by avoiding or denying information that might be threatening. However, prediction from such trait measures as to how the person actually will cope with specific threat situations has been poor (8). One can, alternatively, assess how an individual copes with diverse specific stressful encounters, in effect, measuring the coping process as it occurs rather than seeking to measure a trait. In such a case we would be in a position to determine how much coping changes with the nature of the encounter, and how stable any given coping pattern is for that individual.

Too often, particularly in laboratory or "trait" research, results observed are assumed to be typical of all such relationships. To take an obvious example, the pattern of physiological responses to a stressful circumstance among a group of college students should not necessarily be expected among a group of retired or ill persons. Similarly, patterns of appraisal, coping, and emotional response probably vary not only in different contexts but also in different age, sex, and cultural subgroups. This concern with the issue of who is being studied is particularly critical in a research area as complex as the study of stress.

Similarly, we can measure the social network or support systems generally available to an individual. The usual assumption is that this aspect will be a stable feature of the individual's life setting (a structural property), which may or may not be true. In fact, the social environment can change greatly from one period of life to another, or as a function of illness, divorce, or other forms of crisis. Even adaptational outcomes are changeable things, with morale, social functioning, and illness patterns differing from time to time or from occasion to occasion. In short, to understand the mechanisms—at any or all levels of analysis—that are involved in adaptational outcomes such as health and illness, it is just as important to examine flux and change as it is to study stable structures.

The advantage of a process orientation is nicely illustrated in a study by Kasl et al. (29) of changes in blood pressure associated with job loss. In this often-cited study, a group of men who were being laid off from their factory jobs were studied longitudinally and prospectively. The study began in the months preceding the closing of the factory, when the men were anticipating the loss of their jobs, and continued with repeated follow-ups at regular intervals up to 2 years later. The men were studied with a variety of social psychological and physiological measures, including blood pressure. A control group of men with stable employment showed no consistent changes in blood pressure over this period of time. The men who were laid off experienced a significant drop in blood pressure from the anticipatory phase to a period of 8 to 12 months after job loss. The magnitude of the change in blood pressure was correlated with subjective measures of disturbance and personality attributes such as ego resiliency, rather than with an objective measure of the actual length of unemployment. Kasl and colleagues did not include in their analysis men who failed to find work within 12 months after losing their jobs; it would be interesting to know what their blood pressures were in comparison to that of those who did find jobs. At any rate, we think this study serves as an excellent example of the kind of understanding that can be achieved when subjects are followed in such a way that longer range consequences of a stressful life event can be understood in terms of the mechanisms which bring them about.

*As noted earlier, the mechanisms leading from a disturbed physiological state to enduring changes in function are unknown. One might speculate that highly stable or repetitive patterns of emotions, appraisals, or coping, whether related to a chronic stressful situation or simply characteristic of the person in many situations, would demonstrate such mechanisms as well as the sought-after connection between acute and chronic changes. This would require repeated and concurrent measurement of all these relevant variables across a period of time sufficient for such chronic changes to become manifest, or for changes such as exacerbation or remission to occur in those who already have disease.

INTRAINDIVIDUAL EMPHASIS IN RESEARCH DESIGN

All that we have said above concerning research design and measurement culminates in one major design contrast, namely, between within-individual and across-individual comparison (5,35,37,46). Most research, including epidemiological studies of social conditions or personality and morbidity or mortality as health outcomes, focuses on a single antecedent factor, measured once as a stable structure or trait, and some outcome factor, such as risk of illness or death, expressed in probability terms. This involves large samples and comparisons made strictly across individuals. Processes as they occur across occasions or time, that is, within individuals, cannot be examined in this type of research since only one assessment of the antecedent causal factor is made. Nor can the mechanisms—social, psychological, or physiological—be identified in this style of research, since what is happening when any individual gets sick, worsens, or improves cannot be known.

What is needed in order to study such mechanisms, and to relate the divergent levels of analysis as we have proposed, is concurrent examination of social, psychological, and physiological processes in the same individuals across encounters or situations, and over time. Only in that way can we show how short-range physiological changes associated with stress, coping, and emotion can eventuate in disease or other negative adaptational outcomes in susceptible individuals. And only in that way can we begin to identify the effective and ineffective patterns with which people cope with life-threatening illness, such as cancer, once it has occurred. Ultimately, if we are not to continue whistling in the dark, our interventions to help the ill person, to prevent people from becoming ill, and to prevent such illness from worsening unnecessarily or from producing unnecessary incapacitation must be based on knowledge of such effective and ineffective patterns. We need to show as much interest in psychological and social adaptation to illness as we now do in seeking ways of preventing or curing it at the cellular level.

ACKNOWLEDGMENT

The writing of this chapter was supported in part by a research grant from the National Cancer Institute (CA 19362).

REFERENCES

1. Aldrich, C. K., and Mendkoff, E. (1963): Relocation of the aged and disabled: A mortality study. *J. Am. Geriatr. Soc.,* 11:185–194.
2. Alexander, F. G., and Selesnick, S. T. (1977): *The History of Psychiatry.* Harper & Row, New York.
3. Berne, E. (1964): *Games People Play.* Grove Press, New York.
4. Bower, E. M. (1977): Mythologies, realities, and possibilities in primary prevention. In: *Primary Prevention of Psychopathology. Vol. 1: The Issues,* edited by G. W. Albee, and J. M. Joffe, pp. 18–23. University Press of New England, Hanover, N.H.

5. Broverman, D. M. (1962): Normative and ipsative measurement in psychology. *Psychol. Rev.*, 69:295–305.
6. Cassel, J. (1976): The contribution of the social environment to host resistance. *Am. J. Epidemiol.*, 104:107–123.
7. Clark, M. M. (1967): The anthropology of aging, a new area for studies of culture and personality. *Gerontologist*, 7:55–64.
8. Cohen, F., and Lazarus, R. S. (1973): Active coping processes, coping dispositions, and recovery from surgery. *Psychosom. Med.*, 35:375–389.
9. Cousins, N. (1976): Anatomy of an illness (as perceived by the patient). *N. Engl. J. Med.*, 295:1458–1463.
10. Dember, W. N. (1974): Motivation and the cognitive revolution. *Am. Psychologist*, 29:161–168.
11. Ellis, A. (1962): *Reason and Emotion in Psychotherapy.* Lyle Stuart, New York.
12. Engel, G. L. (1974): Memorial lecture: The psychosomatic approach to individual susceptibility to disease. *Gastroenterology*, 67:1085–1093.
13. Engel, G. L. (1977): The need for a new medical model: A challenge for biomedicine. *Science*, 196:129–136.
14. Erikson, E. H. (1956): The problem of ego identity. *J. Am. Psychoanal. Assoc.*, 4:69.
15. Fenichel, O. (1945): *The Psychoanalytic Theory of Neurosis.* W. W. Norton, New York.
16. Folkman, S., Schaefer, C., and Lazarus, R. S. (1979): Cognitive processes as mediators of stress and coping. In: *Human Stress and Cognition: An Information-Processing Approach,* edited by V. Hamilton and D. M. Warburton, pp. 265–298. John Wiley & Sons, London.
17. Frankenhaeuser, M. (1976): The role of peripheral catecholamines in adaptation to understimulation and overstimulation. In: *Psychopathology of Human Adaptation,* edited by G. Serban, pp. 173–191. Plenum Press, New York.
18. Frankl, V. (1955): *The Doctor and the Soul.* Alfred A. Knopf, New York.
19. Frankl, V. (1963): *Man's Search for Meaning.* Washington Square Press, New York.
20. Glass, D. C. (1977): *Behavior Patterns, Stress and Coronary Disease.* Complex Behavior Series. Halstead Press, New York.
21. Hackett, T. P., and Cassem, H. (1975): Psychological management of the myocardial infarction patient. *J. Hum. Stress,* 1:25–38.
22. Hackett, T. P., and Weisman, A. D. (1964): Reactions to the imminence of death. In: *The Threat of Impending Disaster,* edited by G. H. Grosser, H. Wechsler, and M. Greenblatt, pp. 300–301. MIT Press, Cambridge, Mass.
23. Hamburg, D. A., and Adams, H. E. (1967): A perspective on coping: Seeking and utilizing information in major transitions. *Arch. Gen. Psychiatry,* 17:277–284.
24. Herd, J. A. (1977): *Cardiovascular Correlates of Psychological Stress.* Paper presented at Conference on the Crisis in Stress Research, Boston University School of Medicine, Boston, October 20–22.
25. Hofer, M. A., Wolff, C. T., Friedman, S. B., and Mason, J. W. (1972): A psychoendrocrine study of bereavement. I and II. *Psychosom. Med.,* 34:481–504.
26. Holmes, T. M., and Masuda, M. (1974): Life change and illness susceptibility. In: *Stressful Life Events,* edited by B. S. Bohrenwend, and B. P. Bohrenwend, pp. 45–86. John Wiley & Sons, New York.
27. Janis, I. (1968): Stages in the decision-making process. In: *Theories of Cognitive Consistency: A Sourcebook,* edited by R. Abelson, E. Aronson, W. McGuire, T. Newcomb, M. J. Rosenberg, and P. Tannenbaum, pp. 577–588. Rand McNally, Chicago.
28. Janis, I., and Mann, L. (1977): *Decision Making.* Free Press, New York.
29. Kasl, S. V., Gore, S., and Cobb, S. (1975): The experience of losing a job: Reported changes in health, symptoms and illness behavior. *Psychosom. Med.,* 37:106–122.
30. Katz, J. L., Weiner, H., Gallagher, T. G., and Hellman, L. (1970): Stress, distress, and ego defenses. *Arch. Gen. Psychiatry,* 23:131–142.
31. Lacey, J. I. (1967): Somatic response patterning and stress: Some revisions of activation theory. In: *Psychological stress,* edited by M. H. Appley and R. Trumbull, pp. 14–37. Appleton-Century-Crofts, New York.
32. Lazarus, R. S. (1966): *Psychological Stress and the Coping Process.* McGraw-Hill, New York.
33. Lazarus, R. S. (1968): Emotions and adaptation: Conceptual and empirical relations. In: *Nebraska Symposium on Motivation,* edited by W. J. Arnold, pp. 175–265. University of Nebraska Press, Lincoln.

34. Lazarus, R. S., (1977): Psychological stress and coping in adaptation and illness. In: *Psychosomatic Medicine: Current Trends and Clinical Applications,* edited by Z. J. Lipowski, D. R. Lipsitt, and P. C. Whybrow, pp. 14–26. Oxford University Press, New York.

35. Lazarus, R. S., (1978): A strategy for research on psychological and social factors in hypertension. *J. Hum. Stress,* 4:34–40.

36. Lazarus, R. S., Averill, J. R., and Opton, E. M., Jr. (1970): Toward a cognitive theory of emotion. In: *Feelings and Emotion,* edited by M. Arnold, pp. 207–232. Academic Press, New York.

37. Lazarus, R. S., and Cohen, J. B. (1976): *The Study of Stress and Coping in Aging.* Paper presented at 5th WHO Conference on Society, Stress and Disease: Aging and Old Age, Stockholm, June 14–19, 1976.

38. Lazarus, R. S., and Cohen, J. B. (1977): Environmental stress. In: *Human Behavior and the Environment: Current Theory and Research, Vol. 1,* edited by I. Altman and J. F. Wohlwill, pp. 89–127. Plenum, New York.

39. Lazarus, R. S., Kanner, A. D., and Folkman, S. (1980): Emotions: A cognitive-phenomenological analysis. In: *Theories of Emotion,* edited by R. Plutchik and H. Kellerman, pp. 189–217. Academic Press, New York.

40. Lazarus, R. S., and Launier, R. (1978): Stress-related transactions between person and environment. In: *Perspectives in Interactional Psychology,* edited by L. Pervin and M. Lewis, pp. 287–327. Plenum Press, New York.

41. Lazarus, R. S., Speisman, J. C., and Mordkoff, A. M. (1963): The relationship between autonomic indicators of psychological stress: Heart rate and skin conductance. *Psychosom. Med.,* 25:19–30.

42. Levi, L., and Kagan, A. (1971): Adaptation of the psychological environment to man's abilities and needs. In: *Society, Stress and Disease, Vol. 1,* edited by L. Levi, pp. 395–404. Oxford University Press, London.

43. Lipowski, Z. J. (1977): Psychosomatic medicine in the seventies: An overview. *Am. J. Psychiatry,* 134:233–244.

44. Luborsky, L., Docherty, J. P., and Penick, S. (1973): Onset conditions for psychosomatic symptoms: A comparative review of immediate observation with retrospective research. *Psychosom. Med.,* 35:187–204.

45. Mandler, G. (1975): *Mind and Emotion.* John Wiley & Sons, New York.

46. Marceil, J. C. (1977): Implicit dimensions of ideography and nomothesis: A reformulation. *Am. Psychologist,* 32:1046–1055.

47. Marmot, M. G., and Syme, S. (1976): Acculturation and coronary heart disease in Japanese Americans. *Am. J. Epidemiol.,* 104:225–247.

48. Mason, J. W. (1975): Emotion as reflected in patterns of endocrine regulation. In: *Emotions: Their Parameters and Measurement,* edited by L. Levi, pp. 143–181. Raven Press, New York.

49. Mason, J. W., Maher, J. T., Hartley, L. H. Mougey, E., Perlow, M. J., and Jones, L. G. (1976): Selectivity of corticosteroid and catecholamine response to various natural stimuli. In: *Psychopathology of Human Adaptation,* edited by G. Serban, pp. 147–171. Plenum Press, New York.

50. Moos, R. H. (1974): Psychological techniques in the assessment of adaptive behavior. In: *Coping and Adaptation,* edited by G. V. Coelho, pp. 334–399. Basic Books, New York.

51. Nuckolls, K. B., Cassel, J., and Kaplan, B. H. (1972): Psychosocial assets, life crisis, and the prognosis of pregnancy. *Am. J. Epidemiol.,* 95:431–441.

52. Ostfeld, A. M. (1967): The interaction of biological and social variables in cardiovascular disease. *Milbank Mem. Fund Q.,* 45:13–18.

53. Parkes, C. M., Benjamin, B., and Fitzgerald, R. G. (1969): Broken heart: A statistical study of increased mortality among widowers. *Br. Med. J.,* 11:740–743.

54. Rosenman, R. H., Brand, R. J., Sholtz, R. I., and Friedman, M. (1976); Multivariate prediction of coronary heart disease during 8.5 year follow-up in the Western Collaborative Group Study. *Am. J. Cardiol.,* 37:903–910.

55. Roskies, E., and Lazarus, R. S. (1980): Coping theory and the teaching of coping skills. In: *Behavioral Medicine: Changing Health Life Styles,* edited by P. O. Davidson and S. M. Davidson, pp. 38–69. Brunner/Mazel, New York.

56. Sapira, J. D., Scheib, E. T., Moriarty, R., and Shapiro, A. P. (1971): Differences in perception between hypertensive and normotensive populations. *Psychosom. Med.,* 33:239–250.

57. Schacter, S. (1966): The interaction of cognitive and physiological determinants of emotional

state. In: *Anxiety and Behavior*, edited by C. D. Spielberger, pp. 193–224. Academic Press, New York.

58. Schwartz, G. E., and Weiss, S. M. (1977): What is behavioral medicine? *Psychosom. Med.*, 39:377–381.

59. Selye, H. (1974): *Stress Without Disease*. J. B. Lippincott, Philadelphia.

60. Selye, H. (1976): *The Stress of Life*. McGraw-Hill, New York.

61. Singer, M. T. (1974): Presidential Address—Engagement-involvement: A central phenomenon in psychophysiological research. *Psychosom. Med.*, 36:1–17.

62. Stahl, S. M., Grim, C. E., Donald, S., and Neikirk, H. J. (1975): A model for the social sciences and medicine: The case for hypertension. *Soc. Sci. Med.*, 9:31–38.

63. Syme, S. L. (1977): *Psychosocial Determinants of Hypertension*. Paper presented at Hahnemann College 5th International Symposium on Hypertension, San Juan, Puerto Rico, January 9–12.

64. Syme, S. L. (1977): *Epidemiologic Research in Hypertension: A Critical Appraisal*. Paper presented at the Conference on the Crisis in Stress Research, Boston University School of Medicine, Boston, October 20–21.

65. Syme, S. L., and Berkman, L. F. (1976): Social class, susceptibility and sickness. *Am. J. Epidemiol.*, 104:1–8.

66. Von Kugelgen, E. (1975): *Psychological Determinants of the Delay in Decision to Seek Aid in Cases of Myocardial Infarction*. Unpublished doctoral dissertation, University of California, Berkeley.

67. Weiner, H., Singer, M. T., and Reiser, J. F. (1962): Cardiovascular responses and their psychological correlates. I. A study in healthy young adults and patients with peptic ulcer and hypertension. *Psychosom. Med.*, 24:477–498.

68. Weisman, A. D. (1972): *On Dying and Denying*. Behavioral Publications, New York.

69. Weisman, A. D., and Worden, J. W. (1975): Psychosocial analysis of cancer deaths. *Omega*, 6:61–75.

70. Wolff, C. T., Friedman, S. B., Hofer, M. A., and Mason, J. W. (1964): Relationship between psychological defenses and mean urinary 17-hydroxycorticosteroid excretion rates. I. A predictive study of parents of fatally ill children. *Psychosom. Med.*, 26:576–591.

Psychosocial Aspects of Cancer,
edited by Jerome Cohen et al.
Raven Press, New York © 1982.

Chapter 16

Discussion of "Stress and Coping as Factors in Health and Illness" by Lazarus

Arthur H. Schmale

Psychosocial Medicine Unit, University of Rochester Cancer Center, Rochester, New York 14627

In the preceding chapter Dr. Lazarus has touched on many if not all of the difficulties and dilemmas in the field of what he calls stress and coping and what others of us have been calling the problems of measuring psychosocial variables and their significance for cancer patients, their families, and the health professionals caring for cancer patients as well as the interested and involved behavioral scientists.

Dr. Lazarus states that there has been a remarkable revival of interest and activity in the study of the relationship of stress, coping, and disease in recent years. The discipline, he says, having suffered in "popularity and credibility" through the middle 1950s and 1960s, again appears to be on the threshold of making important advances in understanding the complex relationships between stress process and adaptational outcomes. It must be pointed out, however, that one's evaluation or cognitive appraisal (to use Lazarus's term) of the work of those decades would vary with the vantage point and what one was doing at the time. From a clinical psychosomatic researcher's point of view, those years were exciting but ultimately frustrating, triggering, so to speak, the emotional reaction that influenced the coping response.

Anyone interested in the natural setting of disease onset had to be fascinated by the clinical material collected during this period, and by the results of the pilot studies undertaken by Engel (3), Fischer and Dlin (5), Graham et al. (7), Greene (8), Hinkle and Wolff (10), Knapp and Nemetz (11), Silverman et al. (15), and Weiner et al. (17). But there was clearly a need to operationalize observations into testable hypotheses and to develop means to measure what a person was thinking, feeling, and doing at various points in time—to make, as Dr. Lazarus describes it, an assessment of the coping process.

Today, faced with similar problems, we have a clearer understanding of why this previous work did not progress, why it lost "popularity and credibility."

Today's experts, looking back, say there was a lot of theory and few confirmatory data. No one disagrees with that view, least of all the investigators who are involved in the work. Many of the patient data were gathered retrospectively rather than prospectively—to which, again, we can offer no argument. Observations had to start somewhere, and the systematic confirmation of isolated clinical observations was a first step. The next step—the prospective study of individuals considered at risk for whom prediction of the occurrence of specific reactions would lead to the clinical appearance of disease—was a big step, and one that proved to be impossible, at least in the sense that there were few identifiable high-risk groups of individuals available for longitudinal study, and there was little or no research support available for the type of large-scale, long-term studies that were required. Thus these researchers were forced to turn to other areas of research and to other academic pursuits.

By now, however, our biological and medical science peers are again interested and even concerned about psychosocial variables, and they want answers, results. They want convincing evidence of predictive relationships achieved by means of simple, brief, quick and clear-cut procedures or instruments. These are the standards by which they judge each other's work.

The psychosocial issues are somewhat better identified today even though the investigators in the field are still trying to understand how to define, assess, and then test coping patterns to see which work for whom and when. As Dr. Lazarus says, again or still we are in the position of being asked to design interventions in clinical situations before we know how to measure the problem or in the absence of rational guidelines. We need support for naturalistic field studies which will include the capacity to measure multiple levels or areas of coping.

The National Cancer Institute, through the Division of Cancer Control in particular, has indicated its interest in and commitment to support for research efforts. We who seek to investigate psychosocial issues must nurture, protect, and educate these interests so that our patrons, our supporters, will not expect instant results. They must appreciate the magnitude of the assessment problems we face and be willing to make the larger, longer term commitment which requires the collaborative efforts of the several behavioral science subdisciplines and the combined populations of more than one cancer center. If we are unable to get this kind of support, we will hear the story of the 1950s and 1960s repeated: "Interesting theories but they could not be tested. . . . Promised a lot but delivered little." This prospect should be seen not only as a threat, but as a challenge to change the situation by direct action so that research in this field can fulfill its potential and make a real contribution toward understanding the role of psychosocial factors in diagnostic, treatment, rehabilitation, and even preventive areas.

Dr. Lazarus' theory applies to illness in general as well as to cancer specifically. However, there are a number of reasons why cancer is an excellent disease model for the study of stress, coping, and psychosocial relationships and their influence on such factors as the course, treatment of the disease, side effects, sense of well-being, and survival—what Dr. Lazarus calls adaptive outcomes. The public thinks of cancer as the number one health menace, a killer. The first association we make to the word cancer is death. If there is any one situation in life that can be anticipated as creating high levels of distress, it is to be given a diagnosis of cancer, a disease for which we do not know the cause or the cure.

Cancer, because it is a disease of high incidence and prevalence, is readily available for study. A standard nomenclature for identification of the disease and the many complicated and extended treatment programs provide independent observations of physical condition and physiological parameters which are then available for correlational and outcome comparisons. Because of the elaborate diagnostic procedures, the frequency of recurrence and extension of the disease, plus the dramatic reactions and side effects of the treatments designed as curative, adjuvant, palliative, or "comfort care only," patients, families, and health professionals are faced with frequent changes necessitating repeated psychological and social as well as physical adjustments.

Let me now raise some specific questions about Dr. Lazarus's theory even though it makes clinical and research sense in its main direction. In presenting his point of view he raises a number of issues about differentiating threat versus challenge, real versus defensive reactions, role of specificity versus general psychosocial patterns of somatic and disease effects, the possible somatic effects of positive versus negative emotions, and the possible adaptive importance of ambiguity or uncertainty versus reality orientation. All are provocative issues which appear more important relative to the vantage point, training, and experience of the observer-investigator and state of the science rather than to the processes of coping and adaptation related to health and illness. Dr. Lazarus himself states: "Further, the same event or set of circumstances (e.g., an examination) could clearly be seen as a 'good' stressor by one person and a 'bad' stressor by another." To this should be added the change that occurs over time within individuals. What constitutes a "good" or "bad" stressor may become more or less of the quality first observed, and many observations about quality are usually difficult to specify in terms of the extremes of good or bad. Here again, Dr. Lazarus would probably agree that individuals are not seen in terms of coping or noncoping, but are usually observed as demonstrating varying degrees of distress or coping. Under what combinations of circumstances does the process become dysfunctional, and how if at all do such reactions relate to changes in somatic functioning and disease? These are difficult questions which obviously require the consideration of multiple variables and an understanding of several frameworks of reference going from the biological to the psychological, social, and cultural (4).

To be more specific, Dr. Lazarus's point about differentiating threat and challenge is interesting, but what may be a challenging position on one day may be a threat for the next week or phase of treatment. Cognitions change over time, although not as rapidly as emotions. Individuals who are feeling challenged tend to be positive in mood and morale. The question as to whether the positive appraisal is defensive is not of great importance: if it is, so be it. The defense may be obvious to the observer from its exaggerated qualities or by how ineffective it is in serving to maintain a consistent and positive stance. If it is effective, then it is doing what it is meant to do and the defensive nature of the reaction may not be obvious. Since coping is a process, time will tell if the defense is effective and supportive or is becoming ineffective, threatening, and harmful. Defenses in and of themselves are not necessarily harmful, uneconomical, or unrealistic in meeting the needs of the individual and the demands of the environment at a specific point in time.

In regard to emotions, Dr. Lazarus indicates they are intricately interwoven with processes of cognitive appraisal and coping. The emotions are the royal road to understanding what is unique about man and his behavior, and as such provide the best window for observing these processes as well as adaptive outcome. The verbal and nonverbal expression of emotion is the *QED* of the mind's involvement in man's transactions with his environments. An emotion both reflects the current state and may be the signal which precedes the change to another state. To say, as Dr. Lazarus does, that strong emotion can (a) interfere with adaptive thought and skilled performance, (b) alter the appraisal significance of what is happening, or (c) serve as rewards or punishments that have current emotional as well as developmental significance is to attribute to the emotions an independence and existence that go beyond their role of being the measuring stick or thermometer of how one is doing. It is not the strong emotional reaction which interferes with adaptive thought and skilled performance but the cognitive appraisal of the involvement or arousal of the whole organism which is reflected by the emotional expression.

In regard to specificity or generality about emotions and their physiological concomitants or reactants, Dr. Lazarus needs to decide whether one is more correct than the other. It is my view that there are some events, either unexpected or unwanted, that produce an immediate or initial reaction of orienting or hypervigilance. This reaction, which may fit with the behavior of what has been called startle or shock, is in turn followed by one of disbelief and denial, ultimately leading to a series of actions with accompanying feelings, each having a somatic profile in terms of autonomic, somato-sensory and motor, endocrine, and immune system functions. Such profiles probably differ across individuals and across different phases of the life cycle within a single individual—like the problem of the blind man feeling the elephant, and like our need to think of linear or simple profiles of physiological, endocrinological, or immunological reactions or effects. The interpretation of environmental demands on the self and the individual's solution to the perceived demands will determine which and how much of the several levels or systems will be activated to accomplish the desired result. The individual's prior experiences, his current social, psychological, and physical environments or supports, and his somatic predispositions will determine the outcome.

In such a framework, it is difficult to speculate that the anger expressed in an acute emergency situation which may give rise to an elevation in blood pressure is the culprit in the chronic disease state of idiopathic or essential hypertension. On the other hand, anger which the individual is forced to defend himself against and hide and which he thus is inhibited from expressing may leave the body physiologically prepared for action with no action being allowed—or as Gellhorn (6) calls it, physiological collision: the body may be prepared to go in two directions at the same time.

This formulation concerning defended-against anger could lead the biologically predisposed individual to experience dysfunction or what may be associated with the disease state of hypertension. This then brings us to the issue of what Dr. Lazarus terms the palliative mode of coping, which often requires accepting ambiguity or uncertainty and implies a need to hold back strong natural actions in the interest of other, more important values. He makes it sound as if emotions, inhibition of actions, and intrapsychic modes were completely under our conscious control, or if not that they could become so. Even though he says that defenses are self-deceptive mechanisms, he gives the impression that he thinks the individual has a conscious choice in these matters. Here is one area where psychoanalytic thinking makes a clear distinction: emotions, symptoms, and defenses are part of the autonomous adaptive controls built in to warn and protect the individual from excessive overload or activity. They are automatic and not under the conscious control of the individual. Individuals can be trained to modify their behavior to some extent but they must be able to understand the dynamics of the behaviors before they can have control over and redirect the forms of coping involved.

As indicated elsewhere (13), I think the perception of failure or of not succeeding in reaching a goal and its associated feelings of helplessness or hopelessness signal a need to disengage and withdraw from an active involvement with the external environment. If such disengagement is not allowed or considered possible, here again there may be specific consequences of somatic dysfunction (12). If one is in need of further support for a specificity of variables which relate to disease susceptibility, there is a growing animal literature to turn to for confirmation (1,9,18). To be out of control or unable to cope psychologically may be the final common pathway to somatic or psychological disease. In a systems hierarchy, if the sense of self-worth and control cannot be protected or achieved at the psychological level, the dysfunction may spill over and affect the adjacent systems, those of environmental or social support and/or physiological functioning. If these are ineffective in helping the individual cope, then still other systems will be involved.

In regard to positive or negative emotions, I believe that neither have specific and special constructive or destructive effects at the physiological level the way they may have at the social and psychological levels of interaction. What is important in Norman Cousins' account of his recovery from what was assumed to be a chronic progressive systemic autoimmune disease is his belief in himself and the course of action which he and his physician agreed on, not his program of forced laughter (2). His positive feelings about what he had to do and then did, along with his expectations of recovery, were emotional measures of how well he was coping and would ultimately adapt.

It is difficult to know which is the chicken and which the egg in such a situation. The fact that Mr. Cousins was determined to get better and felt he had to take things into his own hands may have already been the cognitive and emotional signaling, the somatic awareness, that things were better, or that he had the option to participate in this process of helping himself get better. Here I would like to refer to a piece of data that turned up in our research and that also fits with some findings related to the reported predictive outcome of patients who have had a myocardial infarction. One of the predictors of outcome in regard to whether a patient who has had a myocardial infarction will be back at work in 1 year is the patient's response to the question of how well he thinks he will do at the first follow-up visit after the infarction (16). In our research we followed a group of cancer patients who received radiation therapy. There was a statistically significant consistence with what the patients anticipated would happen at 1 month into treatment and what they were able to do at 6 and again at 18 and 24 months later, although the patient group went from 60 subjects to 46 and then to only 24 subjects for observation at the 18- to 24-month observation period (14). It was humbling to say the least: after all our efforts and testing of specific items and attempts to build a scientific instrument to assess outcome, the straightforward method of asking the patient what he anticipated proved to be an important predictor of outcome or adaptation, an example of self-report in assessing the coping process. As Dr. Lazarus has indicated, we need both self-report and observer evaluation to piece together or correlate the meaning of the sources of information about coping.

The issue that Dr. Lazarus raises about the need for ambiguity or uncertainty in some situations rather than insisting on reality orientation for effective coping seems confusing. What is important to me is the same as with the positive affect issue: not whether the feeling is real or defensive, but what the results are of such feelings and their associated or resulting behaviors. Again, one person's reality may be another's fantasy or psychosis. The only problem of being in a fantasy or psychotic state is that the environment may not be able to transact effectively for individuals with such beliefs and behavior for any length of time. To me it is a misuse of the term "uncertainty" when it is applied to the individual who is spared the detailed information of his disease and prognosis. To "fail" to provide technical or detailed information when not solicited is not a matter of affording a patient uncertainty, doubts, or skepticism, but one of providing the certainty of having only as much information as is wanted, that is, the certainty to cope with whatever information, fantasy, and beliefs the individual may find important in helping him adapt. If the individual needs more information or finds that what he has been told is inadequate or puzzling, he should feel free to ask for more information, and again he should be given as much as is wanted and needed in order to enable him to cope.

As indicated in the introduction to these remarks, there are many ideas and formulations, and in general there is considerable agreement, as to what is important in coping and adaptation. The task at hand is to test these ideas by means of a new assessment technology that will be used to measure process, as proposed by Dr. Lazarus. Let us hope that enough of the right people will heed what we have been saying and will be convinced of the importance of this research.

ACKNOWLEDGMENTS

This chapter is based on research supported in part by Grant No. 3-R18 CA 19681, Cancer Center Core Support Grant No. 4-P30 CA 11198–09, and Cancer Education Grant No. 2-R25 CA 17988 awarded by the National Cancer Institute, DHEW. It was first presented at the Psychosocial Study Group, ACS, California Division, Inc., September 25, 1978, San Diego, California.

REFERENCES

1. Ader, R. (1976): Psychosomatic research in animals. In: *Modern Trends in Psychosomatic Medicine,* edited by O. W. Hill, pp. 21–41. Butterworths, London.
2. Cousins, N. (1976): Anatomy of an illness (as perceived by the patient). *N. Engl. J. Med.,* 295:1458–1463.
3. Engel, G. L. (1958): Studies of ulcerative colitis. V. Psychological aspects of their implication for treatment. *Am. J. Dig. Dis.,* 3:315–337.
4. Engel, G. L. (1977): The need for a new medical model: A challenge for biomedicine. *Science,* 196:129–136.
5. Fischer, H. K., and Dlin, B. M. (1964): Emotional factors in coronary occlusion. II. Time patterns and factors related to onset. *Psychosomatics,* 5:280.
6. Gellhorn, E. (1957): Physiological collisions and psychological conflicts. In: *Principles of Autonomic-Somatic Integrations,* pp. 173–182. University of Minnesota Press, Minneapolis.
7. Graham, D. T., Lundy, R. M., Kabler, J. D., et al. (1962): Specific attitudes in initial interviews with patients having different "psychosomatic" diseases. *Psychosom. Med.,* 24:257–266.
8. Greene, W. A. (1965): Disease responses to life stress. *J. Am. Med. Womens Assoc.,* 20:133–140.
9. Henry, J. P., Stephens, P. M., and Santisteban, G. A. (1975): A model of psychosocial hypertension showing reversibility and progression of cardiovascular complications. *Circ. Res.,* 36:156–164.
10. Hinkle, L. E., and Wolff, H. G. (1957): The nature of man's adaptation to his total environment and the relation of this to illness. *Arch. Intern. Med.,* 99:442–460.
11. Knapp, P. H., and Nemetz, S. J. (1957): Sources of tension in bronchial asthma, a study of forty patients. *Psychosom. Med.,* 19:466.
12. Schmale, A. H. (1972): Giving up as a final common pathway to changes in health. *Adv. Psychosom. Med.,* 8:20.
13. Schmale, A. H. (1973): The adaptive role of depression in health and disease. In: *Separation and Depression: Clinical and Research Aspects,* edited by J. P. Scott and E. C. Senay, pp. 187–214. American Association for Advancement of Science, Washington, D.C.
14. Schmale, A. H., Morrow, G. R., Davis, A. K., et al. (1978): *Psychosocial Adjustment of Cancer Patients. I. Search for Clinical Predictors.* Presented at the American Psychosomatic Society, March 31.
15. Silverman, A. J., Cohen, S. I., and Zuidema, G. D. (1957): Psychophysiological investigations in cardiovascular stress. *Am. J. Psychiatry,* 113:691–693.

16. Stern, M. J., and Pascale, L. (1977): Life adjustment postmyocardial infarction. *Arch. Intern. Med.,* 137:1680–1685.
17. Weiner, H., Thaler, M., Teiser, M. F., and Mirsky, I. (1957): Etiology of duodenal ulcer. *Psychosom. Med.,* 19:1–10.
18. Weiss, J. M., (1972): Influence of psychosocial variables on stress-induced pathology in physiology, emotions and psychosomatic illness. *Ciba Found. Symp.,* 8:253–280.

Psychosocial Aspects of Cancer,
edited by Jerome Cohen et al.
Raven Press, New York © 1982.

Chapter 17

Work and Cancer Health Histories

Frances Lomas Feldman

School of Social Work, University of Southern California, Los Angeles, California 90007

That work holds special and profound meaning in the lives of adults in our culture is a truism. We have only to witness the lineal space devoted daily by the press to examining levels of employment, the legislative efforts to cope with fluctuations in the labor force or to develop training resources that will lead to productive employment, the demands on every side that work replace dependency on "welfare" for those not economically self-supporting, the insistence of the 1946 Full Employment Act and later statutes that work is a right, and other constant reminders that the work ethic is alive and well in contemporary America.

That discrimination in the work place is not to be tolerated in a democratic society has also come to be widely accepted as a moral truth. This societal view has found its way into the fabric of social policy, and its violation carries the threat of explicitly defined sanctions.

The possibility, then, that either concept might be flaunted tends to be regarded as outrageous. Thus, when correspondence from individuals to the California Division of the American Cancer Society began to mount, and increasing numbers of news reports appeared that cited the poignant and often bitter experiences of individuals who attributed discrimination in the arena of work to their cancer health histories, the Division was responsive. These were self-selected and generally unverified or unverifiable situations; the aggrieved individuals took the initiative in bringing their plight to the attention of the Division or the communication media. But how representative were they? Would a random sample of recovered cancer patients—that is, patients currently reasonably symptom-free and capable of working—offer some clues to the nature and extent of discrimination experienced by cancer patients in finding or retaining work? Would exploration disclose a relationship between the cancer patient's work adjustment and the quality of his post-cancer diagnosis life?

Little systematic examination of this kind had ever been undertaken. The Metropolitan Life Insurance Company had conducted an important study among

its own employees which disclosed no differences in absenteeism and work performance between those with cancer histories and employees with other health
histories (5). The American Telephone and Telegraph Company had also done
some exploratory work along these lines among its own employees (4). But in
each study the experiences and outcomes centered on a single employing establishment. Were the findings generalizable?

The California Division of the American Cancer Society funded a trilogy of
Work and Cancer studies intended to yield some answers to the above questions.
The first study in this group focused on white collar workers and selected professionals (teachers and nurses) (1). The second centered on the work experiences
of blue collar workers (2). The third study, in process at this writing, is concerned
with the work experiences and expectations of young people with cancer histories
(13 to 23 years old at diagnosis).

The course and findings of the completed studies revealed not only the nature
and probability of occurrences of discrimination; they also disclosed a cluster
of work-related psychological, social, and economic problems that hold profound
import for the prevention, treatment, and control of cancer. Delineated first
in the following pages are the data sources of the blue collar study. Next, we
explore some of the findings from the study followed by some of the implications
of these findings for individuals endeavoring to cope with the reality of the
cancer diagnosis—individuals like the study respondent who remarked:

> I received a death sentence twice, once when the doctor told me I have cancer,
> and then when my boss asked me to quit because the cancer would upset my
> fellow-workers. Except for my wife, that job was my whole world!

THE BLUE COLLAR STUDY

As also was the case in the study of white collar workers, the blue collar
study sought data that might be useful for determining the need for new social
policy or for modifying existing policy employment opportunities and experiences
of work-able individuals with a history of cancer, for developing or stimulating
the development of relevant service or counseling programs, and for devising
appropriate public and professional education measures and content with regard
to cancer patients in the world of work.

The central focus of the study of blue collar workers was on their work-
related needs and experiences. The reconnaissance preliminary to the white
collar study, and that study itself, had revealed at least three dimensions requiring
consideration. One was the patient's own perceptions of the interface of work
experiences and cancer history, and its implications in terms of economic and
social well-being. Another was the impact of employer attitudes, policies, and
practices on work experiences and opportunities. And the third consisted of
economic and legal considerations impinging on the employment situations of
such work-able employees. The white collar study suggested the advisability
of looking at two additional facets: the effect of trade union membership on

continuity in employment and employee benefits, and the role of the physician's comments in shaping patient or employer work decisions. Hence all five dimensions were incorporated into the blue collar study design.

RESPONDENTS

With the prior agreement both of the hospitals reporting to a central cancer data collection center[1] and of the physician of record, 111 patients were interviewed[2] who met the following criteria for inclusion in the study. At the time the cancer diagnosis was made, they were 23 to 50 years old and were employed in an occupation classified by the Bureau of the Census as blue collar service. The site of the cancer was breast, head/neck, or rectum/colon, and the diagnosis had been made from 2 to 4 years prior to the scheduling of the interview. All of the respondents resided in Los Angeles County, although they were widely distributed among urban, suburban, and rural areas.

These specific cancer sites were chosen for three reasons. One was that their frequency rendered them among the most compelling for early attention. Second, survival rates were high enough to suggest that a number of these patients would remain attached to the labor force for many years. And third, the three groups of patients included some with overt evidence of surgical treatment (for example, voice box or facial disfigurement) whereas with others no sign of the health history would be apparent to the ordinary observer.

The fact of actually being employed at the time of diagnosis was regarded as pragmatic evidence of employability at that critical juncture. The age range selected was one that allowed for the probability that the patient had acquired some qualifying experience while precluding a challenge to employability on the ground that the individual was "too old." Moreover, the upper age limit indicated that the individual could ordinarily anticipate a work life of at least 10 more years.

A frequently heard complaint had been that employers and prospective employers sometimes expected cancer patients to have been symptom-free for 5 years as a condition of employment. Consequently, the postdiagnosis span of 2 to 4 years was established because it not only enabled the patients to have some postdiagnosis experience in working or seeking work, but also provided opportunity to find out if the "5-year cure" had been broached in their cases.

The patient-respondents represented a wide spectrum of occupational classifications, from highly skilled technicians to low-paid hourly workers in menial

---

[1] Approximately 200 public and private hospitals in and near Los Angeles County report cancer diagnoses to the Cancer Surveillance Program (CSP), a National Cancer Institute-funded activity that is part of the Regional Cancer Research Center, School of Medicine, University of Southern California.

[2] An additional 14 individuals with the same characteristics were also interviewed, but were not drawn from CSP; their participation was volunteered by their physicians. These interviews were analyzed separately but the experiences described were found to be quite representative of those included in the sample obtained from CSP.

service or laboring jobs. The employing establishments selected for interview were those which generally employed persons in such occupations or where respondents had either worked or applied unsuccessfully for work. If the patient had been in contact with an organization, it was approached only with his written consent. In 12 dyads, the good or bad experiences of the patient were tracked with the employer or potential employer in an effort to ascertain the congruence of the patient and employer perceptions about the specific cancer and work-related experiences. In all, interviews were conducted with 39 individuals in 31 employing establishments.

In addition, 13 individuals in seven unions were interviewed, the unions in some instances representing substantial networks of union locals or several hundred companies. Although these had members among the patient-respondents, not all of the patients who were union members (roughly 25%) were affiliated with the seven unions approached.

A total of 37 doctors were interviewed with three separate objectives: 10 who had declined to permit their patients to be interviewed were queried as to their reasons, which had not been stated in the denial; some were approached to confirm the cancer diagnosis, for in 9 instances the doctor had signed his authorization to contact a patient who had subsequently denied having had cancer; and in the remainder, in which prior consent was obtained from the patient, the purpose was to learn the kinds of responses made—and by whom—to inquiries from employers about the patient's employability and prognosis.

SOME FINDINGS

> I'm work-oriented and I'm feeling desperate when I'm not working. I can't lean over and die at my age [44]. So I've HAD two bouts! I'll be back at my job soon; they're holding it for me.

> You learn to hide what you can hide.

Variations on these themes were heard over and over as patients described their efforts to cling to a place in the world of work, to demonstrate to themselves and others they were still "useful," able to care for themselves and to retain mastery over a major aspect of their lives in spite of the disease that had challenged this control and autonomy. Various work-related excuses were disclosed that had been used to avoid consulting or following initial medical advice when symptoms were suspected, and various successful and unsuccessful coping devices came to light that had been utilized in the simultaneous struggle to follow a treatment regime and to remain attached or to return to a job. With the exception of a very few who had retired (some quite reluctantly) or were living more or less comfortably with the help of disability benefits and with no serious expectation of working for the present, the patient-respondents were full- or part-time members of the work force (85%) or were struggling to rejoin it.

Whether they were men (one-third of the respondents) or women, members of an ethnic minority (one-third of the sample), unskilled (one-fourth of the sample), or in skilled occupations (nearly half of all the interviewees), the respondents stressed the importance of work for psychological as well as economic reasons. This theme was pervasive, whether the respondents were younger or older (at interview, one-third were under age 45), regardless of education (more than half had not finished high school), and whether they were alone or had families (three-fourths were married and more than one-third had children at home under age 18).

The findings yielded answers to the questions initially posed in formulating the study. They were of different orders, centering on job retention and job changes, the work setting, absenteeism and task performance, work problems, and the course of health care. Some were supported by facts; others were in the realm of patterns of attitudes perceived or encountered in the work setting, some voluntarily affirmed by other sources. Thus the data showed that:

1. A total of 84% of the respondents had experienced work problems they associated with their cancer (demotions, loss of benefits and upward salary adjustments, dismissals, overt negative behavior on the part of co-workers and/ or supervisors, rejection for jobs or promotions, and so on);

2. There were 46 separate instances of discrimination alleged, some of which were confirmed and some of which were found to be baseless;

3. Some of the work problems resembled those that might confront any person who has had a serious illness, but some appeared uniquely to stem from the cancer history and others to be exacerbated by this particular illness;

4. Some positive experiences were reported by 59% of the respondents (warmly supportive attitudes of fellow workers and supervisory personnel, promotions, accommodations in tasks or hours as physical conditions indicated the desirability, and so on);

5. After the initial absence at time of diagnosis (the median absence for diagnosis and treatment was just under 9 weeks), 44% of the respondents had no absences at all, women were significantly less likely to be absent on sick leave or disability, and it was not uncommon for the clinically cured cancer patient to avoid being absent even for reasons that ordinarily would have been accepted as normal;

6. In all, 69% of the respondents did or would have liked to change jobs, mostly for cancer-related reasons, but many were frightened about the future and clung to dissatisfying jobs because they feared jeopardizing seniority, insurance benefits, and pension rights, or had been rebuffed elsewhere when the health history became known.

These findings, and many others not enumerated here, emerged from both the statistical and the qualitative data to underscore the patient's reliance on his work connection not just in order to earn a livelihood but also as a means of enabling him to deal with the fact of his cancer and with its threatened or actual impact on the quality of his life.

IMPLICATIONS FOR PSYCHOSOCIAL RESEARCH

The blue collar study, like the white collar study before it, provided a number of insights into the interrelationship of attitudes about cancer, the role of work, and the patient's life style. Both studies established that discrimination existed in several guises, some only implied but some verifiable. It is important, however, to recognize that as long as work-able individuals with cancer perceive their experiences in the work force as reflecting discrimination, whether or not the change is founded on fact, these perceptions *ipso facto* may serve to impede the work and other life adjustments of persons already under stress because of the nature of their illness.

Both studies revealed the vulnerability of the cancer patient to the stress produced by his own attitudes and feelings and those of others. Both pointed to the need for greater understanding of the psychological and social factors that influence the way the patient and his family and friends react to a threat or diagnosis of cancer. Such understanding, going beyond the medical prevention or treatment of the disease, is essential in order to facilitate utilization of measures to prevent contraction of the disease or, if already diagnosed, to follow the prescribed regimen with a fair degree of success. The two studies, by addressing themselves to certain aspects of work behavior affected by the cancer patient's health history and by some of the attitudes that influenced his work adjustment, revealed valuable clues as to how psychological, social, economic, and cultural elements impinge on each other and combine to influence the individual's own functioning as well as his relationships with others. This was particularly evident, for example, with respect to the mythology about and attitudes toward cancer and work and their combined impact on life styles.

DISPELLING MYTHOLOGY

I worried why my sister would not visit me at the hospital—but my parents said, "Put it out of your mind; sister did not visit you because she was afraid to catch the same thing from you."

I was unprepared for the loss of my voice and the attitudes of other people about my problem. My friends tried to avoid me. I was depressed because I couldn't project my voice on the job. . . . I was demoted.

An aura of mystery surrounds cancer because its cause seems murky and elusive and its course remains undetected until "too late." The mystery is deepened when the diagnostic elements are invisible to the naked eye; X-rays or electrocardiograms are clear enough, but the idea of viewing biopsies under a microscope evokes a different reaction. To this mystery is added a fateful quality when the doctor conceals the cancer diagnosis from the patient, as occurred in several instances in the blue collar study, or when the doctor routinely avoids ever using the word, as one physician-respondent said of himself in refusing to permit an interview with his patient.

This aura of mystery, combined with a not infrequent equation that cancer equals death, hints at a malevolency threatening not just the patient but the bystander as well: *anyone* can catch it! And isn't there "proof" of contagion in the news reports of cancer as a "virus"? Moreover, the idea that cancer is intractable, shameful, invidious, and punishing, is centuries old, surviving in literature and metaphor to frighten the unwary. Even the 1966 Freedom of Information Act specifically exempts only one disease, "treatment for cancer," from disclosure as "an unwarranted invasion of personal privacy."

The blue collar study contained ample evidence that fear, shame, and secrecy characterized many of the patient-respondents and were also displayed by those with whom they came in contact not only in their place of work but also in their personal lives. How much do such vestiges of ancient mythology affect the behavior of individuals in checking the nature of symptoms, in pursuing treatment plans, in maintaining accustomed and satisfying life styles? To what extent is a superstitious response to old beliefs manifest in the avoidance of cancer patients by friends or co-workers, or in defensive behaviors that take other forms? What dynamics were operating in the quotations noted immediately above, or in three cases in the blue collar study of foremen with severe voice impairment whose subordinates openly mimicked them, with the consequence that all three were demoted, one later attempting suicide and another giving up the job?

Much needs to be learned about the negative import of such precipitators of hostile defenses in terms of the functioning or adjustment or self-perception of the cancer patient. To be sure, not all persons with similar cancer histories respond in the same ways as the three men just cited. In a fourth instance, the foreman returned to work with the laughing announcement that he was undergoing a belated adolescent voice change; everyone laughed with him and the situation remained in his control. What behavioral clues can be gleaned that could lead to models for coping with hostile or other defensive behavior?

Beliefs of other kinds associated with cancer also surfaced repeatedly in the blue collar study. A common one appeared to be that even when the cancer has been successfully treated, inevitably physical limits prevent the patients from fulfilling all the functions and responsibilities of which they formerly were capable. A correlative one is that this frailty results in curtailed performance at work, leading to inordinate absenteeism and overutilization of sick leave and long-term disability benefits, and creating discomfort among fellow workers whose own sense of mortality is involved and who are uncertain how to behave with an individual whose capacity may be diminished by a life-threatening ailment. These beliefs were found among employers and co-workers as well as patients. One patient-respondent, for example, knew she would be viewed as a "burden" by her fellow workers and would be avoided as "unclean"—attitudes she herself had held about others who had returned to work after "catching it." Would actual examination of the experiences of returning cancer patients reinforce these beliefs or belie them, as was shown in the studies by Metropolitan Life Insurance Company and American Telephone and Telegraph Company?

WORKING AND INDEPENDENCE

The fears and anxieties stirred up by the possibility or actuality of cancer are compounded by internalization of a cluster of societal attitudes that cast a cloud on self-perceptions about the quality of the patient's social functioning, namely, his ability to remain independent and fulfill obligations to dependents, to "carry my own weight," "to be worth my own salt." Dependence—that is, the reduction or disappearance of the accouterments of independent functioning (as with loss of job or earnings, and curtailed management of household and children)—and frailty (short or long-term reduction in physical capacity) are evidence of failure, visible to self and others, and contribute to reduction or loss of self-esteem, a vital ingredient in effective social functioning.

In *The Greening of America,* Reich (3) remarks that "The majority of adults in this country hate their work." However, in the blue collar study (and this had also been found in the white collar study) the content analysis repeatedly underscored the impressions gained by individual members of the research team that work was held in high esteem by the patient-respondents. Although not all the respondents exhibited a strong drive to hold on to or find a job, it was an underlying theme that appeared to be fed by two streams. One was the societal attitude stressing adherence to a work ethic that has long equated adequacy and self-worth with work; morality with the independence that is symbolized by good management of financial resources, self-support, and general economic self-sufficiency; and strength with health and with overcoming the weakness that assumes the facade of illness. In the minds of many, morality and adequacy, as represented by work, fiscal solvency, and health, have remained practically synonymous. Having and holding a job is a daily reminder to the worker that he is independent, that to a considerable degree he retains mastery over his own affairs, meeting his needs and obligations. By "earning" the respect of others he merits self-respect.

Often more important than the work itself is the status derived from it in the human community. Thus one blue collar worker averred, "I was ready to climb the walls before I got back to work; it isn't that I liked the *job* so much; it's that it was a *regular* job and my friends were there!" This example refers to the second feeder-stream: namely, that the fact of having a job, regardless of its nature or their affection for it, had basic significance for the respondents in these studies. It was an element in establishing their sense of worth and also a means of proving to others that their ability to function was not impaired by the cancer, that they could "carry their own weight." Some appeared to struggle to stay on a job that was no longer within their physical capacity to maintain comfortably; many found it essential to work longer and harder than co-workers. Several worked on two or even three jobs each for very long hours each week. Some were angry at doctors who said "Don't work!" without awareness of the meaning of the work to the patients. Was it, in the long run, beneficial to the patient's health and well-being to stay on the job? What needs to be known in order to assess what would or would not be helpful to the patient, what options might be open to him, how to help him select from among these to advantage? The paucity of research in the arena of work and illness begs for correction.

LOVING AND WORKING

Interviews with blue collar workers about their work experiences subsequent to the cancer diagnosis not infrequently moved from the impact on the patient of job threat or loss to the consequences for those close to the patient, particularly the spouse or some other significant individual. There were reports of marital conflict, broken engagements or marriages, with the precipitating factors attributed to the combination of cancer and problems in the work setting. These outcomes were not surprising in light of the long-known fact that the universal task of working is closely linked to that of loving. Indeed, not uncommon is the perception that, to a considerable degree, being loved is reward for adequacy in functioning as a worker and provider. This was dramatically discernible in one situation in which the young husband with rectal cancer encountered delay in becoming re-established in a job and, for the same long period, had no sexual relations with his wife. When she spoke about this to her family physician, he told her to "find a lover," the flippant response reinforcing the husband's belief that job loss meant changes in conjugal relationships as well. Neither had sufficient trust in the family doctor or the oncologist to share their concerns.

On the other hand, the blue collar respondents cited situation after situation in which, instead of reacting as if to a threat to family and life style, the family members had closed tightly around the patient to sustain and encourage him, to share their strength. The opposite situation was apparent especially among individuals who fearfully postponed checking suspicious symptoms or declined to follow medical advice because the work function might be temporarily or permanently affected; and among persons who envisioned cancer as inevitably resulting in pain, physical incapacity, or body loss. More than one blue collar worker said, "I didn't think anyone would love me under the circumstances."

Scant research has been directed to applying findings about human interactional needs to the functions of the prevention or treatment of cancer. It is hardly a new idea that there is a reciprocal relationship between disease and social and psychological environment and functioning. Beginning with William Osler, Adolf Meyer, and Richard C. Cabot at the turn of the century, and Franz Alexander, Hans Selye, and others more contemporary, a steady stream of medical writing has stressed the importance of such features in health and disease. That the psychological and social support and treatment of the patient with cancer constitute a significant dimension of an effective and humane treatment program has been more recently demonstrated in studies by those who have focused on the problems displayed by patients late in the course of illness, when death is near. However, despite the dramatic incidence and implications of cancer in our society, remarkably little research has been undertaken or supported that aims to yield the insights so sorely needed to understand the impacts of social, economic, and emotional elements in the prevention or treatment of cancer in those who will live. The several studies reported here on work and cancer are a modest contribution to learning along these lines. They constitute, however, a beginning response to the wish voiced by a patient-respondent in the blue collar study who said:

> I have been probed and cut and medicated. But no one has *talked* to *me* or *asked* *me* what I think I should do to live my remaining life better. Everyone worries about the *cancer,* but no one sees that it is only one part of *me.* It is time someone looked at me as a whole person. Perhaps then I could think of myself that way.

REFERENCES

1. Feldman, F. L. (1976): *Work and Cancer Health Histories: A Study of the Experiences of Recovered Patients.* California Division, American Cancer Society, San Francisco.
2. Feldman, F. L. (1978): *Work and Cancer Health Histories: A Study of the Experiences of Recovered Blue-Collar Workers.* California Division, American Cancer Society, San Francisco.
3. Reich, C. A. (1970): *The Greening of America,* p. 243. Random House, New York.
4. Stone, R. W. (1975): Employing the recovered cancer patient. Presented at the Georgetown University Medical Center Cancer Symposium, Washington, D.C., Jan. 18. *Cancer* [*Suppl.*], p. 36.
5. Wheatly, G. M., Cunnick, W. R., Wright, B. P., and Van Keuren, D. (1972): *The Employment of Persons with a History of Treatment for Cancer.* Metropolitan Life Insurance Co., New York.

Psychosocial Aspects of Cancer,
edited by Jerome Cohen et al.
Raven Press, New York © 1982.

Chapter 18

Psychological Factors and Cancer Outcome

Daphne M. Panagis

West Coast Cancer Foundation, San Francisco, California 94133

The role of psychological factors in the pathogenesis of cancer has been a subject of inquiry and controversy for centuries. Most of the interest has been in identifying premorbid personality attributes or feeling states of persons who contract the disease. Such pursuits can be traced from the time of Galen, who believed women with melancholic humor were more susceptible to cancer than those of sanguine disposition (24,26). In recent years, attention has also been directed to a second but related problem, that of understanding the effects of psychological variables on the course of the disease once it is manifested. This latter study seeks to explore how dispositional and mood factors might depress or exacerbate tumor growth. It is to this topic that the present chapter is addressed.

Fox (10) has presented a thoughtful and comprehensive discussion of issues concerning the effects of psychological and stress factors on cancer etiology. Others have ably reviewed and critiqued the literature on the relationship between mental events and both the onset and the progression of cancer (34,46). The intention of this chapter is to complement these thorough summaries by considering why psychological factors have so often been related to cancer outcome and how studies of these relationships might be more clearly conceived. Three themes guide the discussion. First, the nature and allure of this psychosomatic approach is examined. Next, a number of limitations in the approach are enumerated. Finally, there is a section offering suggestions as to how we can proceed to test the relationship between the mind and cancer. Although the emphasis throughout is on the relationship of psychological variables to the growth of cancer once it exists, the discussion will rely to some extent on research into the psychosocial etiology of the disease.

STATE-TRAIT APPROACH

The study of the interaction between mental and bodily events has traditionally been termed psychosomatic research by medical investigators. In psychology there is, however, another name for the same field of inquiry, the so-called state-trait paradigm. Basically, the state-trait approach is an individual differences paradigm that entails the search for differences between individuals that are associated with particular outcomes. In the case of cancer, this type of study involves identifying characteristics of an individual's disposition or emotional state that relate to the onset of the disease or its progression.

States Versus Traits

States are differentiated from traits as less stable and more transient attributes of a person's subjective experience. Traits, conversely, are conceived of as more enduring characteristics of the person. Some theorists have argued that the manifestation of a trait in overt behavior is governed by a neurological structure (1), although a more prevailing opinion is to consider traits as configurations or sets of behaviors (5,7).

One of the most thorough discussions of state-versus-trait dynamics is Spielberger's (44) distinction between anxiety as a transitory state and as a personality trait. In this framework, state anxiety is conceived as varying within the person from situation to situation, whereas trait anxiety (e.g., proneness to feel anxious) is viewed as remaining fairly constant within the person but varying between individuals. In other words, states are used to describe how a person feels at a given moment in time, whereas traits describe how a person tends to respond across a wide range of situations.

Study of States and Traits in Cancer Etiology

Early state-trait studies in cancer were designed to look at various psychological characteristics of individuals that might increase their susceptibility to contract the disease. A common pursuit has been to determine the frequency with which emotional trauma preceded, and presumably precipitated, the onset of cancer. Most research in this area has focused on loss, especially loss of a loved one by death (13,27,28,37,41). The feeling of hopelessness is another state factor that has been used to distinguish persons who develop cancer from those who do not (36).

The contribution of dispositional factors to the etiology of neoplasia has been a second area of exploration. Those qualities considered have included the tendency to suppress affect (16,20–22); body physique (34,38); the personality trait of extroversion (6); and body image (8). Some clinicians have also argued that the tendency to use denial as a coping strategy is associated with the development of cancer (3).

Study of States and Traits in the Rate of Cancer Growth

The line of research most relevant to the present discussion is that aimed at identifying mental characteristics of the individual that influence the course of cancer once it is manifested (17,23,45). The classic study, although criticized for its methodology (25), was performed by Blumberg and associates (4). They attempted to find personality attributes that differentiated cancer patients with slow- and fast-growing tumors. To do this they administered the Minnesota Multiphasic Personality Inventory (MMPI) and other tests to male patients immediately following their initial medical treatment for cancer. All patients had an inoperable malignancy and were ambulatory at the time of testing. Scores were then maintained for a number of years until patients could be divided into two groups based on the length of their survival. Patients who had died within 2 years (less than the 25th percentile of survival) were placed in the fast-growing tumor group and were matched on age, stage of cancer, and intelligence to patients with slow-growing tumors who had survived more than 6 years (beyond the 75th percentile). It was found that the fast-growing tumor group differed significantly from the slow-growing tumor group in being more anxious, having less emotional outlet, and acting out fewer emotional feelings. A few years later Krasnoff (25) tried to replicate these findings in a better controlled study, which nonetheless suffered from a small sample size; he did not substantiate the Blumberg findings.

Stavraky (45) performed a similar study with a much larger group of 204 cancer patients of both sexes. By controlling for the site and stage of the disease, she found that patients with a good prognosis were significantly more hostile yet emotionally controlled than patients with a poor chance of survival.

One could go on and on citing findings that have been reviewed elsewhere (46). If we examine instead the reviews of the literature, we find repeated statements about the conflicting findings and poor methodologies that pervade this area of study (34). The previously cited work by Kissen (20,21) and Greer and Morris (16) on the role of the suppression of affect in lung and breast cancer patients, respectively, is exceptional to most investigations in their methodological rigor. Yet these studies, too, suffer from the problems endemic to the field of research (10). Despite these flaws, and despite the problems to be encountered in designing new investigations, we find interest in the area has prevailed. There is renewed attention to the role of mental factors on disease pathogenesis, particularly through psychophysiological pathways (15), and many investigators are concerned with the role of psychological factors as antecedents rather than precedents of cancer (46). For this reason it is important for us to re-examine the paradigm that searches for psychological correlates of tumor growth in the personality and feeling states of the cancer victim. In doing this, we will seek to better understand the appeal of the paradigm, its inherent weaknesses, and methods by which scientific inquiry can be more effectively carried out to answer questions about the role of psychological states and traits in cancer outcome.

ATTRACTIVENESS OF THE STATE-TRAIT APPROACH

Several reasons probably underlie the persistence of attempts to uncover those characteristics of the psychological make-up of individuals which relate to their physical state. First, it is obvious that mind and body processes interact. This is at the core of the ancient mind-body dualism and the psychosomatic approach in medicine. What is not so obvious, however, is how this interaction occurs.

Part of the reason for suggesting that psychological states or traits affect the onset or progression of cancer may be due to the tendency for persons to attribute causality to features of the actor in a given situation (19). Social psychological research has shown that whether viewing the behavior of individuals (18) or moving objects (31), we tend to make statements about the course of observed effects, such as, "John broke the cup because he is hostile," or "The large block bit the small block because it is aggressive." Thus we may tend to infer that a particular effect, such as a fast-growing cancer, is the result of some characteristic or attribute of the person, such as feeling self-destructive or guilty for past actions.

In science, this tendency to relate specific outcomes (e.g., fast-growing tumors) to specific characteristics of the process, event, or individual under study (e.g., anxiety) has been termed an "aristotelian" mode of thought (29). It is aristotelian in concept because features of the person or phenomenon under study are viewed as defining and limiting various outcomes, such as illness. Lewin contrasted this type of thought with a more dynamic conception of inquiry that he labeled "galilean." Galilean thought conceives of events as continual interactions in time between internal and external events. Lewin noted that in most realms of science, aristotelian paradigms have preceded galilean approaches. In medicine, the classic germ theory is an example of an aristotelian paradigm, whereas a holistic position that recognizes the interplay of biological, social, and psychological forces in disease etiology and progression is exemplary of galilean thought.

The tendency to begin scientific inquiry with aristotelian concepts, resulting in the historical primacy of the germ theory, may account in part for efforts to locate the origin of a disease in psychological features of the individual sufferer. That is, the inability of basic researchers to discover a single "germ" cause for cancer may have given impetus to a search for disease correlates in the individual's personality or emotional state.

Finally, it is important to point out that much of the allure of the paradigm is due to the benefits that would come from establishing consistencies between psychological variables and cancer outcome, regardless of the direction of causality. For instance, if we can demonstrate that a mental state or trait is repeatedly associated with a disease state, we may be able to use these factors as marker variables in planning medical and psychosocial treatments. And perhaps more importantly, we may be able to intervene to affect psychological factors in a way that leads to biological changes.

In summary, there are several aspects of human cognition and scientific investigation that might account for the appeal of the state-trait approach. First is the undeniable connection between mental and physical events. Second is a tendency in humans to perceive an effect and to then make attributions about cause based on characteristics of the agent in the situation. Third is the characteristic of scientific theorizing to go through a stage of conceptualization in which a phenomenon is depicted by its characteristic features (e.g., a specific illness is linked to a specific germ, or a specific medical outcome is portrayed as a function of specific personality traits). If we concede that the approach is alluring and of potential value in cancer care, we must next look at it more carefully to apprise ourselves of its shortcomings. By so doing, we can elaborate the paradigm and plan more sensibly for future investigations.

LIMITATIONS OF THE STATE-TRAIT APPROACH

Although there is much to be gained by correlating the psychological characteristics of patients with the course of their disease, there are a number of pitfalls open to the investigator or enthusiast who seeks to relate emotional states and personality traits to cancer outcome. To begin with, one must recognize the biological complexity of the disease. Cancer is not one but actually many diseases that may have different causes. Therefore, a psychological factor may relate to cancer of one site but not another.

Cancer varies not only in kind but also in degree. One must recognize that mental attributes may be associated with early (e.g., stages I or II) or late (e.g., stages III and IV) stage cancers, but not both. Thus, as Fox (10) noted, it is necessary for investigators to carefully select and describe the population of patients (and controls) utilized in research. When a case-control design is utilized to study the effects of psychological attributes on disease course, it is advisable that patients in the study groups be comparable. This is just as true in psychological inquiries as it is in clinical trials or other physiologically oriented endeavors.

A second potential limitation of the approach lies in the measurement of the dependent or psychological variables. The use of standardized tests such as the MMPI, Eysenck Personality Inventory, or Maudsley Personality Inventory, which were not designed for the chronically ill, might be questioned because we are not yet certain of their validity with cancer patients. That is, an MMPI score might really be measuring an effect of the disease when we believe we are measuring a characteristic of the person (10; Chapter 22). Tryon (49) has warned us of this problem, which he calls the "test-trait fallacy." The fallacy is committed when test scores or measures of a trait, as dependent variables, are said to reflect basic qualities of the individual, thereby converting dependent to independent variables. To offset this fallacy, Fiske (9) has recommended methods for empirically validating personality traits.

Related to measurement difficulty is the fact that many investigators in the area have defined their psychological factors by the "operations" or tests used to assess them. When different investigators use different operations that have not been cross-validated, it is difficult to know whether they have measured the same factor.

Although these disadvantages can easily be applied to most psychosocial research in cancer, there are third and fourth limitations specific to the state-trait approach. The most straightforward of these is that the approach pays no attention to the contribution of factors in the person's social and physical environment. Fox and Goldsmith (11), for example, have discussed the importance of environmental agents in the etiology of cancer. And Bloom (Chapter 13) suggests that a person's social support system may influence disease outcome. It is important, then, for investigators to recognize that situational factors can influence behavior (32) and may interact with personality attributes and disease state. Therefore, one should at least control for the effects of the environment on disease course in state-trait research.

A final shortcoming with the state-trait approach is that it carries with it an assumption of a cause-effect relationship. Given present evidence, we cannot safely conclude that a person's emotional and dispositional make-up facilitate the progression of cancer. For instance, Meerloo (30) and others (10,34) have discussed many of the possible relationships that may underlie an observed association between a psychological factor and cancer outcome. These are discussed in the following paragraphs for the purpose of illustrating the kinds of relationships that may exist between mental states or traits and disease progression, and to point to the fallacy of assuming that the former causes the latter:

1. Coincidence. The easiest explanation of an observed relationship between psychological states or traits and cancer outcome is that the two events are the result of coincidence. That is, each was caused by independent agents.

2. External agent. Another obvious alternative is that a third event, some environmental agent, caused both phenomena to occur. This external agent may be in the physical environment or in the person's social network.

3. Internal agent. A third explanation of the relationship between psychological factors and cancer progression is that heredity or some internal immunological or neuroendocrine activity caused both to result. Greer (15) has reviewed some of the literature relating emotional states or dispositions to cancer, noting several physiological mechanisms that may produce observed associations between mental and physical events. He cites research by Solomon (42) and his associates (43) which implicates, in particular, the immune system.

4. Behavioral agent. A fourth possibility is that a behavior may induce particular emotional states and may also affect one's health status. For example, an observed association between depression and poor prognosis might occur because patients demonstrating both have deficient nutritional intake. Their diet, or eating behavior, may thus underlie both outcomes—depressed mood state and poor health status.

5. Intervening agent. Another alternative explanation, which is actually a set of explanations, is that some event intervenes between the psychological and biological factors which causes them to correlate in a particular way. For example, certain authors have argued that the mental state of the patient can

influence the activity of the immune system, which then affects the course of the disease (40). Moreover, mood states like anxiety may affect behaviors such as prompt care-seeking (2,14) or adherence. These behaviors, likewise, may then affect prognosis.

6. Disease causation. A sixth possibility is that the disease of cancer causes particular psychological reactions, or that psychological consequences are secondary to the disease's progression. Since it is impossible to accurately pinpoint biologically the true onset of cancer, it is always possible that physiological changes precede psychological changes. This will undoubtedly be the case even in well-controlled longitudinal studies, because the biological changes associated with cancer long precede its detection.

7. Psychological causation. The final possibility is that some psychological state or trait does indeed cause the disease to spread.

SUGGESTIONS FOR FUTURE INVESTIGATION

The intent of the preceding discussion was to point to the complex relationships that may exist between a person's emotions, dispositions, social or environmental circumstances, and biological state. This complexity should not discourage one from engaging in psychological research in cancer, but it should alert the investigator to potential confounding variables and areas in which experimental or statistical control may be necessary.

It is strongly advised in studying the relationship between mental attributes and the growth rate of cancer that one (a) take an interactionist position; (b) familiarize oneself with the medical and social science literature to gain a better understanding of how factors other than those under study may influence cancer outcome; and (c) begin with a hypothesis, or at least in the context of a theoretical framework. There are many ways to proceed in hypothesis-generating and theory-building endeavors. One may, for example, review what work has been done, or make personal observations, or examine psychological and medical records that currently exist to look for consistencies between dispositions or feeling states and rate of cancer growth. In any single research one cannot examine everything nor control for all factors, but one can utilize a theoretical paradigm to select which particular variables should be measured, manipulated, or controlled.

In the next several paragraphs four approaches will be discussed which can and have been used appropriately to study the role of psychological factors on cancer outcome. All of these approaches are subject to certain shortcomings that are common to all psychosocial research in medicine. These are discussed in order to enlighten or remind those investigators not so acquainted with experimental procedures of issues to be concerned with in designing a study, and hopefully will not offend those readers more sophisticated in research methodology.

Known Group Approach

One approach is to study known groups of patients, such as those with a good or poor prognosis, and to try to identify factors that distinguish them from one another. This type of approach may be a useful one to employ to gather data for theory building because it can provide the basis for making empirical generalizations about the relationships between a given state or trait factor and cancer outcome. Exemplary of the known-group approach are some epidemiological studies that have attempted to imply the contribution of psychological factors to the genesis of cancer by comparing the incidence of the disease in persons known to vary in terms of their psychological characteristics. A problem with this approach is that the best it can do is to establish consistencies between mental and biological states. That is, if we begin a study with two groups of patients already differing in terms of their prognosis and then take psychological measures, we may find significant correlations between personality attributes and disease course, but we cannot be certain whether one preceded the other.

Experimental Approach

A second approach is to experimentally manipulate one or a set of psychological variables and to then look for changes in the growth of the neoplasia. Clinical work in cancer has, for example, utilized a variety of self-healing techniques that involve mental processes. These include systematic desensitization, hypnosis, and guided imagery (33).

Perhaps the most well-known of these techniques in cancer is the Simonton procedure of guided imagery (40). Basing their treatment on the surveillance theory (42), which points to the depression of the immune system as a factor stimulating cancer growth, the Simontons assume that by affecting the patient's belief system and emotional outlook they can influence the activity of the immune system and thereby the rate of cancer growth. The goal of their treatment, which is psychological but used only in conjunction with standard medical therapies, is to change patients' beliefs, to make the patients feel positive and in control of their disease. The procedure involves familiarizing the patient with the principles of stress reduction. An autogenic relaxation technique is used that teaches the patient to breathe deeply and to imagine, symbolically, that the cancer cells are being destroyed by the body's immune system and by the prescribed medical treatment. Persons are asked to practice this visualization exercise three times a day and to attend group therapy classes. Visualization is continued by the patient once the formal therapy ends.

A sound experimental design to evaluate the efficacy of this procedure would require randomly assigning patients to two groups, one which receives the psychological therapy, the other which does not. Premeasures of each patient's attitudes and psychological states or dispositions would be needed, as would measures of his prognosis and physical state. Post-treatment differences between the two groups would provide strong evidence that the psychological manipulation had an effect on the biological course of the disease.

An obvious problem with the experimental approach is that it is difficult to match patients and to randomly assign them to treatment and control groups. Moreover, because some patients will choose not to participate in whatever psychological intervention is planned, the investigator must always cope with the effects of self-selection. If not taken into account in pre-study planning, these two problems may jeopardize the generalizability of study findings. Even with these shortcomings, the experimental method is a powerful research tool and its application in this area is highly recommended.

Longitudinal Study of Asymptomatic Persons

In trying to examine the role of psychological factors in the pathogenesis of cancer, a desirable approach is to follow over time a sample of individuals at high risk of developing cancer but with no known malignancy. By taking both psychological and physiological measures over time, one can look for changes in both mental and biological states. Premorbid personality characteristics or mood states can thus be associated with cancer at the time of diagnosis and growth changes. Thomas and her associates (47,48) employed this longitudinal approach in their well-documented prospective study of the mental and physical well-being of graduates of Johns Hopkins medical school. Although subsidiary to the original study intent, they related a number of factors to the onset of cancer, including the developmental antecedent of closeness to parents.

The merit of this approach is that it builds the factor of time into the research design, and one can establish the temporal course of both psychological and physical factors. Nevertheless, although one may find that particular mental attributes consistently precede the onset or progression of cancer, the psychological factor may not cause the biological changes. A much more significant problem with this approach is the large sample that would be required to yield a sizable number of persons who actually develop cancer, and the expense of obtaining physiological and psychological measures on these persons.

Longitudinal Study of Symptomatic Persons

A related approach is to follow over time persons who have been diagnosed as having cancer. By so doing, one can identify factors that relate to changes in health status and a poor prognosis. Weisman and Worden (50) utilized this method in their study of terminal cancer patients, reporting several psychological factors associated with short survival time.

CONCLUSION

The major thrust of this chapter has been to argue that although it is alluring to search for psychological correlates of cancer growth, one must proceed cautiously when designing research and inferring causal connections with mental and biological factors. Any person embarking on research in this area is strongly advised to utilize a theoretical paradigm or rationale in selecting study populations and dependent measures. If one decides instead to go fishing for significance by measuring a large number of psychological attributes, it is likely that one will find at least one significant relationship between a state or trait factor and disease progression. However, this is a statistical significance, and it can be affected by the number of measures taken in a given experiment or by the number of experiments conducted. If one takes too many measures or does too many experiments, one will undoubtedly make mistakes in sometimes concluding a particular effect when, in fact, there is none.

By learning more about the biological nature of the disease, and how characterological, mood, and social factors have been associated with the pathogenesis of cancer, we can phrase more parsimonious hypotheses and design more sensible experiments. As Frank (12) has noted, by taking a more holistic conception of illness and healing, without overplaying the role of either mental or physical processes, we may be of assistance in "diagnosing, preventing, and treating organic disease" and its psychosocial concomitants.

REFERENCES

1. Allport, G. W. (1961): *Pattern and Growth in Personality.* Holt, Rinehart & Winston, New York.
2. Antonovsky, A., and Hartman, H. (1974): Delay in the detection of cancer: A review of the literature. *Health Educ. Monogr.,* 2:98–128.
3. Bahnson, C. B. (1970): Basic epistemological considerations regarding psychosomatic processes and their application to current psychophysiological cancer research. *Int. J. Psychobiol.,* 1:57–69.
4. Blumberg, E. M., West, P. M., and Ellis, F. W. (1954): A possible relationship between psychological factors and human cancer. *Psychosom. Med.,* 16:277–286.
5. Cattell, R. B. (1965): *The Scientific Analysis of Personality.* Penguin, Baltimore.
6. Coppen, A., and Metcalfe, M. (1963): Cancer and extraversion. *Br. Med. J.,* 2:18–19.
7. Eysenck, H. J. (1953): *The Structure of Human Personality.* Methuen, London.
8. Fisher, S., and Cleveland, S. (1958): *Body Image and Personality.* Van Nostrand, Princeton, N.J.
9. Fiske, D. (1973): Can a personality construct be validated empirically? *Psychol. Bull.,* 80:89–92.
10. Fox, B. H. (1978): Premorbid psychological factors as related to cancer incidence. *J. Behav. Med.,* 1:45–133.
11. Fox, B. H., and Goldsmith, J. R. (1976): Behavioral issues in prevention of cancer. *Prev. Med.,* 5:106–121.
12. Frank, J. D. (1975): Psychotherapy of bodily disease. *Psychother. Psychosom.,* 26:192–202.
13. Greene, W. A., Jr. (1954): Psychological factors and reticuloendothelial disease: I. Preliminary observations on a group of males with lymphomas and leukemias. *Psychosom. Med.,* 16:220.
14. Greer, S. (1974): Psychological aspects: Delay in the treatment of breast cancer. *Proc. R. Soc. Med.,* 67:470–473.

15. Greer, S. (1979): Psychological enquiry: A contribution to cancer research. *Psychol. Med.,* 9:81–89.
16. Greer, S., and Morris, T. (1975): Psychological attributes of women who develop breast cancer: A controlled study. *J. Psychosom. Res.,* 19:147–153.
17. Hinton, J. (1975): The influence of previous personality on reactions to having terminal cancer. *Omega,* 6:95–111.
18. Jones, E. E., and Nisbett, R. E. (1972): The actor and the observer: Divergent perceptions of the causes of behavior. In: *Attribution: Perceiving the Causes of Behavior,* edited by E. E. Jones, D. E. Kanouse, H. H. Kelley, R. E. Nisbett, S. Valins, and B. Weiner. General Learning Press, Morristown, N.J.
19. Kelley, H. H. (1967): Attribution theory in social psychology. In: *Nebraska Symposium on Motivation,* edited by D. Levine. University of Nebraska Press, Lincoln.
20. Kissen, D. M. (1963): Personality characteristics in males conducive to lung cancer. *Br. J. Med. Psychol.,* 36:27–36.
21. Kissen, D. M. (1966): The significance of personality in lung cancer in men. *Ann. N.Y. Acad. Sci.,* 125:820–826.
22. Kissen, D. M., Brown, R. I. F., and Kissen, M. A. (1969): A further report on personality and psychosocial factors in lung cancer. *Ann. N.Y. Acad. Sci.,* 1964:535.
23. Klopfer, B. (1957): Psychological variables in human cancer. *J. Projective Technique,* 21:331–340.
24. Kowal, S. J. (1955): Emotions as a cause of cancer, 18th and 19th century contributions. *Psychoanal. Rev.,* 42:217–227.
25. Krasnoff, A. (1959): Psychological variables and human cancer: A cross validation study. *Psychosom. Med.,* 21:291.
26. LeShan, L. (1959): Psychological states as factors in the development of malignant disease: A critical review. *J. Natl. Cancer Inst.,* 22:1–18.
27. LeShan, L., and Worthington, R. E. (1955): Some psychologic correlates of neoplastic disease: A preliminary report. *J. Clin. Exp. Psychopathol.,* 16:281–288.
28. LeShan, L., and Worthington, R. (1956): Some recurrent life history patterns observed in patients with malignant disease. *J. Nerv. Ment. Dis.,* 124:460–465.
29. Lewin, K. (1935): *A Dynamic Theory of Personality: Selected Papers,* pp. 1–42. McGraw-Hill, New York.
30. Meerloo, J. A. M. (1954): Psychological implications of malignant growth. *Br. J. Med. Psychol.,* 27:210.
31. Michotte, A. E. (1950): The emotions regarded as functional connections. In: *Feelings and Emotions,* edited by M. I. Reymert. McGraw-Hill, New York.
32. Mischel, W. (1968): *Personality and Assessment.* John Wiley & Sons, New York.
33. Panagis, D. M. (1979): Supportive therapy: Goals and methods. In: *Mind and Cancer Prognosis,* edited by B. A. Stoll. John Wiley & Sons, London.
34. Perrin, G. M., and Pierce, I. R. (1959): Psychosomatic aspects of cancer. *Psychosom. Med.,* 21:397–408.
35. Reznikoff, M. (1955): Psychological factors in breast cancer: A preliminary study of the same personality trends in patients with cancer of the breast. *Psychosom. Med.,* 17:96.
36. Schmale, A., and Iker, H. (1971): Hopelessness as a predictor of cervical cancer. *Soc. Sci. Med.,* 5:95–100.
37. Schonfield, J. (1975): Psychological and life-experience differences between Israeli women with benign and cancerous breast lesions. *J. Psychosom. Res.,* 19:229–234.
38. Sheldon, W. H., Hartl, E. M., and McDermott, E. (1949): *The Varieties of Delinquent Youth.* Harper, New York.
39. Simonton, C. (1975): Belief systems and management of the emotional aspects of malignancy. *J. Transpers. Psychol.,* 7:29–47.
40. Simonton, O. C., and Simonton, S. S. (1978): *Getting Well Again.* J. P. Tarcher, Los Angeles.
41. Snell, L., and Graham, S. (1971): Social trauma as related to cancer of the breast. *Br. J. Cancer,* 25:721–734.
42. Solomon, G. F. (1969): Emotions, stress, the central nervous system and immunity. *Ann. N.Y. Acad. Sci.,* 164:335–343.
43. Solomon, G. F., Amkraut, A. A., and Kasper, P. (1974): Immunity, emotions, and stress. *Ann. Clin. Res.,* 6:313–322.

44. Spielberger, C. D. (1975): Anxiety: State-trait process. In: *Stress and Anxiety, Vol. 1,* edited by C. D. Spielberger and I. G. Sarason. Hemisphere, Washington, D.C.
45. Stavraky, K. M. (1968): Psychological factors in the outcome of human cancer. *J. Psychosom. Res.,* 12:251–259.
46. Surawicz, F. G., Brightwell, D. R., Weitzel, W. D., and Othmer, E. (1976): Cancer, emotions, and mental illness: The present state of understanding. *Am. J. Psychiatry,* 133:1306–1310.
47. Thomas, C. B., and Duszynski, K. (1974): Closeness to parents and the family constellation in a prospective study of five disease states: Suicide, mental illness, malignant tumor, hypertension, and coronary heart disease. *Johns Hopkins Med. J.,* 134:251–270.
48. Thomas, C. B., and Greenstreet, R. L. (1973): Psychological characteristics in youth as predictors of five disease states: Suicide, mental illness, hypertension, coronary heart disease, and tumor. *Johns Hopkins Med. J.,* 132:16–43.
49. Tryon, W. W. (1979): The test-trait fallacy. *Am. Psychologist,* 34:402–406.
50. Weisman, A. D., and Worden, J. W. (1975): Psychosocial analysis of cancer deaths. *Omega,* 6:61–75.

Psychosocial Aspects of Cancer,
edited by Jerome Cohen et al.
Raven Press, New York © 1982.

Chapter 19

Intervention Strategies for Families

David M. Kaplan

Social Services, Stanford University, Stanford, California 94305

It has long been evident that any serious and prolonged illness such as cancer functions as a source of stress demanding a major adjustment not only by the patient but also by family members. Family as well as individual reactions are crucial in coping with acute stress since the family has a unique responsibility for mediating the reactions of its members.

Individuals belonging to families do not resolve their own problems of stress independently, nor are family members immune to effects of stress that may be focused primarily within another member. Vincent (11) states that the family is uniquely organized to carry out its stress-mediating responsibilities and is in a strategic position to do so. No other social institution has demonstrated a comparable capability for mediation that affects as many people in the community.

Because the family has a commitment to protect its members over a wide range of stressful conditions and for long periods of time, physicians, social workers, and other professionals working with a severely ill person must extend their concern beyond the patient, at least to members of the immediate family and to other close relatives. Clinicians must offer help to other family members when they need it in order to resolve specific problems of stress. If stress is great enough and sufficiently prolonged, the role of the family as a buffer for its members can be permanently impaired or even destroyed. To prevent this, more must be learned about effective individual and family coping, and more help must be given to protect and improve coping functions.

MANAGEMENT PROBLEMS

In addition to the demonstrable risks associated with a fatal illness, many critical problems of management involving the family confront medical and health personnel. The following, for example, are among the questions of management raised in childhood leukemia:

1. What should the parents, the leukemic child, healthy siblings, and members of the extended family be told about leukemia, that is, about its course, treatment, and prognosis?

2. Who should give each family member the information deemed appropriate?

3. What advice should be given to parents who consider major family changes after they hear about the child's diagnosis, for example, having another child soon, separating from each other, remarrying, moving to a new community?

4. What should be done to help parents who seriously disagree about the handling of fatal illness in the family?

5. What help can be offered to single-parent families faced with long-term illness?

6. During the period in which the parents are preoccupied with the leukemic child and tend to neglect the healthy siblings, how can the needs of these other children be protected?

7. What should be done to help parents who avoid visiting the leukemic child during hospitalization, and to help the child?

8. How can morbid preoccupation over the lost child be avoided?

Similar issues of management apply to families in which an adult member has cancer. Clearly, effective family coping with illness, whether of a child or an adult, involves a number of common points of reference.

COPING WITH STRESS

Adaptive coping entails above all mastery of the psychosocial problems associated with *acute stress.* For family members confronted by stressful situations it offers the greatest protection and the best assurance that the family will continue as a viable unit, able to meet the changing needs of its members after they have gotten over the stress.

The development of preventive or clinical programs capable of reversing maladaptive responses to illness is contingent on having detailed knowledge of the process of adaptation specific to each illness, including relevant coping tasks and methods of task accomplishment. Because coping tasks vary significantly from one illness to another, it is first necessary to identify the problems posed by each.

A premature birth, for example, requires the family to anticipate possible loss of the infant. If it survives, the possibility of its being defective must be faced. Even when the prognosis is favorable, the parents must prepare themselves to care for an infant with special early needs yielding in time to normal patterns. Most families with premature babies manage these tasks well, but a number do not. This minority continues to think of and treat the premature baby as though it were permanently damaged, even after its development follows normal patterns (6).

The family with a cancer patient is also suddenly confronted with major alterations in its circumstances that threaten cherished hopes and values for all its members and involve drastic changes of life style. Each family member must comprehend these new circumstances and adapt to them by making suitable role changes, despite an understandable reluctance to face painful losses.

There are no simple methods of resolving the problems associated with maladaptive responses to illness, but there is a way of conceptualizing such problems that may lead to effective interventions. This relatively new theoretical approach is concerned with the process of adaptation itself, rather than with premorbid factors (7). In this conception, the process of individual adaptation to change is conceived of as a complex, but decipherable, attempt at problem solving. The problem-solving process is at the heart of adaptation and of effective interventions.

In this approach to human adaptation, individual coping responses to illness are conceived of as attempts to resolve specific and immediate coping tasks posed by an illness, whatever the individual's history may be. These coping efforts are coherent responses that can be identified readily and the efficacy of which can be judged by how well they resolve the problems and tasks of adaptation and by the extent to which they are associated with good rehabilitative outcome.

The substance of this problem-solving model lies in detailed knowledge of the nature of successful coping behavior. The quintessential question to ask about an individual struggling to cope with a serious illness is not, is he psychologically healthy, but are his attempts to cope effective? Personality theory has not shed much light on our understanding of the process of human adaptation to change, nor has it produced effective methods of intervention in these situations.

The concept of "problem solving" may connote, to many, an intellectual exercise having little if anything to do with human emotions. In this presentation, cognition is an important part of the problem-solving process, but so are the emotions aroused by an illness that threatens cherished activities, causes suffering and disability, and involves painful sacrifices. The individual ability to handle the emotions generated by illness is an essential ingredient of effective problem solving. The temptation to avoid disturbing emotions such as sadness, anger, fear, and anxiety rather than allowing these feelings to run their course is a cause of much, but not of all, ineffective coping.

The tasks of coping with stress occur in order and relate to the characteristic sequential phases of the illness, that is, diagnosis, treatment, remission, exacerbation, and terminal state. These phase-related tasks must be resolved in proper sequence within the time limits set by the duration of the successive phases of the illness. Failure to resolve them in this manner is likely to jeopardize the total coping process of the entire family and outcome (6).

Successfully resolving any crisis depends largely on the ability of each individual to experience with minimum delay the immediately painful consequences of a stress-producing event and to comprehend and anticipate, even though dimly, the later consequences—the pain, sorrow, and sacrifice that the trauma will entail. Comprehension in this context means learning to accept one's new life circumstances, however painful, and then acting in accordance with the new conditions that follow the original crisis-precipitating event.

The family, primarily through its adult members, can either facilitate or obstruct individual efforts to master a situation of stress. It is important to identify adaptive and maladaptive coping responses by the family as early as possible after diagnosis. Developing a method of early case finding can make intervention feasible during this crucial period and reduce the incidence of families who fail to cope adequately.

Early identification is important because studies of crises suggest that both the individual and the family reactions to the threat of prolonged illness are fashioned from 1 to 4 weeks after the diagnosis is confirmed (11). The coping responses evident by then, whether adaptive or maladaptive, tend to persist and to be reinforced throughout the course of the illness, which may run for years. Therefore, the ideal time to discover that families are coping inadequately is during this early phase.

STANFORD LEUKEMIC FAMILY STUDY FINDINGS

Families with cancer patients constitute a high-risk group in the sense that the severe stress precipitated by diagnosis of the illness generates many problems in addition to those involved in physically treating it. Both clinical and research observations indicate that a disturbingly large number of families who face this situation fail to cope successfully with the problems it poses (1,8). Binger et al. (2) reported that following this diagnosis at least one member in more than half the families in a 1969 study required psychiatric treatment. Bozeman et al. (4) noted that among families with a leukemic child school difficulties among the healthy children, divorce, and illness occurred frequently. Kaplan and associates (8) reported that 87% of the families in their sample failed to cope adequately with the consequences of childhood leukemia, and that this failure created a variety of individual and interpersonal problems which were superimposed on the stresses posed by the illness itself.

The Stanford postmortem survey of 40 leukemic families included 173 surviving members. Of those survivors, 70% were reported as having at least one serious problem with multiple problems reported among the survivors of 87% of the families. Aggravated marital difficulties were reported in 70% of the families, while 65% reported troubled parent-child relationships and problems among their children at school.

Health problems, including ulcers, colitis, and hypertension, were reported by 95% of the families. Drinking by one parent was listed as a serious problem in 40%. In 88% there were morbid grief reactions, including daily visits to the cemetery, enshrining the effects of the dead child, or inability to make any reference to the diseased child within the family. Someone was under psychiatric care for the first time in 35% of the families.

Adults with major work problems were found in 60% of the families; 43% reported mothers who were having trouble managing home responsibilities. Of particular significance is the fact that 80% of all problems elicited by the survey were not in existence prior to the diagnosis of cancer.

The five families that did emerge intact from the leukemic experience had one characteristic in common: they were successful problem solvers of the demands made on them by the illness. The 35 families that suffered multiple problems were ineffective problem solvers, having made poor decisions in their accommodation to cancer.

What critical behaviors and decisions indicated effective problem solving among leukemic families? There were certain tasks that the successful coping families resolved which the majority of poor coping families did not. Specifically, the successful problem-solving families understood the nature of their child's illness from the outset, i.e., that leukemia is a serious chronic illness with a very guarded prognosis. The parents in those few families were able to communicate this concept of the illness to all members of the family, including the ill child, with appropriate concern and sadness and without inhibiting the expression of similar feelings in any other family member.

This minority of effective problem-solving families were then able to prepare themselves realistically for the long haul during the illness without subterfuge, supporting each other effectively throughout the period. The 35 families, the poor problem solvers, were not able to put the illness experience behind them once the leukemic child died but continued to be plagued by the fallout of problems described earlier, by the residual difficulties characteristic of poor problem solving (8).

It is important to note that ineffective coping need not reflect moral or personality defects in the parents. Poor problem solving more commonly was related to a poverty of social supports within the nuclear family, either because little or no extended family or friends were available, or because, when they were, they were not helpful or supportive.

ADAPTATION TO BREAST CANCER

Here the impetus to problem solving is anything but immediate; the process of adaptation to breast cancer is gradual, beginning with a woman's acknowledgment of the existence of a breast lump.[1] Her awareness or suspicion of a growth constitutes the first coping task.

Not uncommonly, a lump of moderate or of large dimensions may exist for some time without being recognized. Failure to acknowledge a tumor itself

---

[1] This section is excerpted from Kaplan and Grandstaff (7).

constitutes a coping decision: it is one way to deal with the problem. In this instance, further problem solving is obviated until such time as the lesion is acknowledged.

The woman who accomplishes the first task of recognizing the existence of a breast lump goes on to face the second coping task—evaluating the potential risk of her tumor. There are women who have not learned that a breast lump may be cancerous; for them the lump is not a threat and there is no need to evaluate its significance. Further problem solving does not occur for these women until an awareness of the potential threat of the lesion is realized.

For the woman who has learned that a breast lump may be cancerous, an assessment must be made of the potential risk she runs from her lesion. There are basically three kinds of decisions that can be reached in such lump evaluations. One decision is to conclude that the growth is not cancerous. It may be perceived as the result of an infection or associated with the menstrual cycle, or it may be viewed as a benign lump in a woman with a history of noncancerous breast lesions. The second possible decision is to concede the possibility of malignancy but to judge the risk to be only potential and not immediate. Usually this decision is accompanied by a wait-and-see attitude while a home remedy or prayer or other action is resorted to in the hope that the lesion will disappear. Weeks or months may go by before this attitude is changed. The third option is to decide that the lump risk is immediate and requires an early examination by a physician or some other healer. (We will assume for the purpose of this presentation that the patient's contacts are with physicians.)

This process of decision making which first occurs following the discovery of the breast lesion is typically repeated two more times: once after an initial examination by a physician who is not a surgeon, and again after a second examination by a surgeon.

After each medical examination, the physician (or surgeon) makes one of three recommendations that closely parallel the decisions a woman has to make independently upon lump discovery. He may decide (a) that the lump is not cancerous, (b) that the lump needs to be examined again after a specified time interval, or (3) that the tumor should be referred to a surgeon for further examination (in the case of the surgeon, his third choice is to recommend a biopsy). The patient can respond to each medical recommendation either by concurring or by disagreeing and/or seeking another medical opinion.

When the patient decides to go ahead with a biopsy, there are several decisions to be made in the event that the tissue proves malignant: (a) the patient may agree to a biopsy without any further treatment commitment; (b) she may decide against any treatment after biopsy or choose to have only a nonsurgical treatment (e.g., radiation implant, chemotherapy, or radiotherapy); (c) if she elects surgical removal of the cancerous tissue, she may agree to one-stage surgery (biopsy and mastectomy performed in one operation) or two-stage surgery (the first surgery limited to the biopsy, followed, usually after a brief interval, by a second surgery for the mastectomy); (d) she may decide to have the type of mastectomy recommended by her surgeon or elect to have an alternative form of mastectomy; and finally (e) she may or may not accept the recommendations for adjuvant treatment following surgery.

The implications for intervention posed by these decisions are not difficult to infer. Those decisions that ignore or overlook the existence of a breast lump are clearly hazardous. Since each woman is primarily responsible for lump discovery on her own, the appropriate intervention is educational in nature, i.e., teaching women that lumps may be cancerous and urging them to conduct regular self-examinations. Our efforts to educate in this area have not met with outstanding success so far.

Those decisions that dismiss lumps as benign without careful examination and biopsy, or that put off medical examinations for more than a few weeks, are also risky. Again, the task of educating women, family members, and physicians about these risks is an important aspect of breast cancer intervention.

The second concurrent group of decisions that each woman makes as she decides whether or not to recognize a breast lump and what to do about it concerns the other persons she involves in her decision making—specifically, which persons she involves, when she involves them, and how she involves herself with them, i.e., for what purposes. There are many reasons for involving other people in the problem-solving process: (a) to gather the data needed to make decisions, (b) to find support for those decisions that are made, (c) to seek comfort for the many fears associated with breast cancer, particularly the threat of death and disfigurement, and finally (d) to allow others who are close to the patient the time to prepare themselves for the possibility and implications of malignancy, just as the woman with a lesion must prepare herself.

The woman who acknowledges the existence of a potentially cancerous breast lump proceeds to make the decisions described above. Moreover, although there may be variations in how they are reached, the decisions made by each individual fall into identifiable patterns and into recognizable subsets that can be identified as adaptive or maladaptive. Whether or not decisions are adaptive can be empirically verified by subsequent assessment once the crisis is over (5).

There are many issues and fears that may preoccupy a woman once she discovers a breast lump. These critical issues and fears are the essence of the coping tasks whose resolution is the main business of the adaptive process. Pattison (9) lists eight fears of the dying patient—fears of the unknown, of loneliness, of sorrow, of the loss of one's body, of the loss of self-control, of suffering and pain, of the loss of one's identity, and of physical and mental regression. The woman with a breast lesion may be concerned with one or more of these fears and others besides—the loss of her good health to a life-threatening chronic disease, the fear of not surviving surgery, and the fear of the disfigurement following mastectomy. Once surgery is over, there is the additional worry about whether cancer cells will be found in the lymph glands, and if they are, a fear of the effects of adjuvant treatment.

Our study observations indicate that those concerns which center on, first, disfigurement following breast amputation, and second, the loss of one's good health to a disease that may eventually cause death should be confronted and substantially resolved before surgery is performed. Successful resolution implies acceptance of these two concerns as real possibilities that no matter how disagreeable they are, one must be prepared to live with. If these issues are denied or are unresolved prior to surgery, the full rehabilitation of the woman may not be achieved or may be delayed for years even when the prognosis of the illness itself is favorable.

Why is it so important to achieve a substantial resolution of these two problems before surgery? In the course of any crisis, one's normal activities and responsibilities vis-à-vis others are suspended while the individual is given a brief time to solve the new problems, to come to terms with one's new reality, with a new set of circumstances imposed by a serious illness. Whether a woman can achieve the resumption of most of her responsibilities—consistent with the limitations of having a serious disease—depends on how quickly and how successfully she comes to terms with her new self. Many women do resume highly satisfying lives within weeks of lump discovery even though they no longer have intact, healthy bodies and have to live with the knowledge of possible recurrence of a life-threatening disease for the rest of their lives. Many women do not.

If these coping tasks—acceptance of disfigurement and of the disease's threat to life—are not resolved before surgery, it will be extremely difficult for the woman to take up the job of fashioning a new life, part of which involves picking up old responsibilities and activities. The longer one is preoccupied with tasks that need to be resolved effectively and quickly, the greater is the risk that important activities and relationships may deteriorate or be lost altogether. A woman, for example, who cannot accept the fact of disfigurement before surgery will not be able to resume sexual relations with any measure of pleasurable anticipation or satisfaction for herself or her partner. The woman who fails to successfully resolve these particular coping tasks early is apt to be preoccupied and/or inhibited by these problems until they are resolved. She will be unable to pick up the pieces of her life and put them together into a new, viable, and satisfying way of living.

Unfortunately, one does not have unlimited time to resolve threatening and disruptive changes. Nature abhors the vacuum created by an illness and permits only a temporary suspension of the normal responsibilities of being a wife, a mother, and so on. If the vacuum is not filled within a fairly brief period of time, family and community relations that existed prior to the illness may never again be reconstituted, or if they are resumed, may continue only in attenuated and unsatisfying forms.

There are a number of accounts written by women who have had breast cancer describing their particular experiences and their efforts to cope with the disease and its implications. Two of these reports suffice to illustrate the contrasting problem-solving approaches to adaptation described in this chapter.

Mrs. B. reports that she had been in the habit of routinely examining her breasts for years before she discovered a lump. She had grown children at the time. She had just been sworn in as Special Assistant to the President's Council on Environmental Quality and was about to represent the United States in Moscow for the meetings of a joint USA-USSR committee on environmental protection. She immediately saw her personal physician who recommended further examination by a surgeon although he thought the lump was probably benign. Since Mrs. B. had no sense of concern at that time and had a full work schedule, she and the surgeon agreed to do the biopsy after her return in 6 weeks from her European trip. She told no one else about her lump but went on to make the planned trip.

While abroad she experienced pain and burning sensations in her breast and she began to be worried. Surreptitiously, after her return home, she read about breast cancer and asked her brother, a hospital administrator, for information. She did not wish to alarm her family, particularly her mother. She found it difficult to talk to her husband but she felt he should be prepared for the possibility of cancer which she was beginning to think about seriously. She was told in her initial medical examination that the chances of finding a benign lump were 60 to 40 in her favor. But now she began to face the fact, with her husband, that the tumor might be malignant, no longer comforted by the 6 to 4 odds, presumably, in her favor.

By the time she entered the hospital for the biopsy, she felt apprehensive. She recalled several close friends, three of whom had died because the cancer was not found in time and several others who had had a mastectomy and survived. One friend had signed papers without understanding she had given permission for a mastectomy. She expected only a biopsy. Mrs. B. decided to have two-stage surgery in the event of malignancy. Her physicians outlined the surgical choices, favoring a modified radical mastectomy. Mrs. B. elected to have a simple mastectomy with nodal dissection (which is a modified mastectomy) on the assumption that the cancer had probably not spread to the lymph glands and, at this point, in considering the type of surgery she could elect she also faced the possibility that her life might be shortened if the malignancy had metastasized. In that event, she decided she "would live as long as she was supposed to." Her biopsy was positive and when she recovered she began to accept the fact that she had cancer and the imminent loss of her breast. She cried for the first time, alone, and with her two daughters as she recovered from the biopsy surgery in the hospital.

Fortunately, the pathology report following surgery indicated no nodal involvement. After the mastectomy, Mrs. B. decided, with her family's agreement, to write about her experience for the benefit of other women. She concluded her account by attributing her good psychological recovery to her family's support during the "unexpected, traumatic experiences of the last several weeks" (3).

Mrs. B.'s initial decisions to put off surgery so that she might attend the Moscow conference and her failure to inform any family members of her predicament are not what our experience would lead us to identify as examples of effective coping. On the contrary, they reflect her early failure to prepare herself or others for the possibility of malignancy and breast amputation, a failure emanating less from an inability to face an unpleasant reality than from an understandable desire to accomplish an important and unique work assignment. Although she wisely sought medical advice beforehand, her decision not to enlarge the circle of those informed of her lesion at that time certainly served the incidental function of lessening the chances that someone might seek to dissuade her from her trip.

On the other hand, once she returned from abroad, Mrs. B.'s coping efforts improved considerably. She began to prepare herself and others in the family for a possible diagnosis of cancer. She achieved this preparation by electing two-stage surgery, which gave her further time to come to terms with cancer and her disfigurement following surgery. She mourned the loss of her health to a chronic disease with its ever-present threat of death and the loss of her intact body as a result of breast amputation. Had she chosen one-stage surgery instead, Mrs. B. might not have been provided with the time she and her family needed to prepare for her cancer. Fortunately, her family responded with realistic and firm support, to which Mrs. B. correctly attributed an important part of her good psychological recovery from her trauma.

The second personal account of the breast cancer experience is more detailed and gives us the opportunity of reviewing another woman's early coping patterns along with the outcome revealed months after surgery.

Ms. R.'s husband discovered her breast lump during sexual intercourse. She was 38 years old at the time, with no children. She went immediately to her physician who, after examining her mammograms, decided there was no need to worry. He diagnosed the lump as a benign cyst.

Almost a year after her first examination, Ms. R., following her physician's earlier recommendation, returned for a second medical examination. Her decision to return was influenced by the publicity given to Mrs. Ford's and Mrs. Rockefeller's mastectomies and the realization that early detection could save one's life. This time, the mammography examination prompted a physician to recommend that the lump be surgically removed. Ms. R., fleetingly, thought about the word "cancer" but dismissed this diagnosis as a real possibility. She was convinced by her history of excellent health and a strong sense of invulnerability that the biopsy was merely a "nuisance interruption." She did little, if anything, to anticipate possible bad news from a biopsy.

Ms. R. later wondered at her being so "pigheadly unafraid" prior to surgery but she was convinced at that time that "bad things don't happen to me." Prior to seeing the surgeon, she acknowledged that she had not come to terms "with what might happen to me." She could not seriously worry about something that probably would not happen. She reminded herself of the odds, 10 to 1 in favor of the lump being benign.

The surgeon told her, following his exam, that there was a "good chance of a malignancy"; Ms. R. reacted with shock to this news. She came very close to fainting. She cried briefly but after leaving the surgeon's office she reminded her husband that "it still might not happen." During the weekend of waiting for surgery scheduled for the following Monday, Ms. R. decided that keeping busy ("with trivia") would best get her through the waiting period. She shopped and spent time with friends. She left instructions for her husband to tell her parents only if cancer was discovered. She did get as far, psychologically, as fearing the loss of her breast. Her husband, she realized later, had gone beyond that to consider that she might die as the result of cancer. She did not consider any issue other than her fear of breast loss nor did she accept emotionally the possibility of breast loss prior to surgery.

The evening before surgery, her surgeon discussed possible options should the biopsy prove positive. He recommended a "modified radical" and gave Ms. R. the choice of one- or two-stage surgery. She thought two-stage surgery was "stupid" and gave the surgeon permission to do what he thought best. Her uppermost concerns, at this point, were her fears of not surviving surgery and of disfigurement.

In the days of hospitalization after surgery, Ms. R. enjoyed the attention and concern of many friends. She acted bravely and cheerfully, playing the part of Pollyanna with visitors. She enjoyed, particularly, visits from an old suitor who indicated his continued, serious interest in her. But she rejected a visit from a Reach-to-Recovery volunteer.

She refused to look at the breast wound, realizing that to do so would shatter her precarious "tough" pose. In the hospital, she "didn't feel much of anything." In her own words, she realized intellectually what had happened but not emotionally. Even the good news from pathology indicating that her lymph nodes were clear brought little reaction from her—a numbness of all feelings characterized her during the hospital stay of 8 days.

The first night at home was the occasion for an abortive attempt at love-making. She endured sex because her "husband needed it" but the effort ended disastrously when he felt her intact breast. The next day the bottom fell out of her "brave" act. She realized that she was not healthy any more. Her chances for long-term survival had dropped from 96% to 80%. She was very angry that the lump had not been taken out a year earlier. Finally, for the first time since the operation she began to cry. She became acutely aware of the possibility of dying of cancer and sought comfort from her husband; she continued to cry profusely. Finally, Ms. R. realized that the fear of dying must be borne—that there was no alternative to bearing this fear. She felt rage, self-pity, and frailty, feelings she had not experienced earlier.

Sex with her husband was something she continued to dread because she no longer found herself attractive. She felt deformed and that killed any sex urge she might have had. She continued to be unable to look at her wound. She made a tentative visit to obtain a breast prosthesis and was so upset at the prospect of wearing one that a month passed before she could again consider the kind of prosthesis she might prefer.

She returned to work 8 days out of the hospital but this didn't work out; she felt strange and exhausted. Two weeks after surgery, she forced herself to look at her wound and found the experience devastating. She no longer slept naked as had been her custom. While her relationship with her husband was deteriorating, she continued to become seriously involved with her old boy friend. She was unable to let her husband see her wound for a few weeks. When she did show it to him, his attempts to reassure her did not comfort her.

One month after surgery, she left her husband to live with her old suitor. She left stealthily, without any warning or discussion with her husband. She was aware that her marriage had not been perfect. On the other hand, she recognized that it had held real satisfaction for both partners. It was her fear of her husband's infidelity based on earlier incidents that caused the separation. About five months later, despite continued protestations of his continuing love, her husband agreed, reluctantly, to a divorce. It was a painful experience for Ms. R. Soon after the divorce, her relation with her new partner began to go sour over his desire for children which put her at some risk of cancer recurrence. The planned marriage was delayed. Their relationship deteriorated further and finally ended 8 months after it began.

Nine months after surgery, Ms. R. was living with her mother after the unexpected death of her father and because she was lonely. She resumed contact with her ex-husband on a tentative basis, both considering remarriage but neither one being willing to move precipitously to reunite (10).

Ms. R. was unable to prepare herself for the possibility that she might have cancer before her surgery. She did not consider the prognostic implications of having cancer until she left the hospital some 8 days after surgery. She got as far as contemplating breast amputation with considerable repugnance but no acceptance. In the hospital, she repressed successfully almost all unpleasant feelings, only to have these feelings, fears, and frightening thoughts overwhelm her once she came home.

Sexual relations proved totally impossible because she felt herself to be physically unattractive. She did not begin to feel better about herself and her body— a stage which in our observation is attained only after a period of mourning one's losses—some months after surgery. Moreover, she failed to achieve acceptance of her disfigured body before terminating a meaningful marriage and catapulting herself into a new relationship with another man, a relationship which also fell apart after 8 months.

Ms. R.'s decision to terminate her marriage while she was in the throes of coping with cancer and with the results of her surgery violates an important coping principle, namely, that one is better advised not to make major changes in one's life until one resolves an existing crisis. The motto to follow in such situations is "don't just do something; stand there!"

If our observations of the importance of solving the breast cancer problems of disfigurement and life-threatening disease prior to surgery hold up in our continued investigation—and we expect that they will—perhaps the most critical intervention will consist of identifying those women who are unable to achieve this problem resolution on their own in the critical presurgery period, and of developing techniques to resolve these coping tasks as expeditiously as possible.

This goal is not unlike the situation that confronts a physician called on to treat a child with an acute infection—for example, a septic sore throat. He must diagnose the disease and introduce antibiotics during the acute stage to prevent permanent damage to vital organs; if suitable treatment is not instituted rapidly, the risk of complications and sequelae will increase considerably. Some significant treatment time can be gained for those women who have not made progress in their resolution of early coping tasks by electing two-stage surgery. However, the extension of time gained in this manner represents an opportunity rather than a guarantee that the time will be used effectively for problem solving.

FAMILY AND STRESS

As both our case studies illustrate, the breast cancer patient's adjustment to cancer is dependent in part on the behavior of individuals closest to the patient. Initially, the woman tends to report the discovery of the breast lesion to her sexual partner, whose responses are particularly important. If he urges her to get an early medical evaluation he is acting in his partner's best interest; if he fails to do so he may contribute to a risky delay in lump evaluation and diagnosis. Children sometimes play a similar role in urging their mothers to arrange for an early medical examination.

The response of family members, particularly the spouse, to viewing the breast after surgery will reassure the patient when the reaction is positive. By the same token, a negative response—one of shock or revulsion—will increase the patient's difficulty in coming to terms with her disfigurement. Reluctance on the part of the partner to participate in sex relations can have a similar negative effect on the patient.

Troubled responses to the diagnosis and treatment by family members indicate their need for clinical intervention. Children exhibit a good deal of concern about their mother's health and the prognosis of the disease. Even young children should be included in family discussions about the illness and be given honest information about risks.

Daughters, on the other hand, are prone to believe that breast cancer in their mother means such an eventual diagnosis for themselves. Discussion of these fears is important to help them avoid delay in receiving medical care should they find breast lumps of their own at a later point.

It is beyond the scope of this chapter to assess just how applicable our experience with coping responses to breast cancer, and, as explored earlier, to childhood leukemia, is to individuals suffering from other, less familiar forms of disease. To this extent the data we have at our disposal may well represent only the tip of the iceberg. It is thus fortunate that we can record even this much progress in an area of such pivotal importance to the family and to each individual within it.

REFERENCES

1. Bard, M., and Sutherland, A. (1955): Psychological impact of cancer. IV. Adaptation to radical mastectomy. *Cancer,* 8:656–672.
2. Binger, C. M., Ablin, C., Feuerstein, R., Kushner, J., Zoger, S., and Mikkelson, C. (1969): Childhood leukemia: Emotional impact on patient and family. *N. Engl. J. Med.,* 280:414–417.
3. Black, S. T. (1973): Don't sit home and be afraid. *McCall's,* February:414–418.
4. Bozeman, M. F., Ohrbach, C., and Sutherland, A. (1955): Psychological impact of cancer and its treatment, III. The adaptation of mothers to the threatened loss of their children through leukemia, Part I. *Cancer,* 8:1–20.
5. Grandstaff, N. (1975): The impact of breast cancer on the family. *Front. Radiat. Ther. Oncol.,* 11:146–156.
6. Kaplan, D. M. (1969): Problem conception and planned intervention. In: *Families in Crisis,* edited by P. Glasser and L. Glasser, pp. 273–290. Harper & Row, New York.
7. Kaplan, D. M., and Grandstaff, N. (1979): A problem-solving approach to terminal illness for the family and physician. In: *Stress and Survival,* edited by C. Garfield, pp. 343–352. C. V. Mosby, St. Louis.
8. Kaplan, D. M., Smith, A., Grobstein, R., and Fischman, S. (1973): Family mediation of stress posed by severe illness. *Social Work,* 18:60–69.
9. Pattison, E. M. (1978): The living–dying process. In: *Psychosocial Care of the Dying Patient,* edited by C. Garfield, pp. 133–168. McGraw-Hill, New York.
10. Rollin, B. (1976): *First, You Cry.* J. B. Lippincott, Philadelphia.
11. Vincent, C. E. (1967): Mental health and the family. *J. Marriage Fam.,* 29:18–38.

Psychosocial Aspects of Cancer,
edited by Jerome Cohen et al.
Raven Press, New York © 1982.

Chapter 20

Sexuality and Cancer

Joanne E. Mantell

*Division of Behavioral Sciences and Health Education, School of Public Health, University
of California, Los Angeles, Los Angeles, California 90024*

When less sophisticated methods of cancer detection and treatment were extant a quarter of a century ago, cancer patients had limited life expectancy between diagnosis and death. Consequently, coping with day-to-day realities was not given serious attention. Although technological advances have prolonged survival, there remains a preoccupation with the life-threatening aspects of cancer. With an extended lease on life, increased attention to the rehabilitative aspects of treatment is required. The cancer patient population needs help and encouragement in normalizing their daily living patterns so as to achieve an optimal level of physical, psychological, and social functioning.

Cancer is a disease which creates a series of situational crises—economic strain, physical limitations, and disruption to interpersonal relationships. Problems of diminished self-esteem, particularly body image, and feelings of pain, anxiety, and abandonment are not uncommon. Social relationships are often changed because usual role responsibilities are relinquished and new behavioral patterns adopted. Patients are increasingly encouraged, however, to alter their life style—their work schedule, leisure time activities, and social involvements —rather than succumb to the sick role.

Modified physical and social expectations as well as the consequences of treatment modalities can affect the sexual behavior of cancer patients and their partners. Both physiological and psychological factors operate to create sexual problems. Although sexual functioning and interest may diminish during acute episodes of illness, many patients are capable of maintaining their premorbid patterns of sexual behavior when their disease has been stabilized. Unfortunately, taboos and misconceptions of chronic illness tend to lead to denial of the sexual concerns of cancer patients.

Cancer patients are members of what Gochros and Gochros (20) call a "sexually oppressed" group. Health professionals often refrain from providing patients with information because they assume sexual desires are nonexistent. In reality, however, the libidinal drive is probably intact. Patients may be reluctant to inquire about sexual issues and, because they are ashamed, fearful, or unaware of their physical capacity, consequently suppress such feelings. Even if they are bold enough to broach the subject of sex, patients may be brushed aside or receive perfunctory responses. All too many health professionals stress survival and control of the malignancy but ignore that sexuality is an important determinant of enrichment and quality of life.

Sexuality is a multidimensional concept referring not only to such biologic aspects as gender and coitus, but to socioculturally derived phenomena such as self-concept, satisfaction, libido, sex roles, and patterns of interpersonal communication. Recognition of patients' sexual needs and dysfunctions is essential to effective patient rehabilitation and professional practice. Sexual issues should be addressed from a patient perspective to preclude professionals from imposing unrealistic or unwanted expectations on patients.

EFFECTS OF CANCER ON SEXUALITY AND SEXUAL FUNCTIONING

It is important to differentiate anatomic changes from the emotional effects of disease (18). A preponderance of sexual dysfunction may be psychological rather than physiological. Some patients may need to attribute sexual dysfunction to their medical disability because they consider physiological problems to form the basis for a more acceptable rationale for inadequacy than psychological ones. As the Coles (8) point out, however, psychosexual dysfunction can be as disabling as iatrogenic sexual dysfunction. Helping patients alleviate the psychological strains on their sexuality is complex for they are apt to perceive themselves as defective and indulge in self-blame. Treatment should focus on exploring feelings about sexuality, exploration of body-image changes, prior attitudes about sexuality and patterns of sexual activity, and availability of social supports. When the patient has accepted the consequences of damage to a sexual site but does not know what to do, treatment may be limited to apprising the patient of alternative modes of sexual pleasure and expression.

Physiological Responses

The person with cancer undergoes a series of endogenous physiologic changes that often will affect sexual functioning. Exogenous factors such as the side effects of surgery, radiation, and chemotherapy can also create barriers to sexual activity. These endogenous and exogenous factors produce specific as well as systemic physical consequences.

Surgery for colon-rectal cancer among males causes sterility and possibly impotence if parasympathetic nerves, seminal vesicles, prostate glands, or ejaculatory ducts are damaged. For women the fear that a colostomy will interfere with fertility, pregnancy, and childbearing is unwarranted, as the reproductive organs are not situated near the operative site (33); however, intercourse will be painful while the surgical site is healing, and it may be impossible if the vaginal wall is resected without dilatation or vaginal reconstruction (12).

The type and extent of the procedure performed will determine the effect of prostatic cancer on sexual functioning. When a perineal prostatectomy is required, impotence usually occurs, and in cases where the perineal nerves are damaged there may be urinary incontinence (37). Surgery that requires removal of the prostate, seminal vesicles, and the base of the bladder can also result in loss of potency (4). Less radical procedures such as a transurethral or suprapubic resection are most commonly performed today and generally do not interfere with sexual performance; erection, intercourse, and gratification can be achieved, but there is often retrograde ejaculation, that is, semen is deposited in the urinary bladder. Radiation and hormonal therapies can also cause impotence. Thus, because of the threat of impaired sexuality, some men opt to forgo treatment and risk the chance of decreased survival.

A bilateral orchiectomy or lymphadenectomy for testicular malignancies leads to infertility and can result in decreased sexual libido and performance. Fertility is unaffected by unilateral orchiectomy or lymphadenectomy. Irradiation of the testes can result in sterility because of decreased semen volume, but sexual function and ejaculation are preserved (5). Cancer of the penis is particularly devastating because it usually requires surgical amputation. Radical pelvic exenteration to control cancer of the pelvic organs may lead to pronounced contraction or obliteration of the vagina, thus eliminating the capacity for coitus (24), as well as removal of the bladder, rectum, and uterus.

Neurological malignancies such as brain and spinal cord tumors can threaten sexual function, depending on the level and type of lesion. Bors and Comarr (3) found that with complete upper-motor neuron lesions, a male's capacity for orgasm and ejaculation is impaired but erectile ability is retained. In the case of complete lower motor neuron lesions, erectile capacity, ejaculation, and orgasm are infrequent. With incomplete lesions, regardless of location, the vast majority of men experienced erection, and a majority of those with lower motor neuron lesions could ejaculate or reach orgasm (9). Neurological dysfunction, however, does not eliminate coitus and conception among women although some labial and clitoral sensation may be lost (10,25,30). In the case of complete cord lesions, orgastic capacity may be permanently impaired (21).

Various physiological problems arising from cancer or its methods of treatment have systemic effects which curtail sexual functioning. Physical debility, fatigue, and nausea as a result of radiation therapy may precipitate sexual disinterest or decrease enjoyment. Severe chest pain, dizziness, and dyspnea can make it physically difficult for patients to tolerate sexual activity. Breast cancer patients with diffuse bony metastases, such as in the pelvis or spine, may be too fragile to have sexual intercourse in missionary or male-superior positions. Muscle and motor weaknesses can also create mechanical impediments to maneuvering.

Many drugs adversely affect sexual function and performance because of their autonomic side effects. Antidepressants and tranquilizers such as the phenothiazines used to control chemotherapy-induced nausea can reduce sexual drive and produce sexual impotence while the latter can also cause ejaculatory incompetence (28). Narcotics such as morphine and heroin for pain control may inhibit sexual activity (19). Some chemotherapeutic drugs can inhibit menstruation and sperm production (7), whereas others have been associated with decreased desire for sexual intercourse (23).

It is obvious that these surgical, neurological, and systemic factors have varying effects on a patient's physical ability to become involved in sexual activity. For example, a radical pelvic exenteration that obliterates the vagina is objectively immensely more serious than nausea resulting from chemotherapy. The subjective response to cancer and its physical consequences, however, is unpredictable. As Wise (34) states: ". . . neoplasms differ as much in their psychological effects as in their virulence."

Psychogenic Responses

Many sexual problems represent psychological reactions to cancer which will reduce if not repress sexual desires or satisfaction. Bodily changes stemming from medical-surgical therapies can threaten self-esteem and interfere with the enjoyment of sexual relations. From a social interactionist perspective, body image, an integral part of sexual self-concept, is formed by self-perceptions and attitudes as well as by reinforcement of others' evaluations of one's body. These perceptions are based on both objective physical attributes and the subjective meaning of the body part (27). When there is a discrepancy between perception of actual and ideal representation of body, cognitive dissonance may produce a distorted concept of body image, and in turn result in diminished self-worth and dysfunctional social and sexual relationships. Cultural valuation of physical attractiveness has reinforced the importance of body image; any deviation from this ideal tends to be regarded as socially unacceptable.

Even though the effects of a body-altering surgery are not readily visible to the individual or significant others, there may be psychological problems (2). Changes brought about by physiological processes—termination of menses and loss of reproductive capacity—can result in poor emotional adaptation. There is no evidence to suggest that removal of the uterus and/or ovaries will alter sexual desires or capacity for orgasm.[1] Nevertheless, feelings of inadequacy and fears of permanent loss of sexual functioning are pervasive and may lead to postsurgical depression (1,16,17). There is a certain folklore and mystique about the womb. To many women a hysterectomy is perceived to be a mutilation and a symbolic castration that is equated with loss of femininity, youth, physical

---

[1] Sexual intercourse may be restricted for a short time after hysterectomy because pressure on the abdomen and temporary vaginal atrophy can cause intermittent discomfort during coitus. Irradiation to the uterine cervix will reduce vaginal lubrication and cause vaginal stenosis, and subsequently lead to dyspareunia (35). Consequently, dilatation may be required.

attractiveness, and sexual desirability. Fear that the loss of the uterus and cervix results in reduced libido, loss of orgasm, pain, and premature menopause is not uncommon. In addition, women who attribute their cancer as a punishment for sexual promiscuity or infidelity often experience guilt and fear that continued sexual intercourse will lead to disease recurrence. There are also realities accompanying genital cancers that threaten fulfillment of certain female cultural roles. For example, the primacy attached to childbearing tends to depreciate the value of women who have lost their reproductive capacity.

Some women may refrain from sexual intercourse after radical vulvectomy with total removal of the clitoris because they perceive themselves lacking the physical apparatus requisite for a satisfactory sexual response. Cessation of coital orgasm after such surgery is not physiological (11); rather, psychological interference is to blame. Thus, for some women, treatment is as threatening as symptoms of the disease.

Other types of disfigurement, although not external, are highly visible to the victim and can precipitate emotional reactions which interfere with expression of sexuality. A colostomy is often viewed as mutilating bodily appearance. The trauma may be so disturbing that some ostomates will personify their stoma in an attempt to disassociate themselves from it (12). There is concern that the stoma and associated apparatus will reduce physical attractiveness. The unreasonable apprehension that clothing will not adequately conceal the outline of the colostomy appliance is also prevalent. Many patients are repelled by looking at feces and interpret their loss of sphincter control with uncleanliness because of childhood toilet-training experiences. The offensiveness of unpleasant odors, flatulence, and fecal spillage has led some ostomates to fear condemnation and rejection (29). Consequently, barriers to social and physical intimacy may be erected (14,15).

Not only do patients have fear of incurring pain or damaging the stoma, but some have reported sexual fantasies that interfere with sexual functioning. For example, one ostomate eroticized his protruding stoma, viewing this surgically constructed appendage as a penis. For the homosexual male, cancer of the rectum can be especially problematic. Anal intercourse, which is frequently the preferred method of sexual expression, may be too painful to endure or impossible to execute. Consequently, some patients may attempt to use the new orifice for sexual intercourse.

Disfigurement produced by mastectomy can also lead to sexual dysfunction. Since the concept of female sexuality is bound up with cultural emphasis on the breast and an intact body, many women are unable to cope with the discrepancy between cultural expectations and their disfigurement. Feelings of intense anxiety and social unacceptability may be provoked. Persistent lymphadema and the scarred postoperative site reawaken women's emotional pain about their concrete loss. Grieving for the lost breast is part of the normal mourning process that is required to facilitate body reintegration (26) and restore social confidence and sexual health. Physical revulsion and fear of rejection by a partner can interfere with sexual responsiveness and, in the extreme, lead to withdrawal from sexual activity.

Alterations to the sexual organs are particularly traumatic. The mutilating effects of pelvic exenteration may be perceived to cause declining sexual vitality and precipitate feelings of asexuality. Consequently, this perception can result in sexual unresponsiveness. Amputation of the penis almost always leads to depression and anxiety. Even when a penile prosthesis can be constructed, silicone implanted, or vaginal reconstruction performed,[2] these procedures rarely compensate for the sexual devaluation typically experienced after such disfiguring surgery.

Changes in the outward appearance of the body can result in social and sexual maladjustment. The mutilating effects of head and neck surgery serve a damaging blow to a patient's self-esteem. Orbital exenterations, nose resections, and extensive maxillary procedures can result in gross facial distortions, while mandibular surgery presents mastication difficulties and loss of salivary control. Certain surgical procedures may make oral sex particularly cumbersome.

There may be adverse reactions to the severe cosmetic defects wrought by these radical alterations. Some patients may refrain from looking in a mirror because of their inability to tolerate the sight of their disfigurement. At the same time, being stared at whenever venturing into public reinforces the patient's sense of being different and feelings of freakishness. This stigma can be so great that without professional intervention self-isolation will be adopted and social relationships disrupted.

Patients who have undergone a laryngectomy with partial or total neck dissection also need to contend with a visible physical defect. The stoma often remains unconcealed and unprotected and a foul odor may emanate. Some patients frequently need to discharge mucosa from this orifice, especially when communicating with esophageal speech. Observing these necessary body functions may be so physically repugnant to some sexual partners and to the patients themselves that all forms of sexual expression are curtailed or, in the extreme, avoided.

There are other physical distortions that can accompany cancer. Some patients with invasive disease will be confronted with cachexia and a sallow or jaundiced appearance. This excessive weight loss and discoloration may not only decrease sexual interest but limit sexual activity for fear of inflicting pain or further assault to the body. Patients taking steroids tend to gain weight and have a bloated appearance because of the drug's water-retention characteristic. Recurrent hair loss as a result of immunosuppressive chemotherapies is another body-image problem that can threaten self-concept, provoking feelings of sexual unattractiveness and undesirability. In subcultures with narrow, rigid definitions of physical well-being, loss of hair, weight, and robustness could be interpreted

---

[2] Morley et al. (24) note, however, that many women who have undergone vaginal reconstruction report satisfactory sexual readjustment.

as a loss of sexual prowess, whereas in those with a more fluid, elastic concept, the disfigured may not feel compelled to be sexually inactive.

Hormone therapy can produce physiologic side effects which cause psychogenic dysfunction. Men who are given estrogen for carcinoma of the prostate may develop secondary gynecomastia, whereas premenopausal women undergoing androgen therapy may find an increase in unwanted hair (7).

The offensive odors that some patients give off can be a sexual deterrent. In addition to odors associated with the various stomas, certain drugs and side effects of cancer alter the body chemistry and result in unpleasant patient scents, as when there is failure in detoxification and excretion of metabolites. Pain as well as discharge from decubitus ulcers can also put a damper on sexual enjoyment.

Although current medical knowledge indicates that cancer is not sexually transmitted among humans, there is still a lurking fear that it might be contagious. In some cases subtle and often covert tactics will be deployed to avoid such physical intimacy as kissing, hugging, and caressing. Women with radium implants for uterine cancer may limit their sexual interactions if they fantasize that they can contaminate others with radioactivity (13,35).

Regardless of cancer site, it is the patient's perception of disfigurement and how this perception influences self-esteem that determines whether there is psychosexual disability (31). Although some will consider the mutilating effects of body-exterior cancers to be the most crippling defects, others may view extirpation of internal organs to be more traumatic. Thus it is the self-perceptions of being ugly and incomplete that are likely to cause feelings of personal inadequacy. The cultural and emotional significance of the organ may also determine an individual's subjective assessment and reactions or the defect or loss.

Patients who feel that they have been robbed of their sexuality will need help accepting the changes that have occurred and reconstructing a healthy self-image. They may be keenly sensitive to covert gestures that they infer are communicating prejudices about their disability. With support from significant others, self-confidence may be bolstered and self-esteem improved. For example, an involved partner or health professional who views structural changes without revulsion can help put patients at ease and convey that others do not perceive them to be too grotesque. In addition, time is needed before patients can heal their psychic wounds. When a vital body part is altered or removed, mourning should be not only permitted but encouraged. Grieving is essential to resolve loss. Denial of this experience will make integration of a new body-image and subsequent sexual readjustment difficult, if not impossible.

IMPLICATIONS FOR HEALTH PRACTITIONERS

Over the last decade dramatic changes in public attitudes about sexuality, as manifested by increased tolerance of homosexuality and candid discussions of sexuality, have occurred. At the same time, sex education has become part of the curricula for training health professionals. The liberation of people from their sexual shackles has progressed to the extent that in some states professional licensure and certification is contingent on completing courses in human sexuality (32). Despite this increasingly permissive ambiance, there is still sexual disenfranchisement of certain subpopulations. The sexual needs of people afflicted with a life-threatening chronic illness such as cancer are often neglected and denied. Similar to cultural attitudes about the aged, sexual desires of cancer patients are often sublimated because society considers them improper. How can people in the process of dying possibly be preoccupied with sexual desires and fantasies? As long as cultural values discourage such feelings, there will not be candid discussions of sexual matters by patients, their significant others, and professional caregivers. Given this predicament, careful thought must be given to mitigating or circumventing such xenophobia.

Growing recognition among patients of the right to participate in their health care has stimulated some to initiate a dialogue about sexual matters with health professionals. Although patients should assume personal responsibility for health and the medical encounter, professionals are obliged to help patients cope with their disabilities. Discussion of real or imagined limitations on sexual expression is as essential as palliation.

Sex Education

Effective sexual counseling in medical practice is a function of not only professional sensitivity but knowledge of human sexual functioning. A general understanding of sexual responses is not adequate; information about the sexual consequences of diseases must be incorporated into the training of health practitioners. Many professionals resist or gloss over the need for dealing with sexual problems because they are uncomfortable with their own sexuality. In addition to the cognitive elements of sex education, professionals need training to deal with their sexual attitudes and predilections so that they will be prepared to deal with those of their patients. In particular, there are a variety of experiential techniques, for example, role playing and desensitization-resensitization exercises, that professionals can employ to increase awareness of their sexual practices and judgments. The intent of these experiences is to expand the horizons so that their professional biases will not obstruct the quality of patient care. With apprehensions diminished, professionals will hopefully overcome their discomfort and reluctance in dealing with patient concerns. Even among sophisticated and well-educated patients, there are misconceptions about sex that should be addressed by health professionals. Thus it is incumbent on professionals to prepare themselves adequately for this important facet of their helping role.

Guidelines for Sexual Counseling of Cancer Patients

Opportunity for sexual counseling of cancer patients can be offered within the context of other professional services, whether in a hospital or community setting. Health administrators should not feel compelled to support the services of a full-time sexual therapist. Since patients tend to define sexual problems as being medical rather than psychological, all caregivers should share the responsibility for sexual counseling. In most cases, if appropriately handled, referral to a sex therapist will not be required.

Within this framework, the objective is to determine ways in which patients can be helped with their sexual problems. General guidelines relating to salient issues of sexuality of the chronically ill are set forth as a model for intervention:

1. There are individual variations in the amount of information, exploration, and confrontation that patients can tolerate. Although informed consent laws and the Patients' Bill of Rights indicate that patients are entitled to full disclosure of information about their illness, its treatment, and sequelae, a standardized approach to disclosure is not always in the best interests of the patient.

Prior to commencing treatment, physicians should inform patients of the potential for sexual dysfunction and distorted body image when experience suggests the possibility of such damage. At the same time, care must be taken not to program patients for sexual failure since the power of suggestion could precipitate the development of psychogenic dysfunction. The degree of explicitness should be tailored to the individual's emotional status, that is, how much does the patient really want to know? The patients' rights to either refuse a cancer therapy that would violate their sexuality or elect a less intrusive treatment regimen to maintain intact sexual organs must be respected. The professionals' value on life-preservation techniques should not overshadow the importance of the patients' need to maintain dignity and quality of life.

2. Evaluation of the implicit and explicit sexual problems of patients should be a routine part of the initial treatment plan. Since many patients will be hesitant or inarticulate about discussing sex and therefore suppress their concerns, professionals may need to take the initiative. Patients who are threatened will communicate their unease in various ways, for instance, by changing the topic of conversation, squirming, or leg rocking. Particular attention should be paid to patients who ask impersonal information about statistical probabilities of sexual dysfunction or present somatic complaints since this may be their way of tacitly pleading for help. Other patients will barrage professionals with problems or questions about the side effects of their disease. Professionals should not be disarmed by this inquisitiveness but attempt to answer questions with candid, unstereotyped responses. Professionals who convey their willingness to address sexual problems should not be threatened by patients who are not ready for self-disclosure.

A range of attitudinal and behavioral domains can be explored, including degree of marital and overall life satisfaction, self-concept and body image, availability of sexual partner, activity or passivity in the sex role, incongruities between sexual performance and expectations, perceptions and frequency of coital and noncoital forms of lovemaking, and capacity for erection, orgasm, and reproduction. Awareness of variations in sexual practices is essential since patients may condone or condemn certain sexual activities because of incompatibility with religious or other sociocultural convictions.

3. The importance of sexual partners and their role in the patients' recovery and rehabilitation should not be minimized or overlooked. Patient self-confidence, however, is requisite. If a patient does not have a positive concept of self and feel sexually desirable, a satisfactory sexual experience will be difficult to achieve. Traditional psychosexual attitudes and behavioral patterns between patient and partner affect the coping process (26). Patients who have had discordant premorbid relationships will be likely to continue this unsatisfactory existence. This is not to imply that cancer does not precipitate stress in a relationship. It is wishful thinking, however, to believe that discord will dissolve as a result of cancer. In reality such problems may only be exacerbated. Other patients will reap secondary gains from their cancer, using illness as a convenient excuse to either refrain from sex or become hypersexual in reaction to feelings of depression, loss, and perceived asexuality and disfigurement.

Patients should be sensitive to their partners' sexual needs. Even though a patient may be unable or unwilling to obtain full enjoyment from sexual activity, this is not necessarily a valid reason for terminating physical intimacy. For most patients, however, the need for intimacy and human contact continues, even in the face of ravaging, invasive disease. In fact, with the impending threat of social isolation, there may be a direct increase in desire for non-coital forms of physical affection (23). A tender, loving, reassuring partner can bolster a patient's sense of self-acceptance and sexual confidence.

Some patients, however, may be reluctant to express the need for affection to their partner because of poor self-image, feelings of inadequacy, perceived physical unattractiveness, and anxiety about sexual failure or performance. Consequently, they may unwittingly impose psychological barriers which create social distance from their partners. At the same time, partners may communicate their apathy, disinterest, or inhibition in sexual activity because of fear of injuring the patient, physical awkwardness of sexual maneuvers, or the patient's altered bodily appearance. If the adverse feelings of both partners are not acknowledged and addressed, a double bind is likely to result. In this type of situation, each party's weakened ego will feed on the mutual unresponsiveness and rejection; consequently, sexual dysfunction may be precipitated.

Professionals should not assume that patients have available sexual partners. Desire for sex does not necessarily imply opportunity. Patients who are disfigured or have distorted body image may be especially troubled by the prospect of sexual activity. Counseling sessions might focus on helping patients reduce or overcome anxiety about their sexual disability, for example, by role-playing how, when, where, and why they might reveal such threatening information to a prospective partner. In addition, many patients may need tacit encouragement to engage in autoeroticism, with either manual stimulation or the use of vibrators and other dildos.

4. Patients' expectations about sex should be explored and assessed in relation

to their physical condition. Some may be unrealistic about their ability to have sexual relations and need help in accepting their limitations. Questions may also arise as to the appropriate time to reinstate the full repertoire of sexual activities. Professionals can convey that the resumption of sex can be a gradual one, paced at the patient and/or couple's level. Performance anxiety may be mitigated if expectations are not excessive (36).

5. Noncoital modalities of sexual expression need to be emphasized. All patients can achieve some level of sexual functioning. Cultural values have conditioned people to perceive a firm erection and lubricating receptive vagina as the sole indicators of normative sexual performance. For many, however, this ideal cannot be enacted because of physiologic or psychogenic sexual impairment. Professionals can expand patients' awareness of mutual masturbation, caressing, fantasy, and sensate-focus techniques of arousal. New erogenous zones can be developed, for example, the breasts and buttocks among women who have had a radical vulvectomy. Although some sexual activities could be considered perverted or "kinky," professionals should be nonjudgmental and refrain from interjecting their views. It is important for patients to find functional and satisfying ways to express their sexuality and achieve sexual gratification and pleasure. Love is a balance between emotional and physical intimacy.

6. Professionals should not hastily attribute sexual problems to patients. It is important to remember that it is the patient's prerogative rather than the professional's to label a concern as a problem. Not all patients will require or accept treatment and these desires to be respected. Rather, professionals need to be supportive and demonstrate interest in patients while maintaining their objectivity.

7. There are a variety of concrete remedial techniques that may be helpful to patients in their sexual readjustment. For example, ostomates can be counseled to cover their stomas with a decorative apparatus and to irrigate prior to sexual relations. For women with pelvic or spinal lesions, the lateral rather than missionary position may be less painful. The placement of a pillow under the pelvis of women with vaginal foreshortening will cause less physical discomfort because it changes the angle of the penile thrust. Patients with urinary catheters can be advised to detach the plastic tubing prior to sexual activity.[3] The use of fantasy and progressive relaxation techniques may help some patients overcome their distorted body image and perceived asexuality. Although these suggestions may seem simplistic, professionals should not assume that patients are able to realize their options when experiencing extensive stress.

8. Careful attention should be paid to situations that impede physical intimacy. The effects of long-term hospitalization will compound cancer patients' personal difficulties because this environment is not particularly conducive to sexual expression. Hospital conditions generally do not permit "conjugal visiting privi-

---

[3] Women, if necessary, can retain the catheter during sexual intercourse since the opening to the vagina is separate from that to the urethra.

leges" and tend to strip patients of any fascimile of intimacy and privacy. Most patients are not afforded the luxury of a private room. Doors cannot be locked and routine procedures—monitoring of blood pressure and temperature and administration of medications—that are repeated with changes in nursing shifts are intrusive. Consequently, as Jaffe (22) points out, prolonged hospitalization leads to sexual estrangement of patient and partner.

Professionals need to be aware of the ways in which institutional arrangements deprive patients of physical intimacy. Sensitivity to feelings of anger and hostility engendered by this situation is essential if professionals are to be compassionate and competent caregivers. Patients should be encouraged to take pride in their appearance, whether it be grooming the hair, shaving, applying make-up, or wearing attractive bed attire. Autoerotic techniques may be suggested. Professionals should do all in their power to remove any unnecessary burdens imposed on patients as a result of situational constraints, striving for institutional change such as warmly decorated private rooms that can be reserved for intimate encounters.

CONCLUSION

Cancer interrupts the rhythm of life. There are a myriad of disabilities that may beset the cancer patient, and sexual dysfunction is prominent among them. Although some problems can clearly be attributed to physiological alterations, others are psychically or socially constructed, such as misinformation, cultural suppression of candid verbalization of sex, and partner and professional prejudices. Despite improved sex education of health professionals and the clinical interest of some professionals in sexual functioning and chronic illness, sexuality remains secondary to other areas of sociomedical treatment.

Cancer should not be allowed to sublimate or repress patients' sexual expression any more than the physiological limitations warrant. All patients are capable of achieving some forms of lovemaking and intimacy. Myths about sexuality and cancer must be dispelled so that patients will not be deprived of their right to sexual gratification, to many an important dimension for maintaining dignity and quality of life.

REFERENCES

1. Amias, A. G. (1975): Sexual life after gynaecological operations. I. *Br. Med. J.,* 2:608–609.
2. Barker, R. G. (1953): *Adjustment to Physical Handicap and Illness: A Survey of the Social Psychology of Physique and Disability.* Social Science Research Council, New York.
3. Bors, E., and Comarr, A. (1960): Neurological disturbances of sexual function, with special reference to 529 patients with spinal cord injury. *Urol. Surv.,* 10:191–222.
4. Boyarsky, S., and Boyarsky, R. (1978): Prostatectomy, sexual disabilities and their management. In: *Sexual Consequences of Disability,* edited by A. Comfort, pp. 133–152. George F. Stickley, Philadelphia.
5. Bracken, R. B., and Johnson, D. E. (1976): Sexual function and fecundity after treatment for testicular tumors. *Urology,* 7(1):35–38.

7. Calman, K. C., and Paul, J. (1978): *An Introduction to Cancer Medicine.* John Wiley & Sons, New York.
8. Cole, T. M., and Cole, S. S. (1978): The handicapped and sexual health. In: *Sexual Consequences of Disability,* edited by A. Comfort, pp. 37–43. George F. Stickley, Philadelphia.
9. Comarr, A. E. (1971): Sexual concepts in traumatic cord and cauda equina lesions. *J. Urol.,* 106:375–378.
10. Comarr, A. E., and Gunderson, B. (1975): Sexual function in traumatic paraplegia and quadriplegia. *Am. J. Nurs.,* 75:250–255.
11. Daly, M. J. (1971): The clitoris as related to human sexuality. *Med. Aspects Hum. Sexual.,* 5:80 ff.
12. Dericks, V. C. (1976): The psychological hurdles of new ostomates: Helping them up . . . and over. *Nursing 76,* American Cancer Society Reprint No. 3359-P.E.
13. Donahue, V. C., and Knapp, R. C. (1977): Sexual rehabilitation of gynecologic cancer patients. *Obstet. Gynecol.,* 49(1):118–121.
14. Dlin, B. M., Perlman, A., and Ringold, E. (1969): Psychosexual response to ileostomy and colostomy. *Am. J. Psychiatry,* 126:374–381.
15. Dlin, B. M., and Perlman, A. (1971): Emotional response to ileostomy and colostomy in patients over the age of 50. *Geriatrics,* 26:112–118.
16. Drellich, M. G. (1967): Sex after hysterectomy. *Med. Aspects Hum. Sexual.,* 1:62–64.
17. Drellich, M. G., Bieber, I., and Sutherland, A. M. (1956): The psychological impact of cancer and cancer surgery. VI. Adaptation to hysterectomy. *Cancer,* 9(6):1120–1126.
18. Ford, A. B., and Orfirer, A. P. (1967): Sexual behavior and the chronically ill patient. *Med. Aspects Hum. Sexual.,* 1:51–61.
19. Freedman, A. M. (1976): Drugs and sexual behavior. In: *The Sexual Experience,* edited by B. J. Sadock, H. I. Kaplan, and A. M. Freedman, pp. 328–334. Williams & Wilkins, Baltimore.
20. Gochros, H. L., and Gochros, J. S. (1977): Who are the sexually oppressed? In: *The Sexually Oppressed,* edited by H. L. Gochros and J. S. Gochros, pp. xix–xxiii. Association Press, New York.
21. Griffith, E. R., Tomko, M. A., and Timms, R. J. (1973): Sexual function and spinal cord-injured patients: A review. *Arch. Phys. Med. Rehabil.,* 54:539–543.
22. Jaffe, L. (1977): The terminally ill. In: *The Sexually Oppressed,* edited by H. L. Gochros and J. S. Gochros, pp. 277–292. Association Press, New York.
23. Leiber, L., Plumb, M. M., Gerstenzang, M. L., and Holland, J. (1976): The communication of affection between cancer patients and their spouses. *Psychosom. Med.,* 38:379–389.
24. Morley, G. W., Lindenauer, S. M., and Youngs, D. (1973): Vaginal reconstruction following pelvic exenteration: Surgical and psychological considerations. *Am. J. Obstet. Gynecol.,* 116(7):996–1002.
25. Romano, M. D., and Lassiter, R. (1972): Sexual counseling with the spinal-cord injured. *Arch. Phys. Med. Rehabil.,* 52:539–543.
26. Schoenberg, B., and Carr, A. C. (1970): Loss of external organs: Limb amputation, mastectomy, and disfiguration. In: *Loss and Grief: Psychological Management in Medical Practice,* edited by B. Schoenberg, A. C. Carr, D. Peretz, and A. H. Kutscher, pp. 119–131. Columbia University Press, New York.
27. Shontz, F. C. (1975): *The Psychological Aspects of Physical Illness and Disability.* Macmillan, New York.
28. Story, N. L. (1974): Sexual dysfunction resulting from drug side effects. *J. Sex Res.,* 10(2):132–149.
29. Sutherland, A. M., and Orbach, C. E. (1952): Psychological impact of cancer and cancer surgery. II. Depressive reactions associated with surgery for cancer. *Cancer,* 5:857–872.
30. Talbot, H. S. (1971): Psycho-social aspects of sexuality in spinal-cord injury patients. *Paraplegia,* 9(1):37–39.
31. Tyler, E. A. (1975): Disfigurement and sexual behavior. *Med. Aspects Hum. Sexual.,* 9(7–12):77–78.
32. Vasconcellos, J., and Wallace, D. (1978): Legislating sex education for professionals. In: *Sex Education for the Health Professional,* edited by N. Rosenzweig and F. P. Pearsall, pp. 37–45. Grune & Stratton, New York.
33. Weinstein, M. (1978): Sexual function after surgery for rectal cancer. *Med. Aspects Hum. Sexual.,* 12:53–54.

34. Wise, T. N. (1978): Sexual functioning in neoplastic disease. *Med. Aspects Hum. Sexual.,* 12:16 ff.
35. Wise, T. N. (1978): Sexual problems resulting from interactions between medical and psychologic conditions. *Med. Aspects Hum. Sexual.,* 12:71 ff.
36. Zilbergeld, B. (1979): Sex and serious illness. In: *Stress and Survival: The Emotional Realities of Life-Threatening Illness,* edited by C. A. Garfield, pp. 237–242. C. V. Mosby, St. Louis.
37. Zinsser, H. H. (1976): Sex and medicine. In: *The Sexual Experience,* edited by B. J. Sadock, H. I. Kaplan, and A. M. Freedman, pp. 303–318. Williams & Wilkins, Baltimore.

Psychosocial Aspects of Cancer,
edited by Jerome Cohen et al.
Raven Press, New York © 1982.

Chapter 21

A Guide to Psychosocial Field Research in Cancer

John J. Spinetta

Department of Psychology, San Diego State University, San Diego, California 92182

Cancer has extensive psychosocial repercussions. The human cost in suffering and in the deterioration of the quality of life has been extensively detailed. Several areas needing detailed study are readily identified, such as the personality of the patient with cancer and its effects on coping styles, family variables, ethnic status, the relationship of the patient with cancer to health care professionals and to the health care system; the response of the health care system to the sick person; and cause-effect relationships of psychosocial variables on the course of treatment and prognosis. In listing such areas as targets for extensive psychosocial research efforts as in earlier chapters in this book, one fundamental question arises. Can "hard-nosed" research be validly and rigorously carried out in so "soft" an area? The answer is an unqualified "yes." This chapter will address in detail the following four issues: (a) the ultimate goals of a research endeavor, (b) intra-individual versus normative research, (c) methods, and (d) instrumentation. Examples from the author's own research in pediatric cancer will follow.

ULTIMATE GOALS

Field research studies are being conducted with increased frequency to ascertain the psychosocial effects of cancer on the patient and family. Health care professionals deal directly with family concerns and psychosocial repercussions on the family group of the serious illness of one of its members. These professionals recognize the necessity for valid scientific inquiry that takes into account not only the physical aspects of an illness but the psychosocial aspects as well. To measure psychosocial issues, one must first define the ultimate goals of the research pursuit:

1. Is the ultimate goal to document the most frequent psychological and social reactions associated with various types of cancer at various stages, in

order to establish a base rate for future decisions regarding individual intervention?

2. Is the goal to document changes due to interventive efforts?

3. Is the goal to obtain knowledge so that one can plan large interventive
programs?

4. Are research efforts aimed at measuring the effectiveness of ongoing programs?

5. Is the goal to study the role of psychosocial factors in contributing to
the medical aspects of the illness (in outcome, etiology, exacerbation of symptoms)?

All of these and others are legitimate research goals, and the research design
should pinpoint and specify which particular goal is being pursued in the particular research effort. Trying to accomplish too much is the sign both of a poor
research design and of a lack of foresight and planning in carrying out the
research effort. Since there are as many research designs as there are research
problems, each design must be geared to the specific problem under study.
The problem itself must be stated in a precise manner that will allow for empirical
testing. Too often, poorly trained researchers attempt to resolve all of the issues
at one time. The specific delineation of the problem in the context of precise
objectives and in the concise fashion that would allow for empirical testing is
critical to the research endeavor.

INTRA-INDIVIDUAL VERSUS NORMATIVE RESEARCH

One of the major problems encountered in psychosocial research is losing
sight of the individual subject while trying to achieve a universal and generalizable conclusion. Although the effort to achieve a normative sample is necessary,
much information regarding individual subjects is lost in the process. When
one is dealing with coping strategies and attempts to master a situation as
complex as living with a life-threatening or life-shortening illness, normative
conclusions may not be as helpful for interventive efforts as knowledge of the
specific individual's habitual mode of coping. If the goal of a health care professional's work with the families of individuals with cancer is to help strengthen
the adaptive capabilities specific to each family and to each member of the
family, then research must take into account intra-individual strategies. Studying
an individual's reactions over time (longitudinal research) and comparing these
reactions to the individual's base rate of response may prove more helpful in
the long run for ultimate interventive judgments than collapsing data across
individuals (cross-sectional research). What the health care professional needs
is to seek new methods of research that can combine the best qualities of both
intra-individual and normative research strategies in order to avoid becoming
so enmeshed in the individual that one cannot analyze the data, or so involved
with norms and standards that one gathers irrelevant data that cannot be applied
in a helpful manner in judgments regarding individual cases.

METHODS

When one is studying real people interacting in the real world, the traditional experimental model cannot always accommodate the problem. Field researchers use different models. There are two models most commonly used in field research: (a) description and (b) quasi-experiments.

Description

In a field of research as new as that of rigorous application of the scientific method to the psychological aspects of cancer, there is a need for the establishment of base rates for the frequency of psychological and social reactions associated with various types of cancer. The art of description has become so finely tuned over the years that a well-trained observer and/or tester can obtain data of a highly reliable quality and in a numerical form that is computer-analyzable. Well-designed descriptive research is both essential and scientifically legitimate.

Quasi-Experiments

When one is dealing with areas of study in which the independent variables have already occurred, the researcher starts with the observation of dependent variables and then studies the independent variables in retrospect for their possible relation to and effects on the dependent variables. When this happens, we no longer have a truly experimental design, but a quasi-experimental design. In such a design, the control of the independent variable is usually not possible and often not desirable. The investigator doing field research must take into account things as they are and try to disentangle them. Many statistical techniques are available to help the researcher in the efforts, such as a variety of correlation and regression methods, analysis of covariance, multiple discriminant analysis, trend analysis, path analysis, and multidimensional scaling. Life is complex; unidimensional scaling does not always tap the proper elements. A person constantly changes. One's research efforts must be able to take the change into account. The process of coping with cancer involves a whole series of thoughts and acts in many different contexts and at different moments as the illness progresses. The methods one uses must take into account the fluctuations and complexities and sort out those problems which can be studied from those which cannot.

INSTRUMENTATION

There are a variety of instruments for observation and data collection. Instruments range from highly standardized objective forms to lesser standardized formats such as projective methods, rating scales, content analyses, behavioral observation schedules, Q-sorts, semantic differentials, and a variety of sociometric techniques. Instruments differ considerably in what they can and cannot do.

A common problem in the conduct of field research is that instruments that are highly standardized often do not measure the problem at hand. Instruments that measure the problem at hand may not be sufficiently standardized to allow for valid judgments. This is certainly the case in research dealing with the psychosocial aspects of cancer. One instrument may be strong, but ill-suited to the problem; another may be well-suited to the problem but have great weaknesses. The subjects under study in cancer research typically are normal individuals who happen to be undergoing psychosocial reactions to a stress event of large proportions. The use of instruments that have been developed for a pathological subject are inappropriate. Further, the most commonly used and most highly standardized instruments typically measure long-standing qualities of a person, and have been developed from cross-sectional designs. A person with cancer undergoes a variety of stress events that may change over time, depending on disease state or extra-disease factors such as age and level of development. It is essential that instruments be developed which take into account the ongoing process reactions of the person to the stress events associated with the illness. The development of new instruments and the creative application of older instruments is essential for further effective research in this area. Validation of instruments is a basic task for researchers investigating such a complex area.

SUMMATION

In the last analysis, all methods and instruments have the technical purpose of enabling the researcher to make observations in such a way that symbols or numerals can be assigned to the objects or to the sets of objects under study. There is always a mutual interplay of problems and methods. Problems dictate methods to a considerable extent, but methods also influence problems. Some problems cannot be satisfactorily studied because methods do not exist to collect the data implied by the problem, or methods that exist cannot yield the precise detail needed. Users of instruments must know the strengths and weaknesses of the methods used if they are to be able to choose those methods and instruments suited to the problem under study. Even a good problem can suffer from an inappropriate or inadequate method. We have given some guidelines for the research effort. However, the specific delineation of the problem in the concise fashion that will allow for empirical testing must remain the task of the specific researcher.

SAMPLES OF FIELD RESEARCH

The author has been engaged for several years in research into the psychosocial repercussions of childhood cancer, both on the patient and on the other family members. Two detailed examples of the type of rigorous research approach to field variables proposed in this chapter are those of Spinetta and Maloney (5) and Spinetta et al. (6). In the Spinetta and Maloney study (5), the authors attempted to define the role that communication and denial play in the coping efforts of children with cancer. The area of coping has been fraught with anecdote and opinion for years, especially in cancer. Although no conclusions were drawn regarding cause-effect relationships, the authors were able to demonstrate that the level of family communication about the illness, as expressed in the mother's judgment of communication, is significantly correlated with coping strategies in the child. Families in which levels of communication about the illness were high were those families in which the children: (a) exhibited a nondefensive personal posture, (b) expressed a long-range close relationship with the parents, and (c) expressed a basic satisfaction with self. If the goal of work with the families of children with cancer is to help strengthen the adaptive capabilities and coping strategies specific to each family and to each member of the family, to help the family members struggle forward as best they can in a commitment to the value of the remaining months or years of their child's life, and to give them access to the interfamilial sources of support they most need to help them in that struggle, then the rigorously designed study pointing to the relationship between levels of communication and the life-threatening child's adaptive strategies is a step toward that goal.

The second study by Spinetta et al. (6) is a further example of the capability of conducting rigorous research in an area typically considered "soft-nosed." The parents of 23 children who had died of cancer 1 year prior to the interviews shared with the authors their view of what family members go through during the illness and after the death of their child. A 10-page literature-based, semi-structured interview schedule was carefully devised by the authors and presented to the families in interview form by a single interviewer. The results were transcribed and quantified by three independent judges. From the content analysis of the interviews, it was shown that certain behaviors during the course of the life of the child are significantly correlated with how well the surviving family members cope after the death of the child. From the parental interview three behaviors were isolated which correlate significantly with the postdeath adjustment level of the surviving family members. Those parents who were most adjusted 1 year postdeath were those: (a) who had a consistent philosophy/theology/cosmology of life prior to the diagnosis, onto which the family could append the diagnosis and its consequences in a consistent and meaningful fashion, (b) who had a viable and ongoing support system to which they could turn for help during the course of the illness, and (c) who had given their child the information and emotional support needed during the course of the illness at a level consistent with their child's questions, age, and level of development. The results are consistent with the results of the proven study (5) measuring the children themselves during the course of the illness. What needs to be done for further validation is a longitudinal study, of the nature described above, of families going from point of diagnosis through to point of death and after death, to see if the data of the present study can be replicated in a prospective manner, and whether an increased length of time post-death leads to more generalized adaptive recovery. Scientifically rigorous and valid groundwork has been laid for interventive programs that can help strengthen the family's ultimate ability to adjust to life without the child.

The two studies cited are examples of a multiple regression analysis applied to what formerly had been a field replete with anecdotal and contradictory prescriptions for intervention. By building the variables into the design, developing instruments devised specifically for the population under study, and taking into account the child and parent's own base rate of response, the researchers were able to delineate the problem in a manner that allowed for empirical testing. These are but two examples of what can be done with "soft" data.[1] Hard-nosed research can be conducted in an area as "soft-nosed" as that of the psychosocial repercussions of cancer. The ideas discussed in this chapter are not new.[2] Their rigorous application to the field of cancer is long overdue, and necessary.

ACKNOWLEDGMENTS

The author wishes to thank Joseph Cullen, Jay Cohen, Bob Martin, and colleagues of the Research Study Group, California Division of the American Cancer Society, for their support and encouragement, and most especially Richard Lazarus and Joan Bloom of the University of California, Berkeley, for their valuable suggestions.

REFERENCES

1. Blalock, H. M. (1972): *Social Statistics, 2nd Ed.* McGraw-Hill, New York.
2. Campbell, D. T., and Stanley, J. C. (1963): *Experimental and Quasi-experimental Designs for Research.* Rand McNally, Chicago.
3. Kerlinger, B. J. (1978): *Statistical Principles in Experimental Design, 2nd Ed.* McGraw-Hill, New York.
4. Marceil, J. C. (1977): Implicit dimensions of idiography and nomothesis: A reformulation. *Am. Psychologist,* 32:1046–1052.
4a. Spinetta, J. J. (1981): Adjustment and adaptation in children with cancer: A three-year study. In: *Living with Childhood Cancer,* edited by J. J. Spinetta and P. M. Deasy-Spinetta. C. V. Mosby, St. Louis.
5. Spinetta, J. J., and Maloney, L. J. (1978): The child with cancer: Patterns of communication and denial. *J. Consult. Clin. Psychol.,* 46:1540–1541.
6. Spinetta, J. J., Swarner, J., and Sheposh, J. P. (1981): Effective parental coping following the death of a child from cancer. *J. Pediatr. Psychol.,* 6:(in press).
7. Winer, B. J. (1962): *Statistical Principles in Experimental Design.* McGraw-Hill, New York.

---

[1] For further examples of the application of these concepts, see Spinetta (4a).

[2] Some of the issues raised in this chapter are discussed in more detail in Blalock (1), Campbell and Stanley (2), Kerlinger (3), Marceil (4), and Winer (7).

Psychosocial Aspects of Cancer,
edited by Jerome Cohen et al.
Raven Press, New York © 1982.

Chapter 22

Measurement of the Psychosocial Aspects of Cancer: Sources of Bias

Joan R. Bloom and *Robert D. Ross

*Department of Social and Administrative Health Sciences, School of Public Health, University of California, Berkeley, Berkeley, California 94720; and *SRI International, Menlo Park, California 94025*

The purpose of this chapter is to call attention to potential sources of bias that may be inherent in psychosocial cancer research, even in studies that are methodologically sound. When one undertakes any research, tentative assumptions are made regarding the model within which the research will be described: research design and data analysis techniques, instrumentation, and interpretation of results. Although the choices made by the researcher may reveal underlying assumptions in some cases, investigators may not be aware of available alternatives, especially if they are entering a field of research that is new or politically controversial. Failure to recognize the assumptions behind choices, or to consider alternatives, increases the risk for research to be biased, and for those biases to be left unexamined. Well-planned, carefully executed research may determine the amount of funding and the direction of support for programs such as patient and family counseling centers. Biased research, however, can direct funds either needlessly or inappropriately; thus it is important that potential sources of bias be detected and taken into account when research is planned.

This chapter will not examine all potential sources of bias, but will explore several significant ones. First, the frame of reference used to pose research questions about the psychosocial aspects of cancer will be considered. Then, the specific questions asked and the instruments selected to measure research outcomes will be examined. Finally, a discussion of psychosocial research in cancer and the current research environment as a source of bias will be presented.

MEASUREMENT MODELS AND ASSUMPTIONS

In this section, two approaches to the conceptualization of the psychosocial aspects of cancer will be examined: the medical model, with its orientation to

255

disease, and the behavioral science model, with its focus on the alterations in interpersonal relations as a consequence of illness.

Current approaches to medical care have evolved from the nineteenth century discovery of microorganisms and their implications in the etiology of disease. The development of the germ theory has led to an understanding of the course of many diseases, to unlocking the mysteries of their cause, and, ultimately, to their resolution. This theory exemplifies the logic of the medical model. First, abnormal signs and symptoms are measured. These can be observable signs as well as information obtained through various examinations and tests. The data are then classified by the scientist as consistent with one or another disease process. If the data are consistent with more than one disease, further examination and testing are conducted to rule out alternatives until greater certainty of the diagnosis can be achieved. Experience with the diagnosis suggests the course of action (the treatment) to be followed and provides a prediction of future events (the prognosis). The utility of the medical model lies in its reliability in predicting future events.

Another important aspect of this model is its determination of the etiology of the disease. This factor is noncritical because many diseases can be treated successfully even when their etiology is not known. The reverse is also true: the course of disease sometimes may not be halted even when its etiology is known (23).

Joining with physicians in the study of the physiopathology of illnesses such as cancer, behavioral scientists have often conceptualized the psychosocial aspects of cancer from the medical model perspective. From this perspective, the contributions of the individual and of the social milieu to the cause, course, and outcome of his or her own cancer are legitimate objectives of inquiry (7, 25,32,38; Chapter 14). Because its advocates have developed systematic methods for measuring psychosocial aspects of health and disease, this model has been more influential in the field than its alternative, the behavioral science model.

The behavioral science model, however, has long guided clinical intervention and is especially seen in the analyses and approaches promulgated by schools of social work (12). This model views the individual as a being composed of multiple physiological systems—respiratory, cardiovascular, and psychological, for example—and belonging to a system of interpersonal relationships. These systems are in a dynamic equilibrium. Any alteration in the physiological system, such as a diagnosis of cancer, will have consequences not only for the other physiological systems but also for the system of relationships (19). Responses from the individual and from the system of relationships are considered normal and natural, and may affect the individual's moods, attitudes, and patterns of living. A description of the individual does not imply a course of treatment or a prediction of future states, nor does it become the basis for determining the etiological question.

Whether the medical model or the behavioral science model underlies one's conceptualization of the psychosocial aspects of cancer affects the research questions asked and the measurement selected to examine these issues. Yet, the validity of the models' major assumptions is rarely examined. In the case of cancer, the assumption of pathology is different for each model. From the perspective of the medical model, the assumption of physiopathology generally, albeit inadvertently, also includes psychopathology. This can be seen metaphorically in titles of many of the instruments, such as the Brief Symptom Inventory (5) used in studying the psychosocial aspects of cancer (14), as well as in commonly used terminology, for example, psychosocial morbidity. Conversely, those conceptualizing the cancer experience from the behavioral science model assume psychological normality. Perhaps it is time to examine the assumption of psychopathology.

Questions about the validity of the assumption of psychopathology come from the authors' research on breast cancer (3). A consecutive series of 139 women with breast surgery was evaluated using a self-administered questionnaire. The cross-sectional survey provided data on women from 4 to 7 days post-surgery to 2½ years post-surgery. The Profile of Mood States (POMS) (22) was one of the scales used. This is a self-administered adjective check list that measures tension/anxiety, depression, anger/hostility, confusion, fatigue, and vigor. In Table 1, raw data on a usable sample of 133 of these subjects are displayed along with standard score equivalents for comparing these data with those from populations of female psychiatric outpatients and college students. Thus in column 1 of Table 1, which presents the Tension/Anxiety Scale results, the breast cancer population has a standard score of 32 relative to a female psychiatric outpatient population with a mean of 50 and a standard deviation

TABLE 1. *Means and standard score equivalents of POMS for breast cancer patients relative to female psychiatric patients and college students*

| | | Standard scores[a] relative to other populations | |
| | | Female psychiatric | College |
Scale	Raw mean	patients	students
Tension/Anxiety (N = 121)	4.63	32	38
Depression/Dejection (N = 123)	7.73	37	44
Anger/Hostility (N = 126)	5.28	41	44
Vigor (N = 128)	17.91	64	54
Fatigue (N = 124)	8.78	50	48
Confusion (N = 120)	1.77	33	33

[a] Mean = 50; SD = 10.

of 10, or almost 2 SDs below the mean for the female outpatient psychiatric population. This patient population does not look like either a psychiatric or a college population. Similar results are found on each of the other five scales of the POMS for which comparative norms exist (22). On only two scales, Vigor and Fatigue, are the norms similar to those of the female psychiatric or the college population. These findings are contrary to clinical judgment and suggest that one ought to be cautious about assuming that breast surgery (because of its connection to sexuality and damage to feminine body image) automatically implies psychopathology. Whether this assumption holds for other cancer sites should be put to test. Important assumptions of the behavioral science model, such as the impact of the individual's disease on significant others, should also be systematically verified.

CHOICE OF RESEARCH DESIGN

Choice of design is linked to the specific research question asked. There are at least four major areas within which questions are asked regarding the psychosocial aspects of cancer. Table 2 lists the major areas and typical objectives for each. Although there is a large body of literature for each area of study

TABLE 2. *Why measure psychological and social responses to cancer?*

Research area	Objectives
Relate psychological and social factors to etiology of disease	To document the strength of relationships between psychosocial functioning and disease occurrence and/or course To identify specific factors associated with disease onset and/or course
Describe the course of disease	To document most frequent psychological and social reactions associated with various cancer sites To document changes associated with various treatment protocols To establish guidelines for "normal," expected reactions
Plan intervention programs	To identify specific needs of patients and their families
Evaluate need and/or effectiveness of program	To document that the incidence of psychosocial problems is significantly greater for cancer patients than for a comparison group To document responses of cancer patients that differ significantly from those of other patients or healthy individuals To document significant changes in patient responses as a result of participating in an intervention program

listed, the increasing number of controlled, methodologically sophisticated studies is only a recent phenomenon. Most work has been directed toward identifying needs of patients and families and evaluating intervention programs, so examples will be drawn from those areas.

One potential source of bias is in the decision to use either a within-subject or a between-subject research design to identify problems uniquely associated with cancer. A within-subject design is frequently impossible because a longitudinal study tracking healthy individuals before the onset of cancer would be required, and such studies are extremely expensive. Another, more common, approach is to demonstrate differences between cancer patients and other comparison groups on such measures as affective responses (depression, anxiety, anger, sadness, hostility, and so forth), body image, personal habits, and personality traits. In most cases, the comparison groups are healthy noncancer subjects, although in some cases patients with various life-threatening or chronic conditions are studied.

It is not the case that within-subject designs are necessarily better than between-subject designs, or that certain comparison groups are inherently inferior to others. Rather, the point is that these choices represent experimenter alternatives that will be associated with systematic sources of bias. Moreover, the potential for bias is increased when these experimenter choices are combined with selection of instruments (discussed in the next section). Elimination of bias may not be possible, but understanding its role in the outcome of studies is desirable, especially when cancer research is used so frequently for policy decision making.

A hypothetical example will illustrate some of the choices faced by the cancer researcher and how those choices affect results and interpretation. Suppose a question is raised regarding psychological problems faced by women who have had breast cancer and its treatment. A specific hypothesis to be tested might be that women who have had breast surgery suffer psychological trauma that is significantly greater than that experienced by women with no history of disease (or women with other life-threatening disease or disfiguring surgery). Another question might be whether women treated for breast cancer suffer psychological trauma that is different from that experienced by other comparison groups. More generally, one could ask whether any individuals being treated for any kind of cancer experience psychological problems that are either different or greater than those encountered by comparison groups.

Testing whether one group experiences more psychopathology than another may result in significant differences on selected measures. One needs also to address the question of whether such differences are meaningful, especially if the measures for each group are not above some threshold level that represents a problem state reliably. For example, breast cancer patients may score significantly higher than a healthy comparison group on a scale of depression, but scores of both groups should be compared with norms from other populations to determine if either score is in a range representing a problem state.

Another problem with using between-subject designs to look for differences between cancer patients and other groups of people is that the specific questions asked are likely to be motivated toward finding that cancer patients are indeed suffering more and differently. This situation need not exist, but at the present time there is a strong need to use research data to justify development of support programs for cancer patients and their families. When cancer patients are compared with either healthy or other-disease groups, there is always the question of which dimensions should be used for the comparisons. Using cancer-specific dimensions, such as questions specifically referring to breasts in a study with breast cancer patients, is sometimes considered inappropriate and biased because the cancer patients are too likely to respond strongly to such items. Use of cancer-specific items or instruments may bias results in such a way that need for support programs will be a logical inference of the study. Researchers working with individuals in the health care system (not only those with cancer) would do well to avoid having to demonstrate that one group of patients is suffering more than another.

Potential sources of bias lie in decisions regarding the moment in time selected to observe patients being studied and the length of time available for follow-up data. It is possible to measure groups of patients at comparable times post-acute phase of disease (e.g., surgery) and find different results at various points in time. Unless the researcher is careful, the course of diseases and typical treatment programs may interact with other factors being controlled and may produce results skewed systematically in one direction or another.

Consider the possible outcomes of our hypothetical study comparing breast cancer patients to those with another disease. Breast cancer patients will be either higher as a group on certain affective measures, or they may have a significantly greater proportion of respondents higher on affective measures, or there may be no differences at all. Figure 1 is a hypothetical comparison of scores from breast cancer patients with those of a comparison group of patients with other surgeries, over time, from shortly after surgery to 15 months post-surgery. Also indicated on the graph are standardized data from healthy adults. Although this is hypothetical, it seems reasonable to assume that data from similar studies will be reported in this way.

Figure 1 may be used to illustrate the points made above about bias. The only areas of comparison that make sense across all groups are common, general psychological measures such as the affective responses referred to earlier. It would be inappropriate to show how much more trauma breast cancer patients have regarding their breasts, for example—that is too obvious—so the cancer-specific issues are not considered legitimate comparisons across all groups. If that is the case, then the assumption behind this design and resulting analysis is that something unusual happens to breast cancer patients that can be measured on standardized instruments; that is, apart from the disease-specific problems, cancer patients are expected to exhibit elevated levels of affective reponses. That result is highly probable (unless there is denial) for some period of time, because

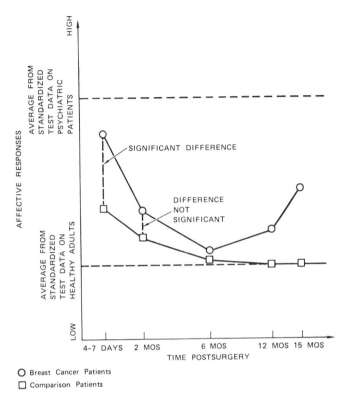

FIG. 1. Hypothetical comparison of breast cancer patients' and comparison group patients' affective responses.

the disease-specific aspects of their lives are not separated within patients as researchers can separate those aspects in sections of a questionnaire package. Still, it does not necessarily mean that when these affective responses approach the level of a healthy comparison group (e.g., at 6 months post-surgery in Fig. 1), the cancer patients are at the same healthy level of affective functioning and therefore are not in need of rehabilitation services. Actually, in designs of this sort, where cancer patients are compared to healthy or other-disease groups, the cancer patients are likely to lose no matter which way the results occur. If elevated levels of psychological disturbance are recorded (e.g., at 4 to 7 days post-surgery in Fig. 1), then the patients are likely to be considered in need of psychiatric services (because the disturbances measured are the general affective ones). However, Fig. 1 suggests that it is possible that elevated levels of affective responses may be greater than those of a healthy comparison population, yet not within the range of a psychiatric population. If such results are found, then patients are likely to be considered in need of nothing more than others going through medical crises. Why do they lose if they are considered in need of psychiatric services? They lose because the elevated levels of psychological measures are usually those that measure psychodynamic problems (the general kinds of conflicts that may be measured across all groups); the specific problems related to the disease and the patients' ability to deal with everyday problems of living are not addressed.

Also illustrated in Fig. 1 is the potential bias associated with choice of time of measurement. One common sense assumption—and one that the authors (3) have argued against—suggests that "time heals all wounds," and that psychological problems are lessened with time post-surgery. If this is indeed the case, then Fig. 1 should show a decreasing level of undesirable affective responses from the time immediately after the acute phase of the disease to any point later. However, it is possible that certain problems associated with living with cancer and its treatment do not appear until several months after the acute phase of disease (at 12 and 15 months post-surgery in Fig. 1). A researcher who subscribed to the notion that time heals all wounds would probably concentrate on looking for psychosocial problems shortly after surgery, perhaps missing times of increased problems. Or, if the researcher were inclined and financially able to follow patients over some time, there would still exist the possibility of selecting inappropriate time periods. Simply not enough is known about changes in responses to cancer throughout the varieties of courses of disease and related treatment programs to justify the assumption that psychological problems measured at one time period represent problems experienced at all time periods. This point is especially important for those responsible for planning intervention support programs for patients and families. It may not be safe or cost-efficient to assume that crisis intervention at the onset of disease is the most appropriate support for cancer patients.

This section pointed to possible problems associated with designing psychosocial cancer research. Particular emphasis was placed on researcher assumptions when choosing a design and measurement timing. Another (and from our point of view the most important) potential source of bias is in choice of instruments used to measure psychosocial problems. This issue is discussed in the next section.

INSTRUMENTATION

Once the research question has been framed, the stage is set for the next phase of the endeavor: instrumentation. Here, assumptions are used about correspondence between the concepts embedded in the research question asked and the indicator that will measure those concepts. Assumptions are also used in selecting the instruments. These assumptions are of at least two types: first, how the subject will respond to a particular item, for example, a forced choice versus a Likert format or a behavior versus an attitudinal item; second, that the instruments may have been constructed from a particular paradigm, for example, the medical versus the behavioral science model. Sources of bias introduced by these assumptions provide the focus for the section that follows.

Definition of Concepts and Selection of Indicators

The value of designing measures specific to cancer versus using standardized instrumentation is frequently debated. Standardized instrumentation has widely recognized benefits. It is psychometrically superior because internal validity and reliability are known. Both accumulated knowledge and generalizability of findings are hampered unless a standardized instrument is used. If the expense entailed in instrument development, including the time needed to complete reliability and validity tests, is also considered, the standardized measure is less costly than its alternative, the specific measure. As behavioral scientists seek to apply standardized instruments to new areas of investigation, however, the general benefits of such use may cause them to overlook some potential liabilities in specific applications.

The solution to these pragmatic concerns is based on the theoretical assumptions that the researcher makes about the correspondence between concepts and the indicators used to measure them. Concepts and indicators can be either global or specific. However, using a specific indicator to measure a global concept introduces bias in the generalization of findings; for instance, an assertion that social support mitigates the effect of stressful life events on psychological distress when only one aspect of social support—social affiliation—has been measured (20). Another source of bias occurs when a global measure is used as an indicator of a specific concept. This is described below in detail.

Because standardized instruments are usually global measures of a concept or phenomenon, it is often difficult to select the most appropriate instrument for a given application. Body image seems an important concept in the study of psychosocial reactions to breast cancer. Available instruments include "Draw a Person" (21) and the Body Image Scale (2). Neither operationalizes the anticipated changes in body image due to mastectomy. A second problem is caused by the indicators used to quantify the concept itself. For example, somatic symptoms such as anorexia and fatigue are often used to quantify concepts such as depression. However, such somatic symptoms are common in cancer as well, confounding many of the available instruments. The obvious solution is to rely on purely psychological symptoms of such concepts when studying their prevalence among the physically ill (8,6,35).

The use of standardized instruments is predicated on the often untested assumption that there are similarities across a variety of health problems; that is, regardless of the illness, the individual's response to the measure will be the same. For this to be true, each item in the scale must be relevant. If not, the irrelevant items add noise to the system, increasing the chance of rejecting a true hypothesis. Thus tests of specific hypotheses can be weakened, confounded, or masked by the use of global measures.

These problems can be illustrated by the previously mentioned study of the psychosocial aspects of breast cancer. An intervention was designed to provide emotional support and information beginning early in the diagnostic/treatment sequence. Interviews with women who had had breast surgery revealed that their initial reactions to the diagnosis were devastating. In addition to feeling as though they were "falling apart," they observed that they were being treated differently. From being normal, healthy individuals they became patients in a matter of minutes; decisions were taken out of their hands; they were treated as if they were ill even though they were feeling quite well (6). Also, because of protocol many of the women were offered adjuvant chemotherapy.[1] To make informed decisions, these women needed to have information about the course of their disease, the different treatment modalities, and the effects of adjuvant chemotherapy. Response to their needs for this information became the second objective of this investigation.

In designing the evaluation for the intervention program, two problems had to be resolved. First, the theory of the program (how it was believed to work) needed to be explicated so that outcomes could be measured. Second, standardized measures needed to be selected so that the concepts could be quantified for testing the theory.

Provision of emotional support and information was predicted to decrease feelings of powerlessness engendered by the diagnosis of cancer and inherent in the role of a patient (3,36). The conceptualization of the process was less problematic than was the selection of indicators.

The best approximation to this conceptualization in the psychological literature is the construct of locus of control. When reinforcement is perceived by the subject as following and contingent on his or her own action, then in our culture it is typically perceived as predictable or subject to internal control. Alternatively, when reinforcement is not perceived as contingent on an action of the subject, then it is typically believed to be unpredictable and externally controlled because it is due to luck, chance, fate, or the control of powerful others (29).

Although the concept deals with both individual differences and situational parameters, most of the studies have been concerned with the former. Locus of control has typically been used as a predictor of behavior; however, increasing evidence suggests that changes in perception of control occur as a consequence of various interventions (1,9,33,40). Even so, conceptually, locus of control only partially captures the sense of powerlessness inherent in the patient situation: discovering one has a life-threatening condition whose outcome is uncertain, and becoming dependent for survival on others.

In the psychological literature, instruments used to measure the locus of control construct include the Internal-External Locus of Control Scale (29), the Health Locus of Control Scale (37), the Personal Efficacy Scale (9), and multiple adaptations of the original Rotter Scale (e.g., 17, 40). The Health

---

[1] Individuals with one or more lymph nodes containing metastases were invited to participate; different protocols were available for pre- and postmenopausal populations.

Locus of Control Scale (HLC) was finally selected. It has an intent similar to that of the Internal-External Locus of Control Scale, with a Likert rather than a forced choice scale. Other apparent advantages included brevity (11 rather than 40 items) and relation to health.

The HLC was administered at a suburban medical center to 115 women who had had breast surgery during the previous 2 years. In order to provide a view of the underlying structure of the data collected, a principal component analysis with a Varimax rotation was computed. The two rotated factor loadings and the scale items are presented in Table 3. When loadings of 0.40 and above are used as a rough index for factor definition, the two factors are interpretable as follows:

Factor 1—Fate: defined by six items involving good fortune, fatalism, luck, and dependency

Factor 2—Self-Blame: defined by four items involving carefulness/carelessness and self-blame

TABLE 3. *Health Locus of Control Items and Varimax factor loading (N = 115)*

Health Locus of Control Items[a]	Rotated factor loadings[b]	
	Factor 1	Factor 2
1. If I take care of myself, I can avoid illness.	−0.27	0.47
2. Whenever I get sick, it is because of something I've done or not done.	0.14	0.68
3. Good health is largely a matter of good fortune.	0.65	−0.07
4. No matter what I do, if I am going to get sick I will get sick.	0.75	−0.02
5. Most people do not realize the extent to which their illnesses are controlled by accidental happenings.	0.56	0.19
6. I can only do what my doctor tells me to do.	0.53	0.14
7. There are so many strange diseases around that you can never know how or when you might pick one up.	0.65	−0.00
8. When I feel ill, I know it is because I have not been getting the proper exercise or eating right.	0.09	0.77
9. People who never get sick are just plain lucky.	0.66	−0.10
10. People's ill health results from their own carelessness.	−0.00	0.61
11. I am directly responsible for my health.	−0.35	0.25
Common Factor Variance accounted for:	60%	40%

[a] Respondents were asked to indicated, on a 6-point scale ranging from "Strongly Agree" to "Strongly Disagree," the extent to which the statement related to their state of health and illness.

[b] Underlining denotes factor on which an item loads.

One item did not load on either factor (item 11). Under scrutiny, however, this item appears to load in an interpretable way on both factors. Responsibility for oneself is positively related to self-blame in that both imply internal attributions; it is negatively related to fate, which implies external attributions. Hence the two extracted factors are easily interpretable. The original global scale seems to be specifically represented by two factor-based variables.

To what extent do the two specific measures reflect what we were trying to measure? The responses of one woman to several items in the Self-Blame scale are indicative of its lack of face validity: for example, "If I did not wear a sweater on a cold day and then got a cold, I would agree with this item; but I know that my breast cancer is not a result of anything I have done." From this and other anecdotal evidence, it was clear that many of the women did not blame themselves for their cancer. Each of the items in this specific measure, if rated by the subject internally, would in fact cause such an inference.

If women do not generally blame themselves for their cancer, are there any conditions under which they will make such attributions? In ongoing analyses of the population referred to in Table 3, some intriguing evidence has been found on which to speculate. A series of regression analyses has been completed by the authors to determine factors and their interrelationships predicting adaptation to cancer. When a number of social and psychological factors are regressed on the HLC and on the two subscales, different factors are found to make important contributions to each. Although sociodemographic factors, such as being employed and of higher social class, are important predictors of both the Fate subscale and the HLC, medical factors such as number of positive lymph nodes and greater life change (13) predict self-blame. These data suggest that women whose disease has progressed further, perhaps due to delay in seeking medical care, do see themselves as responsible for their illness. Regardless, elimination of irrelevant items increases the ecological validity of the scale.

To what extent does the global measure mask the outcomes of the intervention program? Eighteen women who received emotional support and information as part of the primary study and another 18 women who had had surgery in the 4 months prior to that intervention formed a treatment group and a comparison group for this analysis (Table 4).[2] Means were calculated for each measure to compare the results using both the standardized and the more specific measures of locus of control. When means (adjusted for item directionality) are compared, two findings stand out. First, the effect of treatment is most noticeable on the Fate subscale; there is no treatment effect at all on the Self-Blame subscale. Second, the difference is in the comparison group, not in the treatment group. Thus the effect of the intervention was to cancel out what would have been a more fatalistic attitude on the part of treatment group subjects. Added together, these effects partially cancel each other; thus when the means for the total

---

[2] Control data were collected prior to initiating the treatment program to eliminate the possibility of reactivity to its interventions and to prevent unacceptable allocation of subjects, all members of the same prepaid health plan, to either group.

TABLE 4. *Adjusted means and t-test comparisons for Health Locus of Control Scale and Self-Blame and Fate Subscales*

Measure	Condition	Adjusted mean[a,b]	t-Test[c]
Health Locus of Control Scale (11 items)	Comparison (N = 18)	3.71	−2.16[d]
	Treatment (N = 18)	3.25	
Self-Blame Subscale (4 items)	Comparison (N = 18)	3.44	−0.20
	Treatment (N = 18)	3.25	
Fate Subscale (6 items)	Comparison (N = 18)	4.17	−2.63[e]
	Treatment (N = 18)	3.05	

[a] Means adjusted to a common frame of reference. The Health Locus of Control Scale consists of 11 items with a range of scores of 11–66. It is usually reported as a sum of items; however, for comparison with its factor-derived subscales, a mean is calculated and reported herein. After reverse-scoring, means were calculated for the Self-Blame Subscale (range 4–24). The Fate Subscale (range 6–36) was divided by the number of items to form an adjusted mean. Higher values indicate greater externality.
[b] Scale mean is 3.5.
[c] df = 34.
[d] $p < 0.05$.
[e] $p < 0.01$.
From Bloom, ref. 2a, by permission of the American Psychological Association.

scale are compared, the effect of treatment is partially masked. Removing the irrelevant items from the locus of control scale provides a better test of the hypothesis.

We offer a further criticism of studies looking for greater psychopathology in cancer patients than in other patients; that is, the measurement instruments selected are generally designed to be used with patients with psychiatric problems. This makes some sense because if one wants to look for depression, a scale with "depression" items is appropriate; and one that has norms for extreme responses, such as those from a psychiatric population, also makes sense, otherwise it would be too easy to reach a ceiling effect. However, this unintentional bias tends to limit the kinds of things looked for in responses from cancer patients. It tends to encourage use of standardized instruments that are looking for psychopathology that can be measured and may overlook other problems that are actually more important for patients and their families.

Choice of Instruments

In studies with cancer patients, by far the most widely used psychological instrument is the Minnesota Multiphasic Personality Inventory (MMPI) (11).

No other published instrument is cited more than a few times. Its use in a variety of studies with cancer patients may be summarized as follows:

• Studies designed to profile characteristics of the cancer patient (15,31,41).
• Discrimination of patients who delay seeking treatment from those who do not (10,41).
• Relation of psychological factors to the development of cancer (4,8,16, 30,39).
• Relation of psychological variables to adjustment to cancer (31,34).

It is interesting to note that most of these studies use the MMPI as a measure of personality that may predict some future behavior; for example, an unaggressive, acquiescent personality may experience more rapid disease progression (4). Unfortunately, no data are reported that attempt to relate changes in psychological functioning as a result of changes in medical care, disease status, family life, and so forth. In the cited studies, the MMPI is assumed to measure personality traits more likely to cause behavioral change than the reverse. But others, notably Mischel (24), have demonstrated that the relationship between personality factors and future behavior is more complex, encompassing both person and situation factors.

If one wants to compare scores of cancer patients with those of other groups on the kinds of dimensions measured by the MMPI, then it certainly is the instrument of choice. However, such scores are not useful for determining whether cancer patients differ from other groups on the most critical variables, nor do those scores yield much diagnostic information useful for planning interventions. The following represents a summary of the authors' view of the current state of psychological measurement in cancer research:

• The MMPI and most measures of anxiety indicate only the presence or absence of the psychological trait. Use of these instruments for the purpose of planning interventions may be misleading because the measures indicate only the psychological trait of an individual or group, and do not predict behavioral patterns. Moreover, the MMPI clinical scales—hypochondrias, depression, hysteria, psychopathology, masculinity/femininity, paranoia, psychasthenia, schizophrenia, hypomania, and social—are only tangentially related to the everyday problems faced by cancer patients and their families.
• Scales such as the MMPI, measuring general psychological traits, offer easy explanations for behavior and may, in fact, obscure important reasons for cancer patients' behavioral patterns. For example, a patient's response to a test may result in an elevated "depression" score, providing one with the temptation to explain a low activity level with "He doesn't do much because he's depressed." However, the patient's inactivity may actually be due to several factors such as weakness caused by his treatment, the state of his disease, or the attitudes and behavior of staff or family.
• Scales measuring only the presence or absence of particular psychological

traits offer no diagnostic information useful for planning interventions when test results are negative. That is, psychological instruments designed to identify pathology are useful only when they do just that; but when they fail to identify a problem state (or trait), there is little one can conclude or predict.

• Patients with physical disease resent being asked to complete rather long psychological inventories that seem to be looking for psychopathologic states.

• There is no evidence to assume that all cancer patients will experience psychological trauma and/or that they will proceed through an invariant series of stages.

• The experience of cancer patients is better understood by looking at the interactions of multiple factors—the patients' own resources (personal and social, their attitudes and behavior patterns), disease type and stage, medical treatment factors, and relationships with others.

Considering all these problems, understanding and measuring the behavior of individuals diagnosed as having cancer require specifically designed instrumentation. The following criteria for such an instrument are suggested:

• It should reflect both problem and support behaviors most commonly experienced by cancer patients so that the data can be summarized in a multidimensional profile.

• It should reflect changes in behavior over time, and attempt to identify the most probable causes for behavior as perceived by the patients (there is a difference between patients who see themselves as drinking too much because of their disease and those who say that they are drinking too much because it has been typical behavior for them long before their diagnosis).

• It should have high face validity for cancer patients and have a low "mystical" quality—patients should not feel they are being assessed for underlying or subconscious motives.

• It should assume normal functioning but permit extreme responses, especially those considered socially undesirable.

A new approach toward measuring responses to cancer appears necessary. In 1976 the authors established a relationship with the Oncology Department at the Stanford University Medical Center to create an instrument that would meet the criteria listed above. Consequently, the Cancer Patient Behavior Scale (CPBS) (27) was developed to assess the behavioral and emotional responses to cancer within common areas of life function. The scale includes items relevant to all people as well as some items that are disease specific. It also allows the individual an opportunity to indicate whether his or her behavior was caused by the disease, its treatment, or other factors. Originally 170 items were included, but subsequent analyses produced a revised form of 124 more useful and predictive items. It is anticipated that additional revisions will result in fewer items.

The data from pilot studies with Hodgkin's disease patients support the view that understanding the behavior of people with cancer requires less concentration

TABLE 5. *Reliability of Cancer Patient Behavior Scale Subscales in Hodgkin's disease patients (N = 106)*

Subscale	No. of items	Reliability coefficient (alpha)
Problems		
Depression	11	0.91
Interpersonal	10	0.70
Anxiety	13	0.75
Habits	9	0.58
Treatment	7	0.74
Life Disruption	7	0.72
Support		
Activity	19	0.78
Life Satisfaction	14	0.85
Self-Competency	15	0.84
Social Competency	10	0.76

on extreme scores (from any instrument) and increased emphasis on problems that affect behavior frequently. So far, it appears that the CPBS identifies patients who do not necessarily have extreme problems (as would be suggested by the MMPI approach to instrumentation) but differ from a healthy population in the frequency with which they experience more common problems related to everyday functioning. Presently, from the 124 items, 10 subscale scores are computed: Depression, Interpersonal Problems, Treatment Problems, Anxiety, Personal Habits, Life Disruption, Activity, Self-Competency, Social Competency, and Life Satisfaction (alpha reliability coefficients are presented in Table 5).

Preliminary data from the CPBS suggest that it is accepted by cancer patients and is useful because it yields information about frequency of both problem and support behaviors, as well as patient perceptions of the causes of their behavior. Also, it can be used at frequent intervals to provide a record of behavior change, so it may be appropriate for use in evaluation studies.

DISCUSSION

The authors' purpose in this chapter is to call attention to potential sources of bias in psychosocial studies of cancer patients. In particular, it is suggested that researchers and consumers of research (policy makers, patients, families, social workers, physicians, scientists on research study sections, and so forth) be more sensitive to the role that unexamined assumptions may play in influencing research results and their interpretation. It may be useful to distinguish between intentional and unintentional bias because intentional bias is most disguised, and unintentional bias is most overlooked—even by careful design specialists.

Intentional bias in psychosocial cancer research results when researchers write proposals and reports in a manner that suggests more rigorous science than the studies actually deserve. In most cases, researchers proposing a particular study intentionally present their ideas within a scientific paradigm to please reviewers. The resulting proliferation of scientific-appearing but biased reports may have an inappropriately significant impact on funding or policy decisions. These studies may also be motivated by a desire to help cancer patients and their families cope with disease. It is suggested that they may be better described in demonstration or case study reports, which unfortunately have not been in favor with the scientific community.

Unintentional bias comes from well-meaning researchers skilled in design methods, who transfer their research tools from another area to the psychosocial study of cancer. The problem with unintentional bias is not that the studies are conducted poorly or inappropriately, but that the assumptions brought to the research question are unexamined. Consequently, it is possible to find studies that are designed carefully, and conducted and analyzed appropriately, but yield results best interpreted only within the context of the (generally unstated) assumptions behind the hypotheses tested. Ordinarily such studies would be considered good research, be published in respectable journals, and be referred to in subsequent investigations. In a field as new as the study of psychosocial aspects of cancer, well-controlled studies are influential in directing new research and allocation of research funds. For this reason, it is important to stop once in a while and take a critical look at the research being supported and the assumptions behind the research questions asked.

It is important to remember that the psychosocial study of cancer patients is applied research, motivated because of advances in treatment. People are living many years beyond what is generally considered the acute phase of the disease, that is, the diagnosis and initial surgery that frequently follows. Improving the quality of life for patients, their families, and associates is the motive underlying all the studies proposed. This is an important point, because no matter how the motive may be disguised by the use of neutral scientific phrases, it is nevertheless the driving force behind such work. Researchers would be hard pressed to account for their work in terms such as understanding and curiosity—notions generally reserved for research without a definite motive.

People with cancer are different from those who do not have any disease. They are different as well from those who have other life-threatening conditions because the treatment, while potentially lifesaving, is likely to cause body damage. Thus to understand how cancer affects, let us say, a child's schooling, requires more than merely determining whether the child can learn to read. The child may be in and out of school for weeks at a time while undergoing treatment; side effects that may include loss of hair and lack of energy, the resulting peer reactions to the child, and the teacher's attitudes and skill at dealing with such problems all may affect the child's ability to pay attention, make fine discriminations, remember, and reason. Acceptance of the idea that research is motivated toward improving medical care and quality of life increases the likelihood that unintentional bias will be introduced, resulting in null hypotheses that have a low probability of acceptance.

Interestingly, when one takes a close look at some of the areas where major differences between cancer patients and healthy comparison groups would be expected, those differences are not always there. For example, as previously noted, breast cancer patients did not resemble psychiatric patients but were more like a healthy population on such factors as depression, tension, and vigor. Thus the development of psychodynamic support programs for such a population would certainly be open to question.

One mistake is that there really is no reason to suspect that cancer patients are different from other people in personality traits, life events, or problems experienced when coping with a crisis. The notion of predicting behavior by using personality variables alone has been argued against convincingly by Mischel (24). Whether research with cancer patients is research with a special population that negates all the complications involved in understanding human behavior should be questioned. More likely, it is research with a special population that is complicated by the addition of certain variables.

Psychosocial research in cancer will be conducted in a complicated environment, therefore the researcher's questions cannot simply be borrowed from studies in other fields. Nor should investigators be fooled into thinking that classic research methods and data analysis schemes can be directly applied with success. The validity of results cannot be trusted until a large enough body of data exists from which to draw inferences—and this includes research questions and designs that have been modified so as to be relevant to the problems at hand—not taken from other fields simply because scientists in those areas are limited to them. The task is more complex, not more simple, providing a greater challenge to researchers.

REFERENCES

1. Bandura, A. (1977): Self-efficacy: Toward a unifying theory of behavior change. *Psychol. Rev.*, 84:191–215.
2. Berscheid, E., Walster, E., and Bohrnstedt, G. W. (1972): Body image: A *Psychology Today* questionnaire. *Psychol. Today*, 6:57–66.
2a. Bloom, J. R. (1979): Psychosocial measurement and specific hypotheses: A research note. *J. Couns. Clin. Psychol.*, 47:637–639.
3. Bloom, J. R., Ross, R. D., and Burnell, G. M. (1978): The effect of social support on patient adjustment after breast surgery. *Patient Counsel Health Educ.*, 1:50–59.
4. Blumberg, E. M., West, P., and Ellis, F. (1954): A possible relationship between psychological factors and human cancer. *Psychosom. Med.*, 16:277–286.
5. Derogatis, L. R., Lipman, R. S., Rickels, K., Uhlenhuth, E. H., and Covi, L. (1974): The Hopkins Symptom Checklist (HSCL): A self-report inventory. *Behav. Sci.*, 19:1–15.
6. Fitzmaurice, A., and Ross, R. D. (1976): *A Survey of Concerns of Breast Cancer Patients.* DHEW Contract NO1-CN-55313, SRI International, Menlo Park, Ca.
7. Fox, B. H. (1978): Premorbid psychological factors as related to cancer incidence. *J. Behav. Med.*, 1:45–133.
8. Gay, R. L. (1971): The relationship between psychopathology and cancer. *Dissert. Abstr. Int.*, 31:4992-B.

9. Gurin, G. (1968): *Inner-City Negro Youth in a Job Training Project.* Final Report to the Manpower Administration, U.S. Dept. of Labor, and to the Office of Education, U.S. DHEW. University of Michigan Press, Ann Arbor.
10. Hammerschlag, C. A., Fisher, S., DeCosse, J., and Kaplan, E. (1964): Breast symptoms and patient delay: Psychological variables involved. *Cancer,* 17:1480–1485.
11. Hathaway, S. R., and McKinley, J. C. (1951): *Minnesota Multiphasic Personality Inventory: Manual* (rev.). Psychological Corp., New York.
12. Hollis, F. (1964): *Casework: A Psychosocial Therapy.* Random House, New York.
13. Holmes, T. H., and Rahe, R. H. (1967): The Social Readjustment Rating Scale. *J. Psychosom. Res.,* 11:213–218.
14. Jamison, K. R., Wellisch, D. K., and Pasnau, R. O. (1978): Psychosocial aspects of mastectomy: I. The woman's perspective. *Am. J. Psychiatry,* 135:432–436.
15. Koenig, R., Levin, S., and Brennan, M. (1967): The emotional status of cancer patients as measured by a psychological test. *J. Chronic Dis.,* 20:923–930.
16. Krasnoff, A. (1959): Psychological variables and human cancer: A cross-validation study. *Psychosom. Med.,* 21:291.
17. Levenson, H. (1974): Activism and powerful others: Distinctions within the concept of internal/external control. *J. Pers. Assess.,* 38:377–383.
18. Levine, P. M., Silverfarb, P. M., and Lipowski, Z. J. (1978): Mental disorders in cancer patients: A study of 100 psychiatric referrals. *Cancer,* 42:1385–1391.
19. Lewis, F. M., and Bloom, J. R. (1979): Psychosocial adjustment to breast cancer: A review of selected literature. *Int. J. Psychiatr. Med.,* 9:1–17.
20. Lin, N., Simeone, R. S., Ensel, W. M., and Kuo, W. (1979): Social support, stressful life events and illness. *J. Health Soc. Behav.,* 20:108–119.
21. Machover, K. (1949): *Personality Projection in the Drawing of the Human Figure: A Method of Personality Investigation.* University of Michigan Press, Ann Arbor.
22. McNair, P. M., Lorr, M., and Droppelman, L. (1971): *POMS Manual,* pp. 24–25. Education and Industrial Testing Services, San Diego.
23. Mechanic, D. (1962): *Students under Stress: A Study in the Social Psychology of Adaptation.* The Free Press, New York.
24. Mischel, W. (1973): Toward a cognitive social learning reconceptualization of personality. *Psychol. Rev.,* 80:252–283.
25. Panagis, D. (1977): *Perceived Social Support Scale.* West Coast Cancer Foundation, San Francisco.
26. Plumb, M. M., and Holland, J. (1977): Comparative studies of psychological functions in patients with advanced cancer. I. Self-reported depressive symptoms. *Psychosom. Med.,* 39:264–276.
27. Ross, R. D., Stockdale, F., and Jacobs, C. (1978): Cancer Patient Behavior Scale: Scores of cancer patients and healthy adults. *Proc. Am. Soc. Clin. Oncol.,* 19:348.
28. Rotter, J. B. (1966): Generalized expectancies for internal vs. external control of reinforcement. *Psychol. Monogr.,* 80:609.
29. Rotter, J. B. (1975): Some problems and misconceptions related to the construct of internal versus external control of reinforcement. *J. Consult. Clin. Psychol.,* 43:56–67.
30. Schmale, A., and Iker, H. (1971): Hopelessness as a predictor of cervical cancer. *Social Serv. Med.,* 5:95–100.
31. Schonfield, J. (1975): Psychological and life-experience differences between Israeli women with benign and cancerous breast lesions. *J. Psychosom. Res.,* 19:229–234.
32. Simonton, O. C., and Simonton, S. S. (1975): Belief systems and management of the emotional aspects of malignancy. *J. Transpers. Psychol.,* 7:29–47.
33. Smith, R. E. (1970): Change in locus of control as a function of life crisis resolution. *J. Abnorm. Psychol.,* 75:328–332.
34. Sobel, H., and Worden, J. (1979): The MMPI as a predictor of psychosocial adaptation to cancer. *J. Consult. Clin. Psychol,* 47:716–724.
35. Stewart, M. A., Drake, F., and Winokus, G. (1965): Depression among medically ill patients. *Dis. Nerv. Syst.,* 26:479–484.
36. Waitzkin, H., and Stoeckle, J. D. (1972): The communication of information about illness. *Adv. Psychosom. Med.,* 8:180–215.
37. Wallston, B. S., Wallston, K. A., Kaplan, G. D., and Maides, S. A. (1976): Development and validation of the Health Locus of Control (HLC) Scale. *J. Consult. Clin. Psychol.,* 44:580–585.

38. Weisman, A. D., and Worden, J. W. (1975): Psychosocial analysis of cancer deaths. *Omega,* 6:61–75.
39. Weyer, E. M. (ed.) (1966): Psychophysiological aspects of cancer. *Ann. N. Y. Acad. Sci.,* 125:773–1055.
40. Wittes, S. (1970): *People and Power: A Study of Crisis in Secondary Schools.* University of Michigan Press, Ann Arbor.
41. Worden, J. W., and Weisman, A. D. (1975): Psychosocial components of lag time in cancer diagnosis. *J. Psychosom. Res.,* 19:69–79.

Psychosocial Aspects of Cancer,
edited by Jerome Cohen et al.
Raven Press, New York © 1982.

Chapter 23

A Psychological Measure as a Predictor in Cancer

Bernard H. Fox

National Cancer Institute, National Institutes of Health, Bethesda, Maryland 20205

Among the possible roles of psychological factors in cancer, their connection with initiation and physical course of the disease are, perhaps, the most uncertain. A patient's overt emotional or behavioral reaction to cancer, although varied, is to some degree evident, even if one is not sure of its meaning or what may be going on inside the patient. Rarely, however, does it involve the question, "Is there any reaction at all?" Similar reasoning applies to delay in screening or going to the doctor with symptoms. Compliance behavior is a problem of motivation and measurement, not of whether there is such a thing as compliance behavior. Similarly, pain control is a question of a different genre, as are most questions of occupational and other kinds of rehabilitation. But the primary question here, in both initiation and progress of the disease, is whether psychological factors are associated with them at all.

In this brief review I shall examine evidence on the positive and negative sides of that question: (a) *positive*—psychological factors are related to cancer incidence or progress, whether as predictors of greater or lesser incidence than the population or controls, or as predictors of faster or slower progress of disease than those with different psychological characteristics; (b) *negative*—psychological factors are not related to cancer incidence or progress, or they show an inconsistent relationship. Social factors will by and large be ignored, partly because they do not, as yet, help much with a decision on psychological factors, and partly because to deal with them would involve too extensive a discussion for this space. I shall also ignore the fundamental differences between the mechanisms of initiation of cancer and those leading to its faster or slower progression. Lastly, I shall ignore the whole issue of psychosis as a possible precursor to high or low risk of cancer. Instead, statistical and methodological issues will be addressed. Thus the look at the evidence will be incomplete. But it will at least yield perspective on the selected issues.

POSITIVE RESULTS

There is no need to belabor the points made by a number of general reviewers of the question who have paid little critical attention to the experimental and analytic problems: e.g., Baltrusch et al. (13–16), Achterberg et al. (5), LeShan and Worthington (50), Cagossi (21), and Aimez (7). They cite the major studies in the field support of the positive view, and some studies without positive results. Several others have examined the evidence in the literature more critically. These include Abse et al. (2), Bahnson (9), Bahnson and Kissen (12), Crisp (23), Fox (29), McCoy (53), Morrison and Paffenbarger (55), Perrin and Pierce (63), and Wirsching (84). Support for the positive view usually derives from the consistency of results in several studies for each of various personality factors. For example, for the following personality factors, Abse et al. (2) cite the number of references noted below in each case, of which one or two instances each are given here: (a) denial and repression, seven (Bahnson, 10); (b) impaired self-awareness and introspective capacity, five (Abse et al., 1); (c) poor outlet for emotional discharge, seven (Kissen, 42); (d) diminished expression of aggression, five (Thomas, 79); (e) self-sacrificing and self-blaming, six (Nemeth and Mezei, 60); (f) rigid, conventional, five (Bahnson and Bahnson, 11); (g) a "reality" orientation, six (Blumberg, 19); (h) meager but deeply felt object cathexes, three (Booth, 20); and (i) (predisposition for experiencing) hopelessness and despair, four (Greene, 33, Schmale and Iker, 70). To Abse's list a few more can be added: to item (a) above, Henderson (38); to (d), Greer and Morris (34); to (e), Grissom et al. (35); and to (i), Bacon et al. (8). A similar list can be found in Stone et al. (78, p. 105).

Other dimensions and influencers of the psyche have been reported more than once: body-image constriction, e.g., Harrower et al. (37), Fisher and Cleveland (28); extraversion, e.g., Coppen and Metcalfe (22), its equivalent, Hagnell (36); adverse childhood or adult events, e.g., LeShan (49), Kissen (43), Speciani (74), Dillenz (25), Lorenzen (52); diminished sexuality, e.g., Rotkin (69), Stephenson and Grace (77); loss of important emotional object, LeShan (48); depression, many references, e.g., Bieliauskas et al. (18), Achté and Vauhkonen (3). A number of studies, including many of those already mentioned, report positive results on variables not duplicated elsewhere. A good example is that by Reznikoff (64).

In addition, it is important to note the large number of positive results in animals. Some important sources are Riley (65), those of the Russian School (Kavetskii, 40), Ader and Cohen (immune function only) (6), review articles by Rogers et al. (68) and Stein et al. (76), both mostly immune function, and the earlier review article by LaBarba (47). These report both more and earlier tumors under stress appearing both before and after a carcinogen was applied. Stress here means internal effect of a stressor.

NEGATIVE RESULTS

As for negative animal results, we note first a considerable animal literature showing a few studies in which stress failed to affect the time or number of tumors significantly, and a number of studies in which stress actually reduced the number or delayed the onset of tumors (see refs. 39,40,47,65,68). Of course these studies include many types of stressors, carcinogenic agents, times of stressing (e.g., before weaning, hours before the carcinogen, days before the carcinogen), and particularly, many strains of animals, as well as different species.

A fairly respectable list of negative papers on humans can be found. Most of these are negative because the experimental (or case) and control difference, although in the predicted direction, was not significant, usually at the 0.05 level. Some studies, however, showed results in the direction opposite to that hypothesized. For example, Greer and Morris (34) found almost identical proportions of patients and controls with treated depressive illness during the 5 years before breast biopsy (35% and 36%), and similar proportions with loss of a major emotional relationship during that time (18% patients, 16% controls). Finn et al. (27) could show no difference in overall anxiety between coronary patients and cancer patients, both showing more than normals. Grissom et al. (35) reported no significant differences in generally stressful events between cancer patients and normals, although the patients' personality integration was much poorer; neither did Greer and Morris (34), Graham et al. (32), Snell and Graham (73), and, only partially, Weinhold (83). If one contrasts results on the Si scale (social introversion) of the MMPI and the Extraversion dimension of Eysenck's MPI, McCoy (53), in a prospective study, found the former to be high in future cancer patients, and Kissen and Eysenck (44) found the latter to be high in current cancer patients. Earle (26, reported in 16), using the Worthington Personality Test, showed no significant relationship between emotional factors and malignancy, in contrast to LeShan and Worthington (51). Muslin and Pieper (58) showed no excess of separation experiences among cancer patients. Keehn et al. (41), in a most important prospective study, found no relation of psychoneurosis to later probability of dying of cancer. Subjects were soldiers discharged in World War I for psychoneurosis, with average age in the early 20s. About 1,000 cancer deaths occurred.

All of these findings are relatively well known in the literature. New ones have appeared from time to time and deserve attention, particularly new prospective studies (17,18,24,56,59,61,80). Thomas has extended her findings to 48 cases, 20 with serious cancer and 28 with nonmelanotic skin cancer (80). Her original finding of low level of closeness to parents in future cancer patients has remained stable. Betz and Thomas (17) have extended the theory of personality differences found by Thomas (see discussion below). Bieliauskas et al. (18) have reported an excess proportion of people in a future cancer group whose highest MMPI score was D (depression). The cohort was tested in 1958. Watson and Schuld (82) found no prior MMPI differences among psychiatric patients who did and did not later get cancer. Dattore (24) examined the earlier MMPI scores of 75 future cancer patients and 125 with future other diagnoses and found repression and depression among the variables contributing significantly to a discriminant function. Moss (56), examining Human Population Laboratory data in Alameda County, California, found a two- to threefold excess of relative risk of future cancer among deniers. Nemeth (59) predicted with better than chance success from Rorschach records those who would later get breast cancer. And finally, Paffenbarger and colleagues have made a positive finding in their cohort of Harvard and University of Pennsylvania students (61). As the finding is still only tentative, it cannot be detailed here.

THE ISSUES

The basic issues are three, aside from those being ignored (see the beginning of this chapter): (a) How much confidence can one have in extrapolation from animal studies to human? (b) How much can we trust the known prospective studies? (c) How much confidence can we have that positive findings on cancer patients indicate a premorbid state of affairs in general, particularly in the face of parallel negative findings?

Before these questions are addressed, a little theory is necessary. If the true value of the effect of a psychosocial variable is zero, and the distribution of possible effects is not especially asymmetrical, one should expect about as many negative as positive results. We know of the unfortunate tendency of some experimenters to fail to report negative results, so we might have some bias toward positive even if the true value is zero. If the true value is positive, however, our distribution will show more positive than negative results, the excess depending on how strongly positive the mean value is. The issue is clear if the product is number of cases, and chi square is the statistic, since too low a frequency of occurrence will yield a significant chi square as well as too high a frequency. If the yield is a mean test score comparison, however, a value in the direction opposite to the hypothesis' direction is usually reported as "not significant," even if it is truly significant in the reverse direction. For these cases we cannot tell what has happened unless the means and variabilities are given—often not the case.

We now examine the proposed issues.

1. How much confidence can one have in extrapolation from animal studies to humans? To determine the value of stress findings in animal studies, we ask whether there are any controlled human studies of imposition of stress; there is none, except possibly the naturalistic experiment of prisoners of war in whom no difference in cancer incidence was seen (Segal, 72, p. 19). Moreover, none of the human personality studies is relevant to the animal studies. The human studies of stressful events, which could be regarded as a kind of stress, have, when good control groups are used, by and large shown no difference between cancer and control groups (32,34,35,58,73,83) but see Kissen (43). So,

even if one were inclined to set animal stress studies and human traumatic event studies in parallel, the former show mixed results, the latter, negative.

One finding in animals is consistent with a human finding: there exist strains in which particular sites are more susceptible to cancer than others. Although this fact is of help in animal studies, it has been of no help in human work because no studies have been done on stress in human genetic group isolates, and indeed, only a few such isolates are available for such studies without major interference by environmental conditions.

As far as statistics are concerned, the same principles hold as described above, but there is more likelihood of avoiding the "not significant" trap because in almost all cases actual values are reported for animals: days survived, days to first evidence of tumor, average size of tumor, number with tumor, number that died. So far as results are concerned, the problems, some of which are described below in the third issue, are much diminished: animals are usually genetically similar, experimental treatment is uniform, outcome measures are less variable, and animals have more uniform feeding, housing, and environment than humans. Only where laboratory surroundings could involve irregular stresses imposed on the animals, unknown to the experimenter, may there be questionable results [see Riley (66)]. I am inclined strongly to accept the view that in animals, stress under various specific conditions can produce various effects; it can not only increase, but it can be neutral or actually reduce susceptibility to malignancies, both spontaneous and imposed by carcinogenic stimulation. This does not mean that man is thereby subject to the same conclusions. It does, however, incline me to believe more than in the absence of such animal data that stress can, (not "will" but "can") under some restricted conditions, produce a change not only in susceptibility to tumor incidence but also in disease progress in humans. I have used my words cautiously. That belief would have been much more strongly expressed if there did not exist a major discrepancy between, on the one hand, the results of immune suppression in animals, a state which in part some particular kinds of stressors can bring about, and on the other hand, the results of immune suppression in man. In rodents many kinds of tumors are increased with immune suppression, depending on the strain of rodent: lymphomas and tumors of the stomach, ovary, liver, breast, testicles, and others. In man tumors in excess of expected numbers arise mostly in the tissues damaged or influenced by the immune suppression: lymphatic system and sarcomas. In a few cases slightly excess lung and stomach incidence has been seen. In man, moreover, under some conditions immune suppression can inhibit tumor progress. But the tumors that afflict man the most are by and large not affected—breast, colon, rectum, prostate, lung, pancreas, bladder; nor are most other tumor incidences affected. These facts impose limits on any strong conclusions one might draw from animal work.

2. How much can we trust the known prospective studies? Starting from the latest studies, there is only a hint of a positive relationship between psychological factors and increased future risk of cancer from Paffenbarger (61). However,

as yet the data are not fully analyzed. Rogentine et al. (67) predicted 1-year relapse in 33 apparently disease-free melanoma patients at better than chance levels, based on a clinical algorithm and on the coefficients of a discriminant analysis derived from a predictor-development group of 31 similar patients. This study must also stand alone, since the authors (of which I am one) are unwilling as yet to draw inferences about the population of melanoma patients from this sample, let alone those with cancers at other sites. Other predictive studies of disease progress are not cited here because not all the patients were apparently disease free in those studies, and separate analyses were not usually available for those free of disease. The dangers of using patients with overt disease are quite clear, and in a way, preclude confident conclusions about any such study. Moss (56) showed an excess of denial of special kinds (financial troubles and marital troubles) in those destined to get cancer. His finding was inferential, and as he points out, the responses could have been truth, not denial (that is, the reported absence of such troubles could have been real absence, not denial in the sense of a psychological defense mechanism. Watson and Schuld's failure to find MMPI differences (82) is not entirely unexpected, since the groups were neuropsychiatric patients, although it was not clear from their paper whether the tests were given before neuropsychiatric hospitalization or after. Dattore (24) reported low scores in cancer patients on repression and depression scales, although his discriminant analysis is not particularly convincing, nor were his control groups especially attractive (see discussion of Dattore below). Shekelle's group (Bieliauskas, 18) found that an excess number of later cancer patients (all sites) showed depression as their highest MMPI score. Their study was controlled for age, drinking, and smoking. Neither Dattore's nor Watson and Schuld's studies are closely comparable to Shekelle's work, so his data stand alone. They lend support to a positive conclusion. Thomas et al. (80) described the division of cancer sites in their group. There were 20 patients with various serious cancers and 28 nonmelanotic skin cancer patients. Separate analysis for the 20 provides a rather small number to draw conclusions from. The special nature of those prone to nonmelanotic skin cancer almost forces a separate analysis, and an attempt to control for the disposing factors. Betz and Thomas (17), addressing a new personality structuring, described incidence of cancer among those with any of three personality configurations. Among more than 1,000 original subjects, 45 were typed. Unfortunately, only five cancer patients emerged from the group of 45. Five were not enough to draw conclusions from. But even if one uses a chi-square statistic, being aware of the problems with small expected frequencies, the numbers in the three groups did not differ significantly from the expected number, either in a contingency table or using the healthy group to define the expected proportions (my analysis, $p < 0.10$). In the same paper Thomas et al. chose from their cohort a sample of 127 persons with various diseases. A blind retrospective analysis of these persons was done, including 20 cancer patients. Betz allocated the 20 patients to the three personality configurations. When I analyzed these data, the relationship between cancer–no cancer and type of configuration was again not significant ($p < 0.10$). Presumably the above five cases were included in the group of 20, since the same number—20—was reported in the 1979 paper by Thomas et al. (80).

As for the remaining two studies relevant to this section (How much do we trust known prospective studies?), one (Hagnell, 36) has already been examined (Fox, 29), with some basic questions remaining about its conclusions, and the other (McCoy, 53) had inconclusive results (four significant when two were expected, three being related to cancer). That finding, like Bieliauskas' (18), lends support to a positive conclusion but by itself is not sufficiently conclusive.

In sum, we find enough differences and problems among these prospective studies to temper any strong conclusions. Imagine, for judgment on any test measure, that there is a large scale and that to cause it to tip stably we would need a heavy weight on one side. These studies add slight amounts of weight, with consequent instability and uncertainty, to several scales, but not enough to any one scale to tip it stably. The analogy is not far-fetched. Unreliability leads to instability, and we need many such small weights before they can aggregate enough on one side to lead to stable tipping.

3. How much confidence can one have that positive findings in cancer patients indicate a premorbid state of affairs in general, particularly in the face of parallel negative findings? Rather little. We already had strong evidence (see 29) that cancer patients are subject to many and diverse psychic changes due to the cancer, as are people generally who are sick, but more so, except for mental disease. One could thus expect almost any result from studies on cancer patients. This position implies that there are indeed real differences between some cancer patients and controls. I agree that in many cases such differences are there. Exactly which differences to believe as real one cannot tell. Moreover, because such differences can but do not have to appear, one cannot draw population-wide inferences about any single finding in any cancer group. This position removes from consideration of premorbid prediction any studies which merely show that cancer patients differ from noncancer ones.

For purposes of generalization, I think that premorbid states cannot be established from such studies. There are too many conflicting results. This fact leads one to suspect either a null state of affairs, or a mildly positive effect that can add only a little weight (all other things being propitious) to one scale. At present no scale is close to tipping.

In the first place humans have a highly variable mix of genes because of our random mating (within limits). Thus we have little strain purity—surely not even approaching that of animals. Even with selection such as cultural and race isolates (e.g., certain African tribes with practically no Ewing's sarcoma, or the excess of nasopharyngeal cancer among certain Southeast China people—see 57), we can not come close to pure strains such as we have in animals. The differential exposure to carcinogenic environment in humans is poorly controlled, contrary to that in many animal studies. Such variability notwithstanding, we can still search for something common to cancer-prone people, but it must be joined with a fact that often accounts for positive findings: many studies are not well controlled on various factors that could be associated with the cancer group but not with the control group, or vice versa: age, sex, site of cancer, state of cancer, medical or physical findings in the patient, domicile, hospitalization, smoking, knowledge of the presence of cancer, etc.

Perhaps the most important fact to help interpret the overall picture is that most cancer is a chance event, either because there is a stable causative predisposition the physiology of which is not understood, or because the chance event is truly chance in the sense of its being a product of cosmic rays, ambient radiation, casual ingestion or inhalation of a carcinogen, or the like (Miller, 54). The whole picture that Miller describes is one that stresses such chance events, as opposed to persistent predisposition to cancer. This is not to say that such a predisposition does not exist or cannot be imposed by events. But it would be hard to imagine a predisposition as powerful as that suggested by the numbers reported in most studies of psychosocial effect on cancer susceptibility or progress.

MMPI PREDICTIVE STUDIES

I looked at a group of predictive studies that used the MMPI as one measure, or sometimes the only measure, and tried to draw a conclusion about that one test.[1] It was impossible. First I present a short view of each of the 12 cited studies. Then the findings are examined in the light of the above discussion (Tables 1, 2, and 3).

The results of Achterberg et al. (4), predicting disease status 2 months after testing a group with 90% having stage IV cancer (distant metastases), offer no possibility of worthwhile conclusions. Within 2 months a certain number of patients (not specified in the paper) had died. The "mean projected life expectancy [was] 12.6 months." The median life expectancy, not reported, was, of course, even less, since survival time is skewed to the right. One is led to ask what would have happened if the tests had been given 2 months earlier or later. Deriving 11 factors from 35 tests (MMPIs plus others) in 126 patients, most of whom are under the influence of advanced cancer, does not inspire confidence either in the factors derived or in the predictive capability. In any case the contribution of MMPI variables to predictive power was low. The validity scales (F, K, and L) and the experimental control scale loaded on one of the four significant factors and Pa (paranoia) on another. None of the other scales loaded on significant factors.

Bieliauskas et al. (18) analyzed data from a study by Shekelle (National Cancer Institute Grant RO1CA22536), who started with hypotheses that high scores

---

[1] Nonpredictive MMPI studies, e.g., those of Koenig et al. (45) or Pauli and Schmid (62), will not be considered here.

in anxiety and depression would forecast excess risk of death from cancer. Subjects were 2,082 male employees of the Western Electric Co., aged 40 to 55, whose MMPIs were taken in 1958. Results on anxiety were not yet publicly available, but those on D (depression) were. Men with D as highest MMPI subscale score of the nine taken were twice as likely to die of cancer as those with other highest scales. The results persisted when adjusted for age at entry, cigarette smoking, and alcohol consumption. A Mantel-Haenszel analysis was applied to the 82 men who died of cancer and the 2,100 who did not.

Blumberg (19) is perhaps the most widely cited author in respect to psychological factors and rate of cancer progression. He gave several tests, among them the MMPI, to 18 patients, derived a predictive algorithm, and cross-validated on 32 other patients, just as did Rogentine et al. on other measures (67) and Fox et al. (30) on the MMPI, using Rogentine's samples. Blumberg's study, however, is in part pseudo-prospective. Those patients who died quickly were probably labeled as having fast progression—that is, faster progression of disease than the average patient with that cancer—for the most part if their death took place within about a year. This inference is drawn because Blumberg administered the MMPI and used the data on scores and the data on identification of fast and slow cancer progression in his dissertation. In it, he says the judgment by the doctor on rate of disease progression depended partly on patient clinical status, enzyme state (no longer considered a predictor of progression rate), and response to treatment, as well as epidemiologically predicted survival.

In his published paper with West and Ellis (19), only the last element of that judgment, expected survival, was mentioned. In order for expected survival time to be calculated, most of the slow-progressing patients had to have been diagnosed 5 to 10 years earlier, and to have been tested only when they came to the VA hospital, already having survived for a number of years. This fact imposes a formidable probability of bias in the response to any psychological test for the slow progression group.

Moreover, there were probably some patients whose survival would have fallen into the fast-progression group, but whose survival time Blumberg could not observe directly even in that group, if median survival was itself quite long (and hence mean survival even longer); e.g., cancers of the prostate or breast, for which the upper limit of his criterion was about 3½ years. These had to be judged only in terms of their response to therapy, profile clinical status, and the like. Hence the published paper (19) was incomplete in describing the basis of patient allocation for these putative cases and for most of the slow-progression cases, whose survival by Blumberg's definition of slow progression of disease was ≧1.5 times mean survival duration. If we assume a representative sample of cancer patients (excluding those who had no remission after treatment, and whom Blumberg omitted, thereby biasing the estimates of slow and fast progression even further), only for the short-term cancers where most patients die within a year could Blumberg have observed slow-progression cases: for example, cancers of the liver, pancreas, lung, and esophagus, and acute leukemia.

He determined, on 18 cases (dissertation) and 15 cases (published paper), the predictive MMPI structure and cross-validated on 32 or 35, as the case may be. For fast progression he said there should be strongly negative F-K (validity-suppressor) values; high D (depression) without associated high Hs (hypochondriasis) and Hy (hysteria); and low Ma (hypomania). The cross-validation on 32 cases showed $p < 0.01$. Only the data for all 50 were shown in the published paper, and not the breakout into 32 and 18.

Dattore's work (24) was done on VA hospital groups who took the MMPI approximately 4 years before diagnosis. In a true prospective study he attempted to discriminate those groups from each other using the test scores as predictors. The subjects consisted of (a) 75 cancer patients: 25 with lung cancer, 25 with prostate cancer, and 25 with multiple cancers; and (b) 125 controls: 25 with hypertension, 25 with ulcer, 25 with benign tumors, 25 with schizophrenia, and 25 asymptomatic. His work was designed to test portions of the hypotheses of Kissen (43), LeShan (48), and Bahnson and Bahnson (11) that the MMPI could address. Neither Kissen's nor LeShan's hypotheses were supported by his discriminant analyses, but the Bahnsons' hypothesis was partially supported. Because the prostate group was older than the other groups, he attempted a similar discrimination for prostate patients only against an age-matched control group. This procedure separated the prostate and the chosen control group at a significant level, leading him to conclude that age was not the primary discriminator in the first analysis. This conclusion is not necessarily correct (23a), in view of the 8 out of 17 nontrivial—in the sense of Dales and Ury—correlations that he found ($p < 0.13$) between age and MMPI scales. The scales contributing most importantly were Byrnes' R-S (repression-sensitization), D (depression), and HyD (denial of hysteria), an experimental scale. Dattore rejects the latter in view of the scarcity of data on validity and reliability on that scale. Other scales contributing to the overall significance of the discriminant analyses were Pa (paranoia), Mf (masculinity-femininity), Ca (caudality), and Hy (hysteria). The data tend to show that the prostate group contributed most strongly to the discrimination; but the success rate for discrimination was rather low, even though significant; and that by and large the centroids for the different cancer groups and control group lay rather close together, leading to little discriminating power for the MMPI overall. In discussing his results, Dattore (24, pp. 99–103) is properly reluctant to make any claims of importance for his data.

Fox et al. (30) analyzed MMPI data collected by Rogentine et al. (67) in a study of recurrence within 1 year among 64 melanoma patients who were tested during their disease-free interval. Because the state of knowledge was only at the stage of hypotheses, the authors required a significance level of 0.20 in both the first (group A, $N = 31$) and the second (group B, $N = 33$) of two consecutive samples in order for a hypothetical difference not to be lost through a type II error. Out of 38 clinical and experimental MMPI scales, none satisfied this requirement. In group A 14 scales were significant at $p < 0.20$, and one in group B. In the combined groups there were three, none significant at $p <$

0.05. The discrepancy in the two groups points up either the great variability to be expected in MMPI results under these circumstances or the possibility that the two groups were different, for whatever reason.

Gay's study (31) was similar to that of Blumberg in that he used estimates of long and short survival based on clinical state. It was, therefore, a pseudo-prospective study, like Blumberg's. He used 15 patients with "rapid progression" (mean age 57), 15 with "slow" (mean age 54), and 15 patients with bone fracture (mean age 40) as controls. The rapid group (R) scored significantly higher ($p < 0.05$) than the slow group (S) in two of the validity scales, L and K, and lower in the third, the F scale. In the L scale, R scores exceeded those of the controls (C) and in the K scale S > C. As for the clinical scales, S > R for Pd (psychopathic deviate), Sc (schizophrenia), and Ma (hypomania). S or R > C in eight scales and C > R in one. Gay did 45 MMPI scale comparisons of R, S, and C among three groups containing only 15 patients in each group. Because none of the patients was yet dead, actual survival time was not used, in contrast to Blumberg's study, where some of the patients probably died soon enough to measure their survival time (19). Moreover, Gay's only characterization of patients was on age; no other description was given, especially site or stage. In view of the age differences between group C and groups R and S, and the differences in the nature of these groups' illnesses, it is not surprising to find 11 significant MMPI test comparisons involving group C and the other two groups. As for groups R and S, the differences in the patients could easily have been due to stage, with highly probable differences in personality test results if there had been substantial differences in stage. In view of Gay's failure to do multiple comparison tests and in view of unknown site and stage status in groups R and S, I am reluctant to draw any strong inferences as to the predictability of survival from test scores alone in this study.

Krasnoff's study (46) was an attempt to cross-validate the Blumberg criteria (19). However, he used only melanoma patients, the stages were mixed, and knowledge of the nature and severity of disease was mixed, but in his favor. "Slow" membership was based on epidemiologic criteria only: survival <18 months was fast; survival >6 years was slow. No mention was made of differential survival by stage. Prediction using Blumberg's MMPI criteria was poorer than chance. Of 6 fast cases, 3 were called slow; of 16 slow cases, 11 were called fast.

McCoy (53) reported on 16 female and 24 male cancer patients who were one group of four (total $N = 177$) that he analyzed prospectively for disease state after they received a full MMPI at the Mayo Clinic. He did a one-way analysis of variance on each of 23 subtests for men, the four levels for each analysis being whether the group had cancer, hypertension, heart disease, or good health. He did another 23 tests on women, but the subgroups were those with cancer, hypertension, and good health, not enough female heart cases being available. He expected about two tests to be significant at $p < 0.05$, but four were significant. In one, following a Tukey test for multiple comparisons among three groups, cancerous women had significantly higher scores on the Si (social introversion) scale than the health group ($p < 0.05$, two-tailed; $p < 0.01$, one-tailed). Only three other tests gave significant results with the ANOVA: in women, two special scales—HR (Haan Regression) and Crims (critical items)—but the latter was not significant when the Tukey multiple comparisons test was applied; and in men, another special scale, Wb (worried breadwinner), the latter not associated with the cancer. In all three comparisons the extreme group difference was between the cancer group and the hypertension group. The cancer-healthy difference was not significant in any of the three. Thus only two scales are relevant to cancer, Si and HR. Unfortunately, in each sex one-fourth of the cancer patients was given the test less than 2 years before diagnosis, leading to a suspicion of effect of occult cancer in those patients. In addition, one-eighth in each group was tested at an unknown interval before diagnosis, the known range being 0.3 to 12.3 years, with the mean close to 5 years in each sex.

Schonfield (71) examined the power of the Hs (hypochondriasis), D (depression), and L (lie) scales to discriminate 12 breast cancer patients who had experienced a nonmetastatic recurrence within 2 years from 37 who had not. Metastases, when they occurred, did not affect the assignment to the recurrence (A) or nonrecurrence (B) group. Group A had a higher Hs score than group B, but no differences could be found on the D scale. A component of the well-being subscale, physical well-being, was significantly lower for A than for B.

Schonfield's recurrence criterion was peculiar, local recurrence independent of metastases. In fact, he had seven metastatic cases to begin with and 33 cases of regional spread. Tumors reappear locally for different reasons. In particular, though, a certain number appear at the scar of the mastectomy, presumably because of a contamination during surgery, or because infiltration may occur more easily in injured tissue in certain people. For the former, it would not be expected that psychological factors could affect the surgical accident. In the latter, one must postulate a connection between such infiltration probability and personality. Moreover, the number of metastatic sequelae in the whole group, and their distribution among locally recurring and nonrecurring cases, were not given. It would be desirable to see an analysis of such data. As an aside, age control was probably not necessary, since interval to recurrence (including metastases) is not related to age in women with breast cancer.

Stavraky (75) separated their cancer group into most and least favorable survival, assigning the longest survival quartile to most favorable (MF) and the shortest to least favorable (LF). Epidemiologic survival norms by age and stage formed the baseline criterion where there were enough cases to match on those variables. Where not, stage was removed (e.g., lung). Three MMPI measures were taken: means of K (defensiveness), use of profile codes (arranging standard scores derived from K-corrected scores in descending order), and use of Blumberg's criteria. None of the groups differed from any other (MF outcome and controls, LF outcome and controls) on any of the MMPI measures taken. Patients with L scores > 9 or F scores > 15 were not used, their MMPI test scores being deemed invalid.

Viitamäki (81) examined relationship of various psychiatric and psychological measures to malignity stage in 100 Finnish patients, with strongly discriminating results, as expected, and also to survival in 55 patients who completed all psychological tests, using three levels: 0 to 1 year; 1 to 3 years; and more than 3 years. The group was mixed, and no control was exercised on stage when calculating the multiple regression of the variables on survival duration. Only one MMPI variable was significantly related to survival time in the regression, Pt (psychasthenia).

Watson and Schuld (82) used patients at two VA psychiatric hospitals as subjects. There were 17 mixed cancer patients and 17 controls matched for age and MMPI F score, and 26 benign tumor patients and 26 controls, matched on age, F score, and L score. No less than 2 years separated MMPI administration and tumor diagnosis, and mean intervals were 50.4 months for the benign group and 93.4 months for the malignant group. None of the cancer group's MMPI scores differed from those of the control group, although the Hs (hypochondriasis) score almost did. However, the control group's scores exceeded those of the cancer group. Variability among cancer and control group MMPI scores before and after matching was compared, yielding a difference in F score variances at $p < 0.01$. Standard deviation of cancer patients for F was 8.9 in the original 21 patients and 4.0 in the original 21 controls. One or two such significances would be expected by chance, as they observed. After matching, the standard deviations of the 17 pairs were 5.5 and 4.2, respectively. Out of all the mean contrasts, they maintained, two were expected. The Hs difference, they concluded, could not be regarded as especially meaningful, and a psychogenic relationship of MMPI and cancer emergence could not be supported. The findings, of course, are subject to grave question because the subjects all seemed to be psychiatric hospital patients at time of taking the MMPI, although this issue was never addressed by the authors. Whatever was found for them could hardly be extrapolated to individuals without psychiatric diagnosis.

Tables 1 through 3 tell the story. Every MMPI validity and clinical scale appears. Although non-MMPI variables were also used in many of the studies, the MMPI findings are not vitiated by failing to connect them with those other findings. One simply cannot take seriously the results of some of the cited papers. In view of the wide variety of tumors and stages, how can one conclude anything about the MMPI in general, or any single variable in particular? Studies of Blumberg's criteria (19,46,75) do not permit conclusions. His own study (19), as pointed out, was seriously flawed. Krasnoff (46) had too few short-term survivors (six) to draw conclusions from, as he remarked. None of the three studies looking at Blumberg's criteria dealt adequately with the known biological predictors. If, in order to make sure that age is not a more potent variable than the MMPI score, researchers are willing to adjust for age, which,

TABLE 1. *Predictive MMPI studies and their characteristics*

Ref. No.	Cancer sites (stages)[a]	No. with Cancer	No. of controls	Predictor measure	Outcome measure	Analysis
4	Mixed (90% metastatic)	126	None[b]	MMPI scores (and others)	Disease status range 1–5, 5 being "died"	Factor analysis, 34 variables; regression analysis on factors
18	Mixed (almost all healthy)	82	2,100 other	Depression score highest among MMPI scores or not	Cancer death or not	Mantel-Haenszel test, controlled for age, smoking, alcohol; also ANOVA and t-tests
19[c]	Mixed (various stages all inoperable)	18 (32)[d]	None[b]	MMPI score algorithm (see Table 2)	"Fast" vs "slow" progression	χ^2
24	Mixed (various stages)	25 lung, 25 prostate, 25 multiple tumors	25 benign, 25 hypertension, 25 ulcer, 25 schizophrenia, 25 control, 25 age matched to prostates	MMPI scores	Cancer, no cancer (also, several others for various analyses)	Discriminant analysis (also, many others done on different outcomes)
30	Melanoma (stage II except 3 deep Clark level stage I)	31 (33)[d]	None[b]	Did or did not relapse by 1 year	Mean MMPI scores	t-test. Required $p < 0.20$ in first sample, cross-validated in second, test on combined samples also
31[c]	Mixed (not specified; presume various stages)	15 "slow," 15 "fast" progression	15 bone fracture cases	Membership in "slow," "fast," or controls	Mean MMPI scores	ANOVA, confidence band tests
46	Melanoma (various stages)	6 fast, 16 slow progression	None[b]	MMPI score algorithm (see Table 2)	Fast vs slow progression based on actual survival	χ^2

53	Mixed (almost all healthy)	Female, 16 or 14; male, 24 or 23	Female, 16 hypertension, 35 healthy; male, 35 or 36 heart disease, 22 hypertension, 28 healthy	Membership in cancer or other groups	Mean MMPI scores	ANOVA, t-tests, Tukey test
71	Breast (various stages)	49 women	None[b]	Membership in recurrence, nonrecurrence group	MMPI score	t-test
75	Mixed (various stages)	16 most favorable survival, 16 least favorable survival	25 average survival for m.f.; 62 average survival for l.f.	1. membership in the 4 groups 2. membership in the 4 groups 3. Blumberg's criteria (19)	1. Mean differences 2. Profile comparison, but details not given 3. Number satisfying Blumberg criteria in group	1. statistic not given 2. statistic not given 3. statistic not given but presumably χ^2
81	Mixed (various stages)	55	None[b]	MMPI scores	Survival duration	Stepwise regression
82	Mixed (most healthy)	21 men (all mental hospital patients)	21 men (all mental hospital patients)	Membership in the groups	1. Mean MMPI scores 2. Variability of MMPI scores	1. t-test 2. F max test

[a] Status at time of testing.

[b] Controls in the classic sense are not relevant since the discrimination is between types of follow-up status.

[c] These are really pseudo-prospective studies, since the actual survival time—whether short or long—was not observed for all cases. In (19) an unknown number were observed; in (31) none was observed. The short-term survival judgment came from medical estimates based on clinical status and treatment response.

[d] First number is test sample, deriving algorithm or predictor coefficients. (N) is cross-validation sample number.

TABLE 2. *Relation of MMPI scores and outcome in various prospective studies*

Outcome measure	Significant MMPI test	Ref. No.	No. of significant criteria
Signs as in footnotes	L $+^a$, $+^b$; F $-^a$, $+^b$; K $+^a$, $+^b$; Pa $+^a$, $-^b$	4	4
Predicts relative risk	D (highest of all scales for an individual)	18	1
Identifies fast-progression group	F minus K $<$ 0; Ma low; D high; Hs & Hy not high	19	3
Sign of discriminant weight predicts cancer	RS $+$; HyD $+$; D $+$; Ca $-$; Mf $-$; Hy $-$; Pa $+$	24	7
Recurrence within 1 year	None (melanoma only)	30	0
Signs of difference, fast-progression group mean minus slow group mean	L $+$; F $-$; K $+$; Pd $-$; Sc $-$; Ma $-$	31	6
Identifies fast-progression group	None (Blumberg's criteria, melanoma only)	46	0
Sign of score differences among groups with cancer and other conditions	Si $+$ (women, cancer mean minus control mean); HR $-$ (women, cancer mean minus hypertension mean)	53	2
Identifies sign of early recurrence group mean minus late recurrence group mean	Hs $+$ (breast); Comrey's Health Concern (subscale of Hs): t; Physical well-being (subscale of well-being scale) $+$ (breast)	71	2(3?)
Most favorable survival vs least favorable	None (3 measures, including Blumberg criteria)	75	0
Sign of regression weight associated with long survival	Pt $-$	81	1
Associated with future cancer patients	F (high variability only)	82	1

[a] Sign refers to factor loading of the MMPI scale.
[b] Sign refers to beta weight of factor in regression equation for survival prediction.

for different outcomes, is variously a weak and strong biological covariable of survival incidence and other factors, then why not adjust for the other weak and strong biological covariables? Then, again, if one is merely looking for association of psychic states with cancer outcome, not attempting to find the "true" association, why control for anything—age, sex, cancer type, or other variables? One cannot have it both ways.

Of the variables studied, Table 3 shows that no scale or its derivative was cited more than three times, and only one (D, depression) displayed the same relationship in each instance. This pattern of variable results, evident throughout

TABLE 3. Different MMPI scales found significant in different prospective studies

MMPI scale	Ref. No.	MMPI scale	Ref. No.	MMPI scale	Ref. No.
L +[a]+[b]; +[c]	4, 31	Ca −	24	Pt −	81
F −[a]+[b]; −;					
+ (Variability)	4, 31, 82	Mf −	24	F minus K 0; +	19
K +[a]+[b]; +	4, 31	Hy −	24	RS +	24
Pa +[a]−[b]; +	4, 24	Pd −	31	HyD +	24
D +; + with not high Hs & Hy;					
+	18, 19, 24	Sc −	31	HR −	53
Ma low; −	19, 31	Si +	53	Physical well-being +	71
		Hs +	71	Comrey's Health Concern +	71

[a] Sign refers to factor loading of the MMPI scale.
[b] Sign refers to beta weight of factor in regression equation for survival prediction.
[c] Other signs relate to the chances of getting cancer, shorter survival, fast progression, or early recurrence, except Pt, where "−" refers to the beta weight sign associated with length of survival.

both Tables 2 and 3, is further compounded by the inconsistency of experimental designs, samples, outcomes, and analyses shown in Table 1. Of all the studies, that of Shekelle, reported by Bieliauskas et al. (18), is the cleanest and offers the most promise of being free of experimental contamination. Nevertheless, I am still unwilling to take a firm position that any MMPI variable is connected with, let alone has any causative relationship to, cancer outcome—incidence, progress, or survival.

Can one conclude the converse: that because of the failure to produce very strong positive evidence, one is justified in saying that MMPI variables are not forecasters of incidence, progress, or survival in cancer? No. Failure to show a significant difference does not prove the null hypothesis. It is merely not inconsistent with it.

Note that these studies have been called predictive, but some examine the difference in earlier scores, among groups in which cancer appeared or not, or recurrence took place or not, or the patient died or not. If the subjects were chosen on the basis of disease outcome, rather than on the basis of having a test score, independent of outcome, there is a chance of bias because the procedure would be essentially that of a retrospective study, despite the time relations of test and outcome. If every member of the study group who took the test were included in the comparison, however, that kind of bias would not appear. To go back to the main thrust of the discussion, the most worrisome of the positive findings (see p. 276) is the wide variety of variables found to be related to a positive outcome. They should be related to each other, if a parsimonious theory, A, is true. Such a theory demands only a few psychological predictors. With such a theory they must be related, since their amount of explained variance is too high for all the variables to be independent. A second option, a nonparsimonious theory, B, proposes that there are many valid underlying psychological predictors. It is possible that (1) B is true; (2) A is true but there is enough unreliability between samples and conditions for studies to show inconsistent results; (3) B is true, but the latter state of affairs also holds; or (4) a third option holds, namely, C. Under C, there is no predictive power, that is, neither A nor B is true.

My present view is that for predicting incidence of cancer, (3) is correct; but the total psychological contribution is very small. For predicting recurrence or survival, I believe it is even smaller, and it is a toss-up between (2) and (4), in view of the powerful contributions of biological factors. To avoid this conclusion the psychological researcher must show a relationship between psychological variables and these biological factors.

REFERENCES

1. Abse, D. W., Wilkins, M. M., Kirschner, G., Weston, D. L., Brown, R. S., and Buxton, W. D. (1972): Self-frustration, nighttime smoking and lung cancer. *Psychosom. Med.,* 34:395–404.
2. Abse, D. W., Wilkins, M. M., Van De Castle, R. L., Buxton, W. D., Demars, J. P., Brown, R. S., and Kirschner, L. G. (1974): Personality and behavioral characteristics of lung cancer patients. *J. Psychosom. Res.,* 18:101–113.
3. Achté, K. A., and Vauhkonen, M. L. (1971): Cancer and the psyche. *Omega,* 2:46–56.
4. Achterberg, J., Lawlis, G. F., Simonton, O. C., and Matthews-Simonton, S. (1977): Psychological factors and blood chemistries as disease outcome predictors for cancer patients. *Multivariate Exp. Clin. Res.,* 3:107–122.
5. Achterberg, J., Simonton, O. C., and Matthews-Simonton, S. (eds.) (1976): *Stress, Psychological Factors, and Cancer.* New Medicine Press, Fort Worth, Texas.
6. Ader, R., and Cohen, N. (1975): Behaviorally conditioned immunosuppression. *Psychosom. Med.,* 37:333–340.
7. Aimez, P. (1972): Psychophysiologie du cancer: Existe-t-il un terrain psychologique prédisposant? (Psychophysiology of cancer: Is there a cancer-prone personality?) *Rev. Med. Psychosom.,* 14:371–381.
8. Bacon, C. L., Renneker, R., and Cutler, M. (1952): A psychosomatic survey of cancer of the breast. *Psychosom. Med.,* 14:453–460.
9. Bahnson, C. B. (ed.) (1969): Second conference on psychophysiological aspects of cancer. *Ann. N.Y. Acad. Sci.,* 164:307–634.
10. Bahnson, C. B. (1969): Psychophysiological complementarity in malignancies: Past work and future vistas. *Ann. N.Y. Acad. Sci.,* 164:319–334.
11. Bahnson, C. B., and Bahnson, M. B. (1966): Role of the ego defenses: Denial and repression in the etiology of malignant neoplasm. *Ann. N.Y. Acad. Sci.,* 125:827–845.
12. Bahnson, C. B., and Kissen, D. M. (eds.) (1966): First conference on psychophysiological aspects of cancer. *Ann. N.Y. Acad. Sci.,* 125:773–1055.
13. Baltrusch, H. J. F. (1964): Psyche-Nervensystem-Neoplastischer Prozess: Ein altes Problem mit neuer Aktualität. Teil II. Neurale Relationen. (Psyche-nervous system-neoplastic process: An old problem with new topical importance. Part II. Neural relations.) *Z. Psychosom. Med.,* 10:1–10.
14. Baltrusch, H. J. F. (1975): Ergebnisse klinisch-psychosomatischer Krebsforschung (Results of clinical-psychosomatic cancer investigation.) *Psychosom. Med., (Solothurn),* 5:175–208.
15. Baltrusch, H. J. F., and Austarheim, K. (1963): Psyche-Nervensystem-Neoplastischer Prozess: Ein altes Problem mit neuer Aktualität. (Psyche-nervous system-neoplastic process: An old problem with new topical importance.) *Z. Psychosom. Med.,* 9:221–245.

16. Baltrusch, H. J. F., Austarheim, K., and Baltrusch, E. (1964): Psyche-Nervensystem-Neoplastischer Prozess: Ein altes Problem mit neuer Aktualität. Teil III. Klinische Beobachtungen und Untersuchungen zur Psychosomatik der Krebskrankheit mit vorzugsweise psychoanalytischer bzw. psycho-somatischer Methodik. (Psyche-nervous system-neoplastic process: An old problem with new topical importance. Part III. Clinical observations and investigations on the psychosomatics of cancer with predominantly psychoanalytic or psychosomatic methods.) *Z. Psychosom. Med.*, 10:157–169.

17. Betz, B. J., and Thomas, C. B. (1979): Individual temperament as a predictor of health or premature disease. *Johns Hopkins Med. J.*, 144:81–89.

18. Bieliauskas, L., Shekelle, R., Garron, D., Maliza, C., Ostfeld, A., Paul, O., and Raynor, W. (1979): Psychological depression and cancer mortality. *Psychosom. Med.*, 41:77–78. (abst.).

19. Blumberg, E. M. (1952): *The Relationship of Certain Personality Differences to Growth Rate in Neoplastic Diseases: An Exploratory Study.* Ph.D. Dissertation, University of Southern California; Blumberg, E. M., West, P. M., and Ellis, F. W. (1954): Possible relationship between psychological factors and human cancer. *Psychosom. Med.*, 16:277–286.

20. Booth, G. (1965): Irrational complications of the cancer problem. *Am. J. Psychoanal.*, 25:41.

21. Cagossi, M. (1971): La variable psichica nella ricerca oncologica. (Psychological variables in cancer research.) *Arch. Psicol. Neurol. Psichiatr.*, 32:323–337.

22. Coppen, A., and Metcalfe, M. (1963): Cancer and extraversion. *Br. Med. J.*, 2:18–19.

23. Crisp, A. H. (1970): Some psychosomatic aspects of neoplasia. *Br. J. Med. Psychol.*, 43:313–331.

23a. Dales, L. G., and Ury, H. K. (1978): An improper use of statistical significance testing in studying covariables. *Int. J. Epidemiol.*, 7:373.

24. Dattore, P. J. (1978): *Premorbid Personality Characteristics Associated with Neoplasms: An Archival Approach.* Ph.D. Dissertation, University of Kansas, Lawrence.

25. Dillenz, M. (1976): *Lebensveränderungen bei Patienten mit Colon und Rectumcarcinomen im Vergleich zu einer Kontrollgruppe.* (Life changes in patients with colon and rectum carcinoma as compared with a control group.) M.D. Dissertation, University of Heidelberg.

26. Earle, M. J. (1963): *An Evaluation of the Claim that Psychological Factors Are Causally Associated with Cancer.* Ph.D. Thesis, Bedford College, University of London.

27. Finn, F., Mulcahy, R., and Hickey, N. (1974): The psychological profiles of coronary and cancer patients, and of matched controls. *Ir. J. Med. Sci.*, 143:176–178.

28. Fisher, S., and Cleveland, S. E. (1956): Relationship of body image to site of cancer. *Psychosom. Med.*, 18:304.

29. Fox, B. H. (1978): Premorbid psychological factors as related to cancer incidence. *J. Behav. Med.*, 1:45–133.

30. Fox, B. H., Boyd, S., van Kammen, D., and Rogentine, G. N., Jr. (1980): Further analysis of psychological variables in predicting relapse after stage II melanoma surgery. *Proc. Third Int. Symposium on Psychobiologic, Psychophysiologic, Psychosomatic, and Sociosomatic Aspects of Neoplastic Disease,* Bohinj, Yugoslavia, 1978 *(in press).*

31. Gay, R. L. (1970): *The Relationship Between Psychopathology and Cancer.* Ph.D. Dissertation, Michigan State University, East Lansing, Mich.

32. Graham, S., Snell, L. M., Graham, J. B., and Ford, L. (1971): Social trauma in the epidemiology of cancer of the cervix. *J. Chronic Dis.*, 24:711–725.

33. Greene, W. A. (1966): The psychosocial setting of the development of leukemia and lymphoma. *Ann. N.Y. Acad. Sci.*, 125:794–801.

34. Greer, S., and Morris, T. (1978): The study of psychological factors in breast cancer: Problems of method. *Soc. Sci. Med.*, 12:129–134.

35. Grissom, J., Weiner, B., and Weiner, E. (1975): Psychological correlates of cancer. *J. Consult. Clin. Psychol.*, 43:113.

36. Hagnell, O. (1966): The premorbid personality of persons who develop cancer in a total population investigated in 1947 and 1957. *Ann. N.Y. Acad. Sci.*, 125:846–855.

37. Harrower, M., Thomas, C. B., and Altman, A. (1975): Human figure drawings in a prospective study of six disorders: Hypertension, coronary heart disease, malignant tumor, suicide, mental illness, and emotional disturbance. *J. Nerv. Ment. Dis.*, 161:191–199.

38. Henderson, J. G. (1966): Denial and repression as factors in the delay of patients with cancer presenting themselves to the physician. *Ann. N.Y. Acad. Sci.*, 125:856–864.

39. Kališnik, M., Vraspir-Porenta, C., Logonder-Mlinšek, M., Zorc, M., and Pajntar, M. (1980): Interaction of stress and transplanted Ehrlich ascitic tumor in mice. *Proc. Third Int. Symposium*

on *Psychobiologic, Psychophysiologic, Psychosomatic, and Sociosomatic Aspects of Neoplastic Disease,* Bohinj, Yogoslavia, 1978. *(in press).*

40. Kavetskii, R. E. (ed.) (1958): *The Neoplastic Process and the Nervous System.* State Medical Publishing House, Kiev.
41. Keehn, R. J., Goldberg, I. D., and Beebe, G. W. (1974): Twenty-four year follow-up of army veterans with disability separations for psychoneurosis in 1944. *Psychosom. Med.,* 36:27–45.
42. Kissen, D. M. (1963): Personality characteristics in males conducive to lung cancer. *Br. J. Med. Psychol.,* 36:27–36.
43. Kissen, D. M. (1967): Psychosocial factors, personality and lung cancer in men aged 55–64. *Br. J. Med. Psychol.,* 40:29–43.
44. Kissen, D. M., and Eysenck, H. J. (1962): Personality in male lung cancer patients. *J. Psychosom. Res.,* 6:123–127.
45. Koenig, R., Levin, S. M., and Brennan, M. J. (1967): The emotional status of cancer patients as measured by a psychological test. *J. Chronic Dis.,* 20:923–930.
46. Krasnoff, A. (1959): Psychological variables and human cancer: A cross-validation study. *Psychosom. Med.,* 21:291–295.
47. LaBarba, R. C. (1970): Experimental and environmental factors in cancer. A review of research with animals. *Psychosom. Med.,* 32:259–276.
48. LeShan, L. (1961): A basic psychological orientation apparently associated with malignant disease. *Psychiatr. Q.,* 35:314–330.
49. LeShan, L. (1966): An emotional life-history pattern associated with neoplastic disease. *Ann. N.Y. Acad. Sci.,* 125:780–793.
50. LeShan, L., and Worthington, R. E. (1956): Personality as a factor in the pathogenesis of cancer: A review of the literature. *Br. J. Med. Psychol.,* 29:49–56.
51. LeShan, L., and Worthington, R. E. (1956): Loss of cathexes as a common psychodynamic characteristic of cancer patients: An attempt at statistical validation of a clinical hypothesis. *Psychol. Rep.,* 2:183–193.
52. Lorenzen, M. (1975): *Unterschiede in der Beantwortung psychosozialer Fragen zwischen Magenkrebs-Patienten und Kontrollpersonen.* (Differences in answers to psychosocial questions between stomach cancer patients and controls.) M.D. Dissertation, Heidelberg University, Heidelberg.
53. McCoy, J. W. (1974): *Psychological Variables and Onset of Cancer.* Ph.D. Dissertation, Oklahoma State University, Stillwater, Oklahoma.
54. Miller, D. G. (1979): *On the Nature of Susceptibility to Cancer.* Presidential Address, 3rd Annual Meeting, Am. Soc. Prev. Oncol., New York.
55. Morrison, F. R., and Paffenbarger, R. S. (1981): Epidemiologic aspects of biobehavior in the etiology of cancer. In: *Perspectives on Behavioral Medicine,* edited by S. M. Weiss, J. A. Herd, and B. H. Fox. Academic Press, New York.
56. Moss, A. (1979): *Mortality and General Susceptibility: A Study of Heart Disease and Cancer Mortality in Alameda Co., California.* Ph.D. Dissertation, University of California, Berkeley.
57. Mulvihill, J. J., Miller, R. W., and Fraumeni, J. R. (eds.) (1977): *Genetics of Human Cancer.* Raven Press, New York.
58. Muslin, H., and Pieper, W. (1962): Separation experience and cancer of the breast. *Psychosomatics,* 111:230–236.
59. Nemeth, G. (1980): Prospective psychologic and somatic examinations of patients who later developed carcinoma. *Proc., Third Internat. Symposium on Psychobiologic, Psychophysiologic, Psychosomatic, and Sociosomatic Aspects of Neoplastic Disease,* Bohinj, Yugoslavia, 1978 *(in press).*
60. Nemeth, G., and Mezei, A. (1963): Personality traits of cancer patients compared with benign tumors on the basis of the Rorschach test. In: *Psychosomatic Aspects of Neoplastic Disease,* edited by D. Kissen and L. L. LeShan, pp. 12–17. Pitman, London.
61. Paffenbarger, R. S. (1977): *Psychosocial Factors in Students Predictive of Cancer.* Grant No. 1R01CA225 74–01, National Cancer Institute, Bethesda, Md.
62. Pauli, H. K., and Schmid, V. (1972): Psychosomatische Aspekte bei der klinischen Manifestationen von Mamma-Carcinomen. (Psychosomatic aspects in the clinical manifestation of breast cancers.) *Z. Psychother. Med. Psychol.,* 22:76–80.
63. Perrin, G., and Pierce, I. R. (1959): Psychosomatic aspects of cancer. *Psychosom. Med.,* 21:397–421.
64. Reznikoff, M. (1955): Psychological factors in breast cancer. *Psychosom. Med.,* 17:96–108.

65. Riley, V. (1975): Mouse mammary tumors: Alteration of incidence as apparent function of stress. *Science,* 189:465–467.
66. Riley, V. (1981): Biobehavioral factors in animal work on tumorogenesis. In: *Perspectives on Behavioral Medicine,* edited by S. M. Weiss, J. A. Herd, and B. H. Fox. Academic Press, New York.
67. Rogentine, G. N., Jr., van Kammen, D. P., Fox, B. H., Docherty, J. P., Rosenblatt, J. E., Boyd, S. C., and Bunney, W. E. (1979): Psychological factors in the prognosis of malignant melanoma, a prospective study. *Psychosom. Med.,* 41:647–655.
68. Rogers, M. P., Dubey, D., and Reich, P. (1979): The influence of the psyche and the brain on immunity and disease susceptibility: A critical review. *Psychosom. Med.,* 41:147–164.
69. Rotkin, I. D. (1967): Epidemiology of cancer of the cervix. III. Sexual characteristics of a cervical cancer population. *Am. J. Public Health,* 57:815–829.
70. Schmale, A. H., and Iker, H. (1971): Hopelessness as a predictor of cervical cancer. *Soc. Sci. Med.,* 5:95–100.
71. Schonfield, J. (1977): Psychological factors related to recovery from breast cancer. *Psychosom. Med.,* 39:51 (abst.).
72. Segal, J. (1974): *Long Term Psychological and Physical Effects of the POW Experience: A Review of the Literature.* Report No. 74–2. Naval Health Research Center, San Diego, Ca.
73. Snell, L., and Graham, S. (1971): Social trauma as related to cancer of the breast. *Br. J. Cancer,* 25:721–734.
74. Speciani, L. O. (1979): *Pre-morbid Stress Measuring in Psychosomatic Pathology: Reliability and Predictive Power.* Paper given at 5th World Congress, International College of Psychosomatic Medicine, Jerusalem.
75. Stavraky, K. M. (1968): Psychological factors in the outcome of human cancer. *J. Psychosom. Res.,* 12:251–259.
76. Stein, M., Schiavi, R. C., and Camerino, M. (1976): Influence of brain and behavior on the immune system. *Science,* 191:435–440.
77. Stephenson, J., and Grace, W. (1954): Life stress and cancer of the cervix. *Psychosom. Med.,* 16:287–294.
78. Stone, G. C., Cohen, F., and Adler, N. E. (eds.) (1979): *Health Psychology.* Jossey-Bass, San Francisco.
79. Thomas, C. B. (1976): Precursors of premature disease and death. *Ann. Intern. Med.,* 85:653–658.
80. Thomas, C. B., Duszynski, K. R., and Shaffer, J. W. (1979): Family attitudes reported in youth as potential predictors of cancer. *Psychosom. Med.,* 41:287–302.
81. Viitamäki, R. O. (1970): Cancer and psyche. II. Psychological determinants of cancer. Psychometric approach. *Monograph 1, Univ. Center Hosp., Helsinki,* 45–153.
82. Watson, C. G., and Schuld, D. (1977): Psychosomatic factors in the etiology of neoplasms. *J. Consult. Clin. Psychol.,* 45:455–561.
83. Weinhold, M. (1977): *Sozio-psycho-somatische Aspekte bei der Genese von Lungen-, Magen- und Mammakarzinomen.* (Socio-psycho-somatic aspects in the genesis of lung, stomach and breast cancers.) M.D. Dissertation, Heidelberg University, Heidelberg.
84. Wirsching, M. (1975): Zur Psychosomatik des Brustkrebs—Stand der Forschung und neuere Entwicklungen. (Psychosomatic aspects of breast cancer—Present state of research and new developments.) *Z. Psychosom. Med. Psychoanal.,* 25:240–250.

Psychosocial Aspects of Cancer,
edited by Jerome Cohen et al.
Raven Press, New York © 1982.

Chapter 24

Program Planning for Cancer Control: From Theory to Action

Joan R. Bloom

Department of Social and Administrative Health Sciences, School of Public Health, University of California, Berkeley, Berkeley, California 94720

How quickly and to what extent will advances in prevention and control of cancer be adopted in this country? Since passage of the National Cancer Act in 1971, a substantial increase in knowledge with applicability for cancer control has occurred, although the problems associated with its utilization (technology transfer) have received scant attention from either health workers or social scientists. Development of ways to introduce this knowledge successfully in the shortest possible time among the greatest number of people at the lowest cost must have the highest priority (7). Unless this occurs, areas where prevention practices on every level can have the most impact on cancer control will show less than optimum improvement.

Typically, the problem of information utilization has been conceptualized as the process by which knowledge of new products, ideas, or technology diffuses through populations and the decision to adopt this or that new method or product is made. From the perspective of cancer control activities, however, it is fairly clear that this conceptualization has been inadequate. The following inconsistencies between what is known and what is used are evidence for this assertion. We know the strong relationship between smoking and lung and bladder cancer; yet the per capita use of tobacco is greater today than when the Surgeon General made his report (17). We know of the relationship between exposure to the sun and skin cancer and possibly melanoma; however, the use of sun visors and other means of protection has not been subject to as much programmatic effort as smoking cessation. Breast self-examination (BSE), the Papanicolaou smear, the breast Pap smear, and proctoscopic examinations have been shown to be worthwhile efforts in early cancer detection. But 75% of women do not routinely engage in BSE; 35 years after the introduction of the Pap smear not all women routinely receive this test; the breast Pap smear is not widely accepted by physicians; and only a small percentage of men (24%)

and women (22%) have received a proctoscopic examination (6,8). By 1971 over 1,500 studies had been done on the diffusion and adoption of new information (15); why has there not been greater payoff from this extensive investigation?

There are several reasons to account for the lack of fruitfulness of this research (2):

1. Most of the studies in the health field focus on a single technical invention— a new medicine, a new surgical procedure, a new approach to health education— and the factors that cause an *individual* to adopt or reject it.

2. Not only is the adopter always an individual, but the factors that produce innovative outlooks or behaviors are typically individualistic. Factors include demographic characteristics such as age (being younger), position in the community (such as being a leader or being central in the social network), outlook on life (modern rather than traditional), or having relatively high economic or social status (15).

3. Even though innovations[1] are usually used by an organization as a program, rather than by individuals—as either providers or consumers—organizations are rarely considered in the diffusion literature. Although an individual administrator might be the adopter of a new piece of hospital equipment, he or she is firmly enmeshed in a network within an organization, which carries implications for both the adoption and the maintenance of the new practice. In Rogers' monumental work (14), 52 propositions are enumerated regarding the innovation/diffusion process. Not one of these propositions refers to the organization as the adopter or to features of the organization as affecting the process of adoption. The revision of his work (15) is no different.

4. In addition to the individualistic bias of both heuristic models and empirical research, these findings are less useful to an administrator because their focus is on nonmanipulable factors. This is because individuals and their personal characteristics are considered the important determinants of the spread and adoption of social innovations. Thus we could have concluded from our second reason that young, less-experienced physicians from middle-class families are more likely to adopt new medical practices. However, such a statement leaves one with an undesirable alternative: trying to manipulate people to bring about structural changes.

5. Little of the research on innovation has been application oriented. Psychologists have studied personality characteristics of innovators, anthropologists have studied their kinship ties, and sociologists have been concerned with their position within the social network. Although this research has added to the body of knowledge in a given discipline, it has not been problem focused—for example, on cancer control—and therefore does not conclude with the implications for policy formation. Either practical guidelines have not been developed from important research or indifferent research has unduly influenced policy.

6. Finally, the focus of the traditional approach to research on innovation

---

[1] Innovation refers to "any idea, practice or material artifact perceived to be new by the relevant unit of adoption" (21).

has been on the decision to adopt. Problems of its implementation and those of its maintenance within an institution have not been considered.

In the health field, the process of innovation is particularly complex, suggesting the need for an elaborate framework within which to consider the problem. First, a provider of medical care, usually a physician, acts as a gatekeeper. Both the safety and the effectiveness of the innovation must be considered before the innovation is accepted. Only then will the adoption process commence. Second, the adoption of the innovation must be viewed as the province of health care organizations because the new practice or technique is more frequently packaged as a health program to be implemented thereby. The difficulties and complexities of this phase are only too apparent to those who know of the many demonstration programs designed by well-meaning professionals and funded by the government that are never implemented, that are implemented without regard to unique characteristics of local situations and are thus never institutionalized, or that may be implemented successfully but function only as long as the external source of funding continues. Only when a program is implemented can we learn whether the information about a new preventive health practice will be received or adopted by the individual consumer—the target.

A FRAMEWORK FOR KNOWLEDGE UTILIZATION IN CANCER CONTROL

The relationships to be considered in the remainder of this chapter are summarized in Fig. 1. This framework combines a general model of organizational innovation (21) with a general model of diffusion/adoption (14,15) and its adaptation to health care providers (12).

It seems that social science research can contribute in two general areas. Fundamental is the conceptualization of the process of innovation. If we do not understand how new knowledge diffuses through society and is accepted and utilized by the health sector as well as by the general public, we cannot determine how to intervene. The first area of research would necessarily be aimed at specification of a framework. And, second, when we do intervene, we must choose the most promising strategies not only for adoption of the program but also for its implementation and institutionalization. Intervention research must take into account the interaction between type of adopting organization, structure of the adopting unit(s), and whether we are concerned about adoption, implementation, or institutionalization of the program—in our case, cancer control.

Adoption Stage

Adoption by the Provider

The health professional is often the intermediary in the process between the generation of knowledge and its utilization; this is an important interface. Ac-

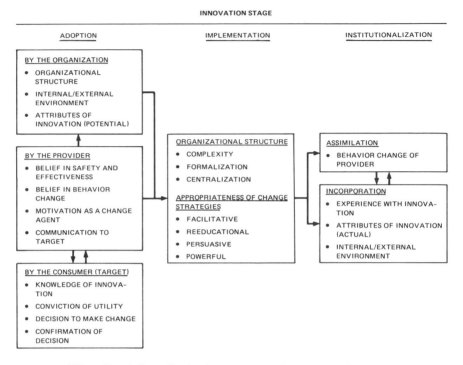

FIG. 1. Knowledge utilization in cancer control programs: a framework.

cording to McQueen (12), there are four key steps in the process between acceptance of new knowledge and communication of the preventive health practice to the target audience. First, the innovation must be *accepted* by health professionals. Its acceptance is predicated on the professionals' certainty that the innovation is safe and effective (16). Second, professionals must believe that they have the *ability* to alter the behavior in question. Two types of ability are of concern: power to effect change, and belief in their own competence to effect change. Prior successful experience with the innovation, or others like it, as well as its attributes will affect these dimensions. For example, a surgeon has more control over changing from a one- to a two-stage breast biopsy procedure than over convincing a woman to do a BSE routinely. Third is the *desire* or motivation to change the behavior in question. This desire may be either internally or externally motivated. A physician's motivation to adopt the Sartorius procedure (breast Pap smear), for example, may result from attendance at a continuing education course or from consumer pressure. As outlined by McQueen, the final step of this process is the *communication* of strong messages from the health professional to the consumer. How convincing the professional is in this communication process will be a factor in determining success.

To assess the probability of success or the location of potential problems, one must consider each innovation separately rather than by type. For example, in changing from the Halsted radical mastectomy to the modified radical,[2] surgeons have found the acceptance stage most problematic. This is probably due to the controversy surrounding the efficacy of the latter procedure. However, in the change from a one-stage procedure (malignant biopsy immediately followed by a mastectomy) to a two-stage (come-and-go biopsy with a second hospitalization for a mastectomy), problems are more likely to be encountered in the motivation stage.

Adoption by the Organization

Three characteristics of an organization's structure (or units within it) appear to be related to the adoption of innovations. Organizations can be characterized by their complexity (the number of occupational specialties, how they work, and their professionalism), by formalization (degree to which rules are codified and enforced), and by centralization (locus of authority and decision making). These structural aspects affect the adoption process mainly by the extent to which they facilitate or impede the generation of new ideas and their transmission to and discussion by decision makers. Thus adoption of new ideas is stimulated when a variety of personnel is available in an organization (high complexity), when rules and procedures regarding appropriate sources and channels of communication of these ideas are not rigid so that new information can reach suitable individuals easily, and when more people participate in a decision-making process that takes place at a lower level so that greater awareness of the innovation opportunity exists (low centralization).

In order to survive, organizations must be able to reduce the uncertainty in their environments (18). Sources of environmental uncertainty are different for organizations primarily supported by public funds, such as health departments, than they are for organizations that are supported by fees billed to a client. The political arena is the source of environmental uncertainty in the former instance; therefore the individual(s) or, for example, consumer groups that can exert political pressure will have the most influence in a publicly supported organization's decision to adopt a preventive health program. The medical staff is the source of environmental uncertainty in the latter case—because physicians refer clients to the organization—and therefore is a persuasive force.

If organizations, depending on their funding, are likely to be influenced by different groups, it seems reasonable to assume that attributes of innovations will appeal differentially to hospitals as compared to health departments. To test this hypothesis, Kaluzney and Veney (9,10) in a nationwide study examined attributes of services adopted and implemented by these two types of organiza-

---

[2] The Halsted radical mastectomy is surgical *en bloc* removal of the entire involved breast, the underlying chest muscles, and the lymph nodes in the axilla. The modified radical mastectomy is surgical removal of the entire involved breast and many lymph nodes in the axilla. The underlying chest muscles are left in place or partially removed after removal of the nodes in the axilla.

tions. Their findings not only confirmed their predictions but also provided useful information for the development of strategies by program planners. For example, they found that the payoff of the innovation (rate at which cost is recovered) is important for adoption by a hospital but less so for a health department. The divisibility of an innovation into separable components and its preventive orientation were attributes of innovations adopted by health departments, where cost recovery was not primary.

Characteristics of the environment will determine not only which groups in an organization are likely to be influential but also the probability that an innovation will be adopted. One such element is the political process itself. For example, pressures toward cost containment embodied in the National Health Planning and Resources Act of 1974 (PL 93–641) and, locally, as an aftermath of Proposition 13 in California (13), will undoubtedly influence organizational decision-makers' assessments of innovative opportunities. Other environmental aspects of importance include changes in technological development which create performance gaps that might affect the organization's competitive position. The move to adopt oncology units in hospitals is an example of this force. Within the organization, changes in personnel or shifts in power relationships between personnel also can have important consequences for adoption of innovations.

Implementation Stage

Although there is little literature in the health field relevant to the importance of the implementation process in cancer control programs, management scientists have given a great deal of attention to the process in other health care areas. Organizations seek their services to develop methods for scheduling hospital admissions or outpatient appointments and to plan complex interorganization information systems for collection of data on client services such as those provided by nationwide drug abuse or alcohol programs. Unfortunately, however, the probability is less than 50% that any solution developed by a management scientist will be implemented (19).

The structure of the unit(s) in which the innovation will be placed and the change strategies of the implementation plan itself are important at this stage.

Organizational Structure

Although organizations that are characterized by high complexity, low formalization, and low centralization are more likely to generate and adopt an innovation, these characteristics work against its implementation. Representation from a lot of different specialty groups generates new ideas, but also may generate more conflict that can delay or inhibit decision-making and ultimately hinder or sabotage the implementation effort. Although highly formalized organizations provide reduced opportunities for information flow into and through an organization, their clearly specified rules and procedures also reduce ambiguity concerning the effect the innovation may have on the individual's job and thus can facilitate implementation. Finally, although a highly centralized organization can reduce awareness of innovations, it can also reduce conflict and ambiguity that may impair the implementation attempt.

Change Strategies

Often an innovation is set up within an organization with little forethought. Because potential sources of resistance are not anticipated, strategies to counteract them are not developed and a low level of implementation results. Zaltman and Duncan (20) refer to this problem as the technocratic bias—overemphasis of the technological aspects of the innovation and underemphasis of its political aspects.

The way in which the innovative cancer control program is introduced to consumers, either individuals or organizations, is critical to its success. Strategies to facilitate this change, whether they focus on attitudes and behaviors of an individual consumer or provider, or on acceptance of a program by a community organization, appear to be an important area of research for those interested in the application of knowledge. A potentially successful approach may not be given an opportunity unless the program designer takes its marketing into account.

A typology of change strategies has been described by Chin and Benne (5) and, more recently, by Zaltman and Duncan (20). The former typology is useful when an individual is the target, whereas the latter is relevant when an organization is concerned, as discussed below.

A first category of change strategies is *facilitative.* They assist the organization by providing resources such as money, staff, and technology. The Ford Foundation has assisted in the implementation of international programs in birth control in this manner, and the American Cancer Society is a facilitator of implementations related to the prevention and control of cancer.

Second is a re-*educational* strategy whereby the relatively unbiased presentation of fact is intended to provide a rational justification for action. This strategy assumes that humans are rational beings capable of discerning fact and adjusting their behavior accordingly. This assumption underlies some health education programs and is often the strategy program designers use with organizational decision makers. The approach is feasible when time is not a pressing factor or when rapid change occurs in the political arena and the re-educative approach may bring attitudes or beliefs in line with the forced behavioral change. Two successful examples of this approach include acceptance of a mobile rural health program in El Salvador (20) and education of New York City residents to the benefits of Medicaid (1). In each case, a re-education effort preceded implementation of the program.

A third category of change strategies utilizes *persuasion.* Persuasive strategies are "strategies which attempt to bring about change partly through bias in the manner in which the message is structured and presented. They attempt to create change by reasoning, urging and inducing. Persuasive strategies can be based on rational appeal and can reflect facts accurately or be totally false" (21). They are useful when the client is not committed to change, when a reallocation of resources from one program or activity to another is being advocated, when time constraints exist, or when the innovation is perceived as risky or socially disruptive. Use of threat appeals such as pictures of cancerous lungs in smoking cessation efforts is an example of this approach (11).

A fourth class of strategies is based on notions of *power*. Power is defined as the ability to change the probability of performance by the target of some behavior by manipulation or threat of manipulation of the target's outcome. The strength of the power is related to goals controlled by the change agent, availability of alternatives, and the cost of these alternatives. The best examples of this approach involve use of the political system in the development of laws with which individuals must comply. The amendments to the Social Security Act of 1965, for example, require hospitals to develop utilization review committees to certify the appropriate levels of care and lengths of stay for patients receiving Medicare benefits. Withholding of payment to the hospitals provides the Health Care Financing Agency with the power to enforce compliance with its provisions. Power strategies are useful when commitment by the client system is low or when a reallocation of resources is desirable to initiate and sustain change. Because the political system has been supporting smoking through subsidies to the tobacco industry (4), power strategies will be necessary in any major smoking cessation attempt.

Institutionalization Stage

Institutionalization of a program, that is, its maintenance by the adopting organization, must be considered when developing a successful implementation strategy because it is not automatic. Although lack of continued funding is a frequently cited reason, programs fail to survive even when funding is guaranteed. Theoretically, two processes are important at this stage: the *assimilation* of the program parts by participants and the *incorporation* of the program by the adopting organization. Each process has different dynamics that are influenced by different factors. Assimilation is primarily an individual learning process, whereas incorporation must be analyzed as an organizational process composed of many decisions made by many actors. Also, assimilation can occur without incorporation, and vice versa; thus an innovation may often survive without institutionalization because of the loose coupling existing between these necessary components. The very act of putting a program into operation constitutes a learning experience that may produce enduring changes in participants' behavior or in use of materials developed by the program. The individual's assimilation of new behaviors or methods means that parts of the program may be institutionalized whether or not the program survives in toto.

A survey of innovations institutionalized by educational organizations indicates that two conditions of the implementation plans were critical to assimilation (3): staff commitment to the program and freedom to modify. Commitment of the staff responsible for carrying out the program after federal funding ceased was crucial. In institutions in which a grant paid for staff training time prior to implementing the innovation, less commitment to the program was found and survival was less likely. However, when staff members volunteered their time for training, commitment to the program was greater; thus the social-psychological principle of dissonance reduction seems to have operated: those who participated without pay justified the program on the basis of its inherent goodness and were more committed to it than those who needed no justification to themselves or others because they were paid.

The other condition related to assimilation was the degree to which staff members were allowed to modify the program to meet local circumstances and, perhaps, their own biases. In programs in which such modifications were allowed, assimilation was greater. Although the opportunity to modify gives the staff members a greater sense of ownership, this strategy can also be problematic. If factors critical to the success of a program are not well understood, the opportunity to modify a program may inadvertently result in decreased effectiveness—the degree to which a program meets its objectives.

The second process that must be completed for full institutionalization is incorporation—integration of the project into the normal operations of the organization. Unless the project sheds its special status, it will remain vulnerable to challenge. Its budget may be trimmed or eliminated; a crisis in leadership that threatens the project's survival may occur if the original staff of the project leaves; or project participants may be denied central support activities. A program is incorporated only if the organization's budget process, personnel allocation, support activities, facilities assignment, and so forth are routinely provided for its maintenance.

In summary, project-related changes are institutionalized only insofar as they are assimilated by providers and incorporated into the organization's standard operating procedures.

The potential of a program, which enhances its attractiveness to particular organizations, often must be realized if the program is to survive. Cost recovery was cited earlier as an important attribute of program innovations in hospitals. If, after a trial period, a program does not meet organizational expectations, its survival will not be assured. For example, a hospital administrator advised me of his willingness to underwrite for 2 years a home care program needed in his community; he added, however, that no program would survive in his hospital unless it was self-supporting. In health departments, the social approval of the agency and its constituency may be a determining factor in survival.

Not all programs should be institutionalized. Sometimes programs are designed to meet specific problems in an organization or community. Once these problems are solved, the program is no longer necessary. Unfortunately, if sunset rules are not incorporated, the program may outlast its usefulness. Examples include an adult drop-in clinic still operating in a major medical center 2 years after expansion of facilities eliminated its need, and the testing of cows for brucellosis even where pasteurization has eliminated it as a human health problem.

FUTURE DIRECTIONS

This review suggests that additional research in the utilization of innovation in the health field is indicated. Payoff for practitioners and planners from research in this area is more likely to occur when the problem is not conceptualized as a unitary process. As described in Fig. 1, we submit that there are three distinct stages—adoption, implementation, and institutionalization—involved in the transfer of new technology. Currently, the adoption of the innovation by the target audience has been the major focus of research efforts. As indicated in Fig. 1, empirical verification of McQueen's model, which describes the process by which health care providers adopt new practices and take on the responsibility for their dissemination to a target audience, is needed. In addition, research that will further our understanding of the factors that predict acceptance of programs incorporating these practices by organizational decision makers is important.

We have indicated here the importance of understanding the implementation/institutionalization sequence of social change efforts and the dearth of research on health programs of any type—let alone programs for the prevention and control of cancer. Consideration of factors which facilitate the acceptance and utilization of programs shown to be effective is necessary if their dissemination is to be assured.

The areas of program implementation and institutionalization are almost totally unexplored for research possibilities. Testing some of the variables suggested by the framework is one possible direction. A fruitful tactic might be to consider the structural characteristics of organizations or differences in change strategies as predictors of program implementation. In the area of program institutionalization, further exploratory work seems indicated prior to hypothesis-testing studies.

CONCLUSIONS

To ensure success, the planner of a cancer prevention or any other health program must include a strategy for implementation in its design. This must take into account individual actors who will be involved—the individuals who will implement the program and the consumers of the program services that have been designed. However, because this is an organizational strategy as well, the political milieu of the adopting organization must be considered. Key decision makers within the organization, for example, are responsible administrators and the physician, who is a gatekeeper in health care innovation. Other factors include the structure of the organization and the interaction between this structure and the stage of the innovation.

Successful consultants and program designers often intuitively understand the process that must be followed to have their innovations adopted, implemented, and institutionalized. The process is an art form for them and for those who perceive the underlying structure. If this process can be conceptualized and described, however, the innovation of cancer prevention programs will no longer appear to be arbitrary or mysterious.

REFERENCES

1. Alexander, R. S., and Podair, S. (1969): Educating New York City residents to benefits of Medicaid. *Public Health Rep.,* 84:767–772.
2. Baldridge, J. V., and Deal, T. E. (1975): *Managing Change in Educational Organizations.* McCutchan, Berkeley, Ca.
3. Berman, P., and McLaughlin, M. W. (1977): *Federal Programs Supporting Educational Change* (R-159-HEW). Rand Corp., Santa Monica, Ca.
4. *Cancer in California* (1978): The choice: Cigarette smoking or the health of Americans. Reference issue. *ACS Volunteer,* 24:2–7.
5. Chin, R., and Benne, K. D. (1969): General strategies for effecting change in human systems. In: *The Planning of Change, 2nd Ed.,* edited by W. Bennis, K. Benne, and R. Chin, pp. 233–254. Holt, Rinehart & Winston, New York.
6. Gallup Organizations (1974): *The Public's Awareness and Use of Cancer Detection Tests.* Summary report.
7. Graham, S. (1973): Studies of behavior change to enhance public health. *Am. J. Public Health,* 63:327–334.
8. Guzik, D. S. (1978): Efficacy of screening for cervical cancer: A review. *Am. J. Public Health,* 68:125–134.
9. Kaluzney, A., and Veney, J. (1973): Attributes of health services as factors in program implementation. *J. Health Soc. Behav.,* 14:124–133.
10. Kaluzney, A., Veney, J., and Gentry, J. (1974): Innovation of health services: A comparative study of hospitals and health departments. *Milbank Mem. Fund Q.,* 52:58–82.
11. Levanthal, H. (1970): Findings and theory in the study of fear communication. *Adv. Exp. Soc. Psychol.,* 5:120–186.
12. McQueen, D. V. (1975): Diffusion of heart disease risk factors to health professionals. In: *Applying Behavioral Science to Cardiovascular Risk,* edited by A. J. Enelow and J. B. Henderson, pp. 71–83. American Heart Association, New York.
13. Proposition 13 (1978): Initiative Constitutional Amendment, State of California—Tax Limitation.
14. Rogers, E. S. (1962): *Diffusion of Innovations.* The Free Press, New York.
15. Rogers, E. S., and Shoemaker, F. F. (1971): *Communication of Innovations: A Cross-Cultural Approach.* The Free Press, New York.
16. Sapolsky, H. M. (1968): Science, voters and the fluoridation controversy. *Science,* 162:427–433.
17. Surgeon General of the Public Health Service (1964): Report of the Advisory Committee on Smoking and Health (DHEW). U.S. G.P.O., Washington, D.C.
18. Thompson, J. D. (1967): *Organization in Action.* McGraw-Hill, New York.
19. Zald, D., and Sorenson, R. (1975): Theory of change and the effective use of management science. *Admin. Sci. Q.,* 20:532–545.
20. Zaltman, G., and Duncan, R. (1977): *Strategies for Change.* John Wiley & Sons, New York.
21. Zaltman, G., Duncan, R., and Holbeck, J. (1973): *Innovations and Organizations.* John Wiley & Sons, New York.

SUBJECT INDEX

Subject Index